Linguistic Varieties in North America

COMMUNICATION DISORDERS ACROSS LANGUAGES

The discipline of communication disorders has made great strides over the last fifty years and more. We now know much more about the nature and causes of breakdowns in speech and language, both in adults and children. We know more about how to classify these breakdowns, how to describe and analyse pathological speech and language, and how to treat communication disorders. Unfortunately, a large proportion of this work is restricted to a small number of European languages; indeed, much of it is on and in English alone.

Research in communication disorders in languages other than English has seen a marked increase in recent years, as has the investigation of such disorders in speakers of more than one language, and communities where bi- and multilingualism is the norm. This series serves to spotlight new and ongoing research in communication disorders across languages. We aim to do this by including studies of communication disorders (including assessment methods and guidelines for intervention) in particular multilingual communities, studies of the manifestations of specific types of disorder in a range of languages (particularly lesser researched languages), and of communication breakdown in bi- and multilingual speakers. Books in the series are used by practitioners, researchers and students, and they address a range of topics, including speech and language disorders in children, literacy, acquired speech and language disorders in adults, fluency, and voice.

All books in this series are externally peer-reviewed.

Full details of all the books in this series and of all our other publications can be found on https://www.multilingual-matters.com, or by writing to Multilingual Matters, BLOCK, The Fairfax, Pithay Court, Bristol, BS1 3BN, UK.

COMMUNICATION DISORDERS ACROSS LANGUAGES: 21

Linguistic Varieties in North America

A Guide for Speech and Language Practitioners

Edited by
Elena Babatsouli, Yolanda F. Holt and Karla N. Washington

MULTILINGUAL MATTERS
Bristol • Jackson

DOI https://doi.org/10.21832/BABATS2682
Library of Congress Cataloging in Publication Data
A catalog record for this book is available from the Library of Congress.
Names: Babatsouli, Elena editor | Holt, Yolanda F., editor |
Washington, Karla N., editor
Title: Linguistic Varieties in North America: A Guide for Speech and
Language Practitioners/Edited by Elena Babatsouli, Yolanda F. Holt and
Karla N. Washington.
Description: Bristol; Jackson: Multilingual Matters, 2026. | Series:
Communication Disorders Across Languages: 21 | Includes bibliographical
references and index. | Summary: "This volume provides insight into the
complex linguistic landscape of North America, from understudied
varieties of English to Indigenous languages and emerging language
varieties. It explores the unique features of each language variety to
aid the identification, diagnosis and treatment of speech and language
disorders in these communities"-- Provided by publisher.
Identifiers: LCCN 2026011416 (print) | LCCN 2026011417 (ebook) | ISBN 9781800412637 paperback |
ISBN 9781800412682 hardback | ISBN 9781800412736 epub | ISBN 9781800412781 pdf
Subjects: LCSH: English language--Variation--United States | English
language--Variation--Canada | Indians of North America--Languages |
Language and languages--Variation | LCGFT: Essays
Classification: LCC PE2808.8 .L56 2026 (print) | LCC PE2808.8 (ebook)
LC record available at https://lccn.loc.gov/2026011416
LC ebook record available at https://lccn.loc.gov/2026011417

British Library Cataloguing in Publication Data
A catalogue entry for this book is available from the British Library.

ISBN-13: 978-1-80041-268-2 (hbk)
ISBN-13: 978-1-80041-263-7 (pbk)

Multilingual Matters
UK: BLOCK, The Fairfax, Pithay Court, Bristol, BS1 3BN, UK.
USA: Ingram, Jackson, TN, USA.
Authorised Representative: Easy Access System Europe - Mustamäe tee 50, 10621 Tallinn, Estonia,
gpsr.requests@easproject.com.

Website: https://www.multilingual-matters.com
Bluesky: @multi-ling-mat.bsky.social
X: Multi_Ling_Mat
Facebook: https://www.facebook.com/multilingualmatters
Blog: https://www.channelviewpublications.wordpress.com

The policy of Multilingual Matters/Channel View Publications is to use papers that are natural, renewable
and recyclable products, made from wood grown in sustainable forests.

Typeset by Deanta Global Publishing Services, Chennai, India.

Contents

Contributors

Shanley Allen, PhD, is Professor of Psycholinguistics and Language Development at the RPTU University Kaiserslautern-Landau in Germany. She is co-editor of the book series Trends in Language Acquisition Research, is on the Editorial Board of the *Journal of Child Language* and is President of the International Association for the Study of Child Language. She has been doing research on children's language development in Inuktitut for over 30 years, with a focus on morphosyntax and the lexicon. Together with colleagues, she has also adapted two early language assessments for Inuktitut.

Joshuaa D. Allison-Burbank, PhD, CCC-SLP, is a Diné and Acoma Pueblo developmental scientist and licensed Speech Language Pathologist who grew up on the Navajo Nation. He is an Assistant Scientist at the Johns Hopkins Center for Indigenous Health and brings interdisciplinary training in communication sciences, public health and Indigenous knowledge systems. He has led several NIH- and foundation-funded studies focused on early language development, developmental delay prevention and equity in early intervention. He is committed to Indigenous data sovereignty, disability rights and culturally grounded care.

Ran An, PhD, is an Assistant Professor of Communication Sciences and Disorders at Fort Hays State University. With over 20 years of international experience as an academic faculty member, she specializes in fluency disorders and multilingual speech-language pathology. Her research investigates the intersection of linguistic diversity and sociocultural factors, with a focus on gender-informed clinical practices in stuttering and cross-cultural considerations in assessment protocols for diverse populations.

Elizabeth Ancel, PhD, CCC-SLP, is a T32 postdoctoral fellow with the Waisman Center at the University of Wisconsin-Madison. She researches how adults' speech characteristics influence children's language and social outcomes in clinical settings in speech-language pathology.

Currently, her work with Dr Sterling in the Research in Developmental Disabilities and Language Lab (RIDDLL) focuses on understanding how the similarity between adult and child speech characteristics reflects ratings of rapport in assessment settings. This work will deepen our understanding of how children process language and make social evaluations of adults in clinical and educational settings.

Martha A. Austin-Garrison, MA, is a Diné (Navajo) educator, language specialist and cultural knowledge holder with decades of experience in Navajo language education and community-based teaching. A fluent Navajo speaker from early childhood, she has served for many years as faculty at Diné college, the tribally controlled college of the Navajo Nation, where she teaches Navajo language, history, and culturally grounded courses rooted in Diné philosophy. She has also contributed to Navajo-language health education initiatives, including the development and translation of culturally appropriate medical and cancer awareness materials. Her work reflects a lifelong commitment to sustaining Navajo language, knowledge systems and community well-being.

Elena Babatsouli, PhD, is Associate Professor and the Blanco/BORSF Endowed Professor in Communicative Disorders at the University of Louisiana at Lafayette in the USA. She is the Editor-in-Chief of the *Journal of Monolingual and Bilingual Speech* (UTP) and Associate Editor of the *Journal of Child Language* (CUP) and of *Languages* (MDPI). She is also on the Executive Committee of the International Association for the Study of Child Language. Elena has also served on the Multicultural Issues Board of the American Speech-Language-Hearing Association. A recent edited volume Elena has published is *Multilingual Acquisition and Learning: An Ecosystemic View to Diversity* (John Benjamins).

Baylee Badawy is a Lebanese-American artist and writer based in New Orleans. She works with the New Orleans Jazz Museum and Gallatin Street Records and previously held communications roles with the New Orleans Jazz & Heritage Foundation and the Louisiana Department of Culture, Recreation, and Tourism. She is a co-founder of The Red Beret Chess Foundation with chess master Jude Acers and founded 'the chess cave' in the French Quarter. She is currently an MA candidate studying Musicology at Tulane University in the USA.

Elaine Ballard, PhD, is Associate Professor (US: Professor) of Linguistics in the School of Psychology at the University of Auckland in New Zealand. Her research explores linguistic and social dimensions of bilingualism and multilingualism in Asian and Pacific migrant communities, focusing on language change and implications for proficiency assessment. Supported by the Royal Society of New Zealand Marsden,

Health Research Council and the EU, her work examines how transplanted languages evolve. Currently, she is investigating ways to adapt standard English language speech-pathology assessments for diverse languages.

Stefanie N. Becerril holds a PhD in Applied Language and Speech Sciences from the University of Louisiana at Lafayette in the USA. She also holds an MA in Communication and Learning Disorders with a Bilingual Certificate. Stefanie has worked as a bilingual (English/Spanish) speech language pathologist (SLP) primarily in public schools. Currently, she teaches in the undergraduate and MA programs at Lamar University in the USA and supervises 1st-year graduate student clinicians working at the on-campus clinic. Her current research and teaching interests include cultural and linguistic diversity, fluency disorders, counseling in communication disorders and the scholarship of teaching and learning.

Wilbur V. Bennett, MA, serves as the Assistant Department Head of the Department of English and is pursuing a PhD in Applied Language and Speech Sciences in the Department of Communicative Disorders at the University of Louisiana at Lafayette in the USA. His research focus is on language variation in Southern Louisiana, Cajun English and resistance to language prejudice. His current collaborative projects are the Louisiana Language Archive and the Cajun English Dialect Project.

Jessica R. Berry, PhD, is an accomplished educator, researcher and nationally certified Speech Language Pathologist from Huger, South Carolina. She holds degrees from Winthrop University, South Carolina State University, and Louisiana State University, in the USA, where she completed doctoral studies in communication disorders with a minor in linguistics. Jessica is a leading expert on Gullah Geechee language, culture and history. She founded The OKRA Soup Foundation, empowering Gullah Geechee youth, and owns Garden City Gymnastics in Orangeburg, South Carolina. A wife and mother of two, she is also a musician, worship leader and lifelong learner.

Helen L. Blake, PhD, is a Senior Research Fellow at Charles Sturt University in Australia and a certified practicing speech pathologist. She is a member of the International Expert Panel on Multilingual Children's Speech and a member of the working party that developed Speech Pathology Australia's national position paper and clinical guidelines for Culturally Responsive Speech Pathology Practice. Helen's research focuses on English proficiency, intelligibility and participation of multilingual speakers. Her work in intelligibility enhancement in multilingual speakers is informed by her previous role as an air traffic control standardisation officer.

Phillip M. Carter, PhD, is Professor of Linguistics and English at Florida International University in Miami in the USA, where he is also Director of the Center for Humanities in an Urban Environment. He is an expert on language in the United States, focusing primarily on the linguistic and social outcomes of contact between Spanish and English. With Julie Tetel Andresen, he is author of *Languages in the World: How History, Culture, and Politics Shape Language.*

Sea Hee Choi, PhD, is an Assistant Professor of Korean Linguistics at the University of Hawai'i at Mānoa in the USA. She has expertise in Korean linguistics, psycholinguistics and second language acquisition. She investigates the syntax-semantics interface and real-time sentence processing in Korean and other languages. Using experimental methods such as eye-tracking and event-related potentials (EEG/ERP), she examines how native speakers, second-language learners and heritage speakers acquire and process different aspects of grammar and meaning. Her work addresses topics such as the count/mass distinction, definiteness, classifiers and bare noun interpretation, integrating theoretical linguistics with experimental approaches across multilingual populations, tasks, and diverse contexts.

Aris Moreno Clemons, PhD, is Assistant Professor of Hispanic Linguistics in the Department of World Languages and Cultures at the University of Tennessee Knoxville in the USA, specializing in the intersections between language, race and identity. Her work spans the fields of linguistics, education, anthropology and Black and Latinx studies with the aim of providing liberatory frames from racial justice. Originally from (all over) the Bay Area in California, she has been steeped in the traditions of anti-racist pedagogies and has dedicated herself to developing and sustaining these practices in her own research and teaching. As such, her research agenda is rooted in social change through an examination of the ways that what appears to be common knowledge is often constructed and ideologically maintained by various social institutions. Overarchingly, Aris questions the linguistic mechanisms – repetitions, stance taking, tropicalizations, etc. – responsible for the (re)construction and maintenance of racializing and marginalizing ideologies.

Richard Compton, PhD, is a Professor in the Department of Linguistics at the Université du Québec à Montréal (UQAM) in Canada. He holds the Canada Research Chair in Knowledge and Transmission of the Inuit Language. His theoretically oriented work has examined phenomena including polysynthesis, lexical categories, modification and agreement in Inuktitut and Inuinnaqtun. His work in language description and documentation includes co-editing a dictionary of Inuinnaqtun with Emily Kudlak and two ongoing projects in partnership with the Kitikmeot

Heritage Society to build a corpus of spoken Inuinnaqtun and create a community grammar.

Jeffery U. Darensbourg, PhD, MLIS, is a writer, performer, multidisciplinary artist, researcher and activist for Indigenous place names and languages. He is a Louisiana Creole whose lineage includes French, West African, Choctaw and Atakapa-Ishak ancestors, and he is a member and tribal councilperson of the Atakapa-Ishak Nation. For over a decade he has spearheaded efforts at reviving the original name of the city where he lives, Bulbancha (Choctaw for the 'Place of Speakers of Other Languages'), which many know as 'New Orleans'. He holds a doctorate in cognitive science and his artistic work and research show a strong linguistic orientation.

Leandra Espeseth, MS, CF-SLP, is a Diné speech-language pathology fellow from Tohatchi, New Mexico. She is an Assistant Research Coordinator with the Johns Hopkins Center for Indigenous Health in the USA. Her work focuses on early childhood intervention and culturally responsive assessment. She brings over 30 years of experience as a registered nurse on the Navajo Nation, along with lived experiences that guide her commitment to giving back through culturally grounded care and advocacy. She is dedicated to bridging community knowledge with research and clinical practice to support Diné children and families.

Ina Fautua, BSLT, is a Speech Language Pathologist (SLP). She is the first person of Samoan descent to graduate from a New Zealand (NZ) university with a degree in SLP. She currently works at the Ministry of Education in Auckland and is one of the few practicing NZ born Samoan therapists working with Samoan communities in the city. She is developing assessments and resources for Samoan children based on Talanoa, a Pacific approach, and integrating it with Samoan indigenous knowledge and other models of clinical practice.

Clive Forrester, PhD, is an Associate Professor (Teaching Stream) in the Department of English Language and Literature at the University of Waterloo in Canada where he teaches courses on academic writing, technical writing, linguistics and Caribbean language and culture. His special area of research is in forensic linguistics which investigates the intersection between language and the law in its broadest sense. In addition to publications on language rights and language advocacy, he has served as expert witness and linguistic consultant on court cases ranging from murder, to threatening speech, to authorship identification.

Davis E. Henderson, PhD, CCC-SLP, is an Associate Professor at Northern Arizona University in the USA. Davis is a bilingual (Navajo-English)

Speech Language Pathologist with extensive clinical experience working with Navajo children with speech and language impairments, as well as those who use Navajo-influenced English. He worked for the Gallup-McKinley County Schools as a Speech Language Pathologist for five years. He is the director of the Indigenous, Culturally and Linguistically Diverse Language Research Lab. His research expertise is in the area of Navajo linguistics, the development of Navajo speech and language assessments and the evaluation of their psychometric properties, and the communication skills of Navajo children on the autism spectrum. As a Navajo researcher and scholar, he has engaged in sustained collaboration for more than 12 years with Navajo Tribal Officials, the Navajo Nation Department of Education and the Navajo Nation Human Research Review Board. He currently serves as Co-Chair of the Native American Caucus.

Yolanda F. Holt, PhD, CCC-SLP, is the Director of PPSS The Holt Lab and is a researcher, educator and Speech Language Pathologist with over 20 years of experience. She researches speech development in culturally and linguistically diverse communities focusing on African American and Standard American English. Her work characterizes dialectal variation and its relationship to developmental outcomes. She is currently investigating the trajectory of speech sound development in African American English to more accurately capture the dynamic relationship between expected and unexpected variation. This work will advance understanding of typical development, inform diagnostic accuracy and reduce misdiagnosis of disorders in diverse communities.

Qiang Li, PhD, CCC-SLP, is Associate Professor in the Department of Communication Sciences and Disorders at the Fort Hays State University in the USA. He has been working in the area of adult neurogenic communication disorders as an instructor, researcher and Speech Language Pathologist with over ten years of experience. He is an active member of American Speech-Language-Hearing Association, Kansas Speech-Language-Hearing Association and Brain Injury Association of Kansas and Greater Kansas City. His current research focuses on clinical application of brain stimulation for interventions of motor speech disorders and cognitive communication disorders among both monolingual and multilingual populations.

Kate Margetson, PhD, is a Lecturer in Speech Pathology at Charles Sturt University in Australia. Her research focuses on multilingual children's speech assessment, Speech Language Pathologists' transcription of unfamiliar languages and diagnosis of speech sound disorders in multilingual children. She has worked clinically with multilingual children in Australia and Vietnam and serves on the board of directors for Trinh Foundation Australia.

Sharynne McLeod, PhD, is a Distinguished Professor and Director of the Children's Voices Centre at Charles Sturt University in Australia. She received Honors of the American Speech-Language-Hearing Association and is a Life Member of Speech Pathology Australia. She is a Board-Certified Member of the American Board of Child Language and Language Disorders and President of the International Clinical Phonetics and Linguistics Association (ICPLA). She has been named Australia's Research Field Leader in Audiology, Speech and Language Pathology and Best in the World based on the 'quality, volume and impact' of her research.

Jessica K. Meese, MS, CCC-SLP, is a Diné Speech language pathologist who grew up in Tohlakai, New Mexico, on the Navajo Nation. She is a research coordinator at the Johns Hopkins Center for Indigenous Health. She identifies as a Navajo woman, a mother, a clinician and a researcher deeply rooted in the communities she serves. Her work spans clinical practice in tribal communities, language nutrition interventions and culturally responsive tools that center Indigenous voices and ways of knowing. Her lived experiences navigating systems of care and working alongside families inform her commitment to family-centered, culturally responsive and community-driven approaches to care.

Monique T. Mills, PhD, is a Professor of Communication Sciences and Disorders at the University of Houston in the USA. She is a Speech Language Pathologist who holds American Board Certification in Child Language. Her research examines the social, cognitive and linguistic correlates of narration in school-age children from culturally and linguistically diverse backgrounds. She directs the Child Language Ability Lab which is currently engaged in a project examining language production and processing in school-age bidialectal and bilingual children.

Benjamin E. Munson (he/him), PhD, is an activist, educator and scholar who has dedicated his career to understanding the intersection of sociolinguistic and psycholinguistic knowledge in speech-sound development and disorders. His work has addressed the co-development of phonology and the lexicon and the ways that gender differences in speech affect children's speech sound development and disorders, among other topics. His work endeavors to transform the field of speech-language pathology to move from a medicalized, commercialized focus on 'disorders' to one that honors linguistic variation and the social functions of language.

Kumiko Murasugi, PhD, is Professor of Linguistics in the School of Linguistics and Language Studies at Carleton University in Ottawa in Canada. Her research encompasses language documentation, linguistic cartography and theoretical and applied linguistics. Her work on

Inuktut, conducted in collaboration with Inuit organizations across Canada, includes a survey of language vitality in Nunatsiavut, consultations on the standardization of the Inuktut writing system and the development of an online cybercartographic atlas of Inuktut in partnership with the Geomatics and Cartographic Research Centre at Carleton University.

Fe D. Murray, EdD, MS, CCC-SLP, is an Associate Clinical Professor in Communication Sciences and Disorders at Northern Arizona University in the USA and a bilingual (Spanish-English) Speech Language Pathologist. She has over 35 years of professional experience, including extensive clinical practice in and around the Navajo Nation. She is a national and international speaker on culturally and linguistically responsive assessment and intervention, multilingual language development and collaboration with interpreters. She has served on ASHA's Multicultural Issues Board and as member and coordinator of ASHA Special Interest Group 14: Cultural and Linguistic Diversity.

Diana Neill is Inuk from the Qikiqtaaluk Region of Nunavut, she is a Speech Language Pathologist and a PhD student at the University of Alberta in Canada. She is on a journey reclaiming her language and is decolonizing her practice of Speech and Language Therapy. Through her research, she aims to uplift Inuit language and knowledge to support Inuktut speaking children with language learning needs.

Ruochen Ning, PhD, is a postdoctoral fellow in the Department of Specch-Language Pathology at the University of Toronto in Canada and holds a PhD in Translation and Language Sciences from Pompeu Fabra University in Spain. Her dissertation examined the acquisition of Catalan as a third language by adult learners of Chinese origin, shaped both by Catalonia's unique sociolinguistic context and their native language and cultural background. Her postdoctoral research investigates the neural mechanisms underlying late talking in toddlers and developmental language disorders (DLD) in preschool-aged children. Her contribution to this volume examines sociolinguistic landscape and bilingualism in Catalonia, offering implications for culturally responsive research and practice with multilingual adults.

Donna Patrick, PhD, is Professor in the Department of Sociology and Anthropology at Carleton University in Canada. Her research has focused on Indigenous and minority language policy, politics, rights and practices and has included work on Indigenous language education, teaching and learning, critical literacies and social semiotics. She has worked with Inuit and on Inuit languages for over 30 years and since 2003 has worked on a number of participatory research projects with Inuit in Ottawa and Montreal.

Shamara A. Peart, BAS, MA, holds an MA in English Literature from Queen's University in Canada. Her research focuses on areas closely aligned with speech pathology, particularly multilingualism and dialectal variation in Jamaican diaspora communities. She translates theory and research into practical insights that support practitioners working with individuals who have communication needs. Peart uses an interdisciplinary and evidence-informed approach to emphasize diagnostic accuracy in Jamaican Creole and Black Canadian English speakers. This work complements clinical practice by highlighting how cross-linguistic assessment can reduce linguistic and semantic barriers while supporting effective and culturally informed treatment.

Ben Phạm, PhD, is an Associate Professor of Special Education at Hanoi National University of Education in Vietnam. Her research focuses on Vietnamese speaking children's speech and language development, disorders and diversity. She has worked clinically with monolingual and multilingual children living in Vietnam.

Raul F. Prezas, PhD, CCC-SLP, is a Professor of Speech and Hearing Sciences at Lamar University in the USA with over 20 years of clinical experience. His expertise includes speech sound disorders, phonological development and bilingual/multilingual assessment and intervention. He has published in leading journals, including the *American Journal of Speech-Language Pathology* and contributed chapters to major scholarly volumes. He currently serves as Chair of ASHA's Continuing Education Board. His scholarship focuses on phonological intervention for multilingual speakers and on advancing access and success for first-generation college students.

Paul E. Reed, PhD Associate Professor, Phonology/Speech Science, Department of Speech, Language, and Hearing Sciences, University of Alabama. His research focuses on the sociophonetic variation and change in the English varieties of the American South, particularly of the Appalachian region. He is the co-author (with Katie Carmichael) of the Cambridge University Press book *Language and Place*. His work has appeared in *PLoS One*, the *Journal of Phonetics*, *American Speech*, the *Journal of the Acoustical Society of America*, the *Journal of Speech-Language and Hearing Research*, *WiRES Cognitive Science*, and in several collections, including *Language Variety in the New South: Change and Variation*, *Appalachian Englishes in the 21st Century*, among others.

Claiborne Rice, PhD, is an Associate Professor of English at the University of Louisiana at Lafayette in the USA and has published articles on cognitive linguistics and poetics and on Cajun English. His work on folk illusions, with folklorist Brandon Barker, is the first study of the traditions of childhood illusion play.

Kevin K.H. So, MSc, is an educator, Speech Language Pathologist and doctoral candidate specializing in speech, language and communication disorders. His investigations focus on the rhythm processing mechanisms underlying developmental language disorder and language impairments associated with autism spectrum disorder. This research aims to elucidate the etiology of language disorders and contribute to the advancement of clinical understanding.

Maria-Sofia Sotiropoulou is a polyglot and a student at Pomona College in the USA. She is interested in languages and linguistics, in the areas of language documentation, language evolution, quantitative linguistics across languages and psycholinguistics. She has presented her research results at the 20th and 21st Applied Stochastic Models and Data Analysis International Conferences and at the 4th and 5th International Symposia on Monolingual and Bilingual Speech. Besides her work in this volume, she has published on the grammatical gender correspondence and semantics of French, Greek and Spanish nouns in conference proceedings and in the *Journal of Monolingual and Bilingual Speech* (UTP).

Mojtaba Taghvafard is a PhD student at the University of Louisiana at Lafayette in the USA and is a researcher in phonetics, phonology and language assessment, with a particular focus on bilingual and multilingual speech. Mojtaba studies Applied Language and Speech Sciences, with a focus on phonetics, phonology and the assessment of spoken language in multilingual, educational and clinical contexts. His work integrates phonological theory, quantitative methods and measurement models, including many-faceted Rasch analysis, to investigate speech production and assessment bias. His research interests also include Persian phonetics and phonology, second language acquisition, language testing and assessment and clinical and educational applications of speech analysis.

Carol K.S. To is an Associate Professor in the Faculty of Education at The University of Hong Kong and a qualified Speech Language Pathologist. Her research focuses on speech, language and reading development and disorders in Chinese-speaking children, with particular interests in speech sound disorders, developmental language disorder, autism spectrum condition and reading difficulties. Her work examines how linguistic, cognitive and perceptual processes support communication and literacy development, drawing primarily on behavioral approaches, alongside emerging eye-movement and neurocognitive methods. She is committed to advancing evidence-based, culturally responsive assessment and intervention practices beyond English-dominant contexts.

Van H. Tran, PhD, is a postdoctoral researcher at Charles Sturt University in Australia and a NAATI-accredited translator. She has been teaching English language and linguistics, translation and interpreting and Vietnamese language at University of Wollongong, Western Sydney University, and Defence Force School of Languages. She hosts SBS Vietnamese's weekly show on maintaining home language for Vietnamese–Australian children. Her research focuses on home language maintenance among Vietnamese-Australian families, multilingualism and multilingual children's speech and language acquisition.

Sarah Verdon, PhD, is a Professor of Speech-Language Pathology at Charles Sturt University in Australia. Her research focuses on children's speech, language and communication development in culturally diverse contexts. She is co-Chair of The International Expert Panel on Multilingual Children's Speech which advocates culturally responsive practice with multilingual children. She oversaw the development the Speech Pathology Australia national position paper and clinical guidelines for culturally responsive practice.

Karla N. Washington, PhD, S-LP(C), CCC-SLP, BCS-CL, is an Associate Professor in the Department of Speech-Language Pathology at the University of Toronto in Canada and directs the PedLLS Outcomes Lab. She is a Canada Research Chair and Fellow, American Speech-Language-Hearing Association. She is also Editor in Chief, Language, Speech, and Hearing Services in Schools, and is an invited member of the International Expert Panel on Multilingual Children's Speech. Her research focuses on speech-language development and disorders in monolingual and multilingual preschoolers which has been supported by Canadian and US Federal Funding. She characterizes language learning and use, with an interest in understanding how the child's contextual factors are related to their outcomes.

Christine P. Weill, PhD, CCC-SLP, is an Assistant Professor in the Department of Communicative Disorders at the University of Louisiana at Lafayette in the USA and Coordinator of the Scottish RiteCare Clinic. She is a Speech Language Pathologist, educator and researcher working in the areas of pediatric language disorders, literacy challenges and autism. Most recently, she is investigating the effects of children reading their own writing as part of evidence-informed language pedagogy and the literacy process from the perspective of people with autism. Her recent research collaborations have expanded to the study of dialect and family culture on expressed identity and social interaction skills.

Tynashia Whitaker is a Speech Language Pathologist in Houston, Texas.

Abbreviations

Chapter 12

1	first person
2	second person
3	third person
4	fourth person
ABS	absolutive case
AP	antipassive
CAUS	causative
CTG	contingent mood
CTM	contemporative mood
DECL	declarative mood
DU	dual
ERG	ergative case
FUT	future tense
ICM	incontemporative mood
IMP	imperative mood
INT	interrogative mood
LOC	locative case
MOD	modalis case
NEG	negation
PL	plural
POL	politeness
PAR	participial/participative mood
PLEON	pleonastic
POSS	possessor
PRSP	prospective aspect
PST	past tense
SEC	secondary case
SG	singular

Chapter 15

art.	article
dem.	demonstrative
erg.	ergative
perf.	perfective aspect
poss.	possessive
pres.	present tense
prog.	progressive aspect
pron.	pronoun
pst.	past tense
top.	topic
1st ps sg.	first person singular
3rd ps. sg.	third person singular

Chapter 18

ACC	Accusative (Marks the direct object)
COMP	Complementizer (Introduces a subordinate clause)
DAT	Dative (Marks the indirect object)
DECL	Declarative (Marks a declarative sentence)
GEN	Genitive (Indicates possession)
HON	Honorific (Indicates respect or politeness)
INST	Instrumental (Indicates the instrument used for an action)
LOC	Locative (Indicates location)
NEG	Negative (Indicates negation)
NOM	Nominative (Marks the subject of the sentence)
PROG	Progressive (Indicates an ongoing action)
PST	Past tense (Indicates past tense)
TOP	Topic (Marks the topic of the sentence)

1 Introduction

Yolanda F. Holt

The Vibrant Linguistic Tapestry of North America

Language stands as perhaps humanity's most remarkable achievement. Language is a complex system of symbols used by community members to create shared meaning and facilitate communication from the most basic to the most complex. These shared systems fundamentally and universally shape the way we understand ourselves, each other, and our world. Language is the vehicle through which we transmit knowledge across generations, express our deepest emotions, and construct the social bonds that define our communities. Beyond serving as a complex tool of functional communication, language is a structural component of human creativity, adaptability and cultural expression. Language describes our environment and our experiences. It is who we are in words. As we breathe and speak our lives, our culture travels to others in our words. With our language, we construct and share our world.

Linguistic diversity is one of our greatest treasures. It allows us to engage with our neighbors and see the world through their eyes. The languages spoken worldwide contain irreplaceable knowledge systems, epistemologies, and cultural insights. They are living archives of human history, repositories of ecological wisdom and the foundation of cultural identity for millions. When we consider that many languages are in danger of extinction due to both a lack of use and a lack of growth through their generational transmission by fluent speakers we can begin to grasp the urgency of documenting, supporting, and celebrating linguistic diversity.

Linguistic diversity includes profound variations in how humans conceptualize everything from time and space to social relationships and the natural world (Boroditsky, 2001; Evans & Levinson, 2009). Research in linguistic relativity continues to reveal how language shapes our perception, cognition, and behavior in subtle yet significant ways (Casasanto, 2008; Wolff & Holmes, 2011). When we embrace linguistic diversity, we preserve not only communication systems but also diverse approaches to problem-solving, environmental stewardship, and social organization that may prove crucial for addressing humanity's collective challenges (Harrison, 2007; Maffi, 2005; Skutnabb-Kangas *et al.*, 2003).

North America: A linguistic mosaic

Within this global panorama of linguistic diversity, North America presents a particularly fascinating case study on a continent where ancient linguistic traditions coexist with recent arrivals, and where continuous processes of language contact, evolution, and innovation create an ever-changing mosaic. Long before European colonization, North America sustained many Indigenous languages representing dozens of language families, often with no demonstrable relationship to languages elsewhere in the world. The Indigenous languages of North America from the Algonquian languages of the Northeast to the Na-Dene languages of the Northwest, from the Uto-Aztecan languages of the Southwest to the Inuktitut varieties of the Arctic evolved over millennia to encode sophisticated knowledge of local ecosystems, social structures, and philosophical traditions.

The colonial era introduced European languages that would dramatically reshape the linguistic landscape. English and French in what would become Canada, and English and Spanish in what would become the United States, established themselves as dominant languages through complex processes of settlement, governance, education and often suppression of Indigenous languages. Yet even as these European languages gained prominence, they did not remain static. Contact with Indigenous languages, with the African languages imported to North America through the forced immigration of Black Africans during the period of chattel slavery, and with languages from successive waves of European, Asian and African immigration transformed French, English and Spanish into distinctly North American varieties.

Today, the linguistic landscape of North America defies simple characterization. It encompasses established regional varieties of English, from the distinctive cadences of Appalachian speech to the evolving urban dialects of major metropolitan areas, including the birth of the recently described Miami English. The North American linguistic landscape includes varieties of Spanish that have been spoken continuously in some regions since the 16th century, to current iterations of Spanish enriched by more recent immigration of Spanish speakers from throughout the Caribbean. North America contains simultaneously unique yet familiar creoles like Gullah Geechee along the southeastern coasts of the Carolinas and Georgia, in addition to the French-influenced Louisiana Creole, which blends African, European and Indigenous linguistic elements. And we must not forget the Haitian Creoles of Florida and the northeastern United States, as well as the Jamaican varieties of Creole spoken throughout Canada and in the States. The linguistic variety in

North America embraces the speech of diverse immigrant communities, from Mandarin and Vietnamese to Somali and Nigerian, which are developing their own distinctive North American characteristics while maintaining transnational connections.

This dynamic mosaic has been shaped by powerful sociopolitical and historical forces: the devastating impacts of colonization on Indigenous languages; the linguistic innovations of enslaved Africans who created new forms of communication under oppressive conditions; the pressures of assimilation and standardization policies that permeated immigrant languages; and the revitalization movements that have emerged to reclaim linguistic heritage. Language variation in North America is influenced by geographical factors, patterns of settlement and migration, urbanization and more recently, digital communication and global media flows.

The need for a deeper understanding and a cause for celebration

Despite this extraordinary richness, North America's linguistic diversity remains inadequately understood, appreciated, and supported by many of its institutions and citizens. Mainstream narratives often present the continent as predominantly English-speaking, with other languages marginalized and receiving scant attention even when the languages in question have existed in the North American linguistic landscape for centuries. Educational systems frequently fail to build upon the linguistic resources that students bring to the classroom. Healthcare and social services struggle to accommodate speakers of languages other than English. Popular culture perpetuates stereotypes about unfamiliar or regional accents and the need for everyone to use 'proper speech' while failing to recognize that everyone speaks with an accent. Even the so-called standard form is itself an accent. It has simply been selected as the acceptable one.

The choices we make as users and teachers of language have real-world consequences. Children who speak non-mainstream varieties of English or who grow up in multilingual households may have their language development misdiagnosed as disordered rather than different. Indigenous language speakers may find their knowledge and perspectives excluded from important conversations about land management or cultural heritage. Immigrants may face barriers to education, employment and civic participation based on linguistic discrimination. And speakers of all backgrounds may internalize harmful messages about the value of their linguistic heritage.

This volume aims to address these gaps by providing a primer, an accessible yet scholarly introduction to the diverse language varieties of North America. By bringing together perspectives from linguistics, education, speech and language pathology, we hope to foster greater awareness, understanding and celebration of the continent's linguistic tapestry. In doing so, we believe our contribution will result in more equitable and effective practices in education, healthcare and beyond, while also encouraging readers to accept that language diversity is not a problem we need to solve but a resource to be cherished.

Purpose, Perspective and Practicality

This volume, *Linguistic Varieties in North America: A Guide for Speech and Language Practitioners*, represents a collaborative effort to document, analyze and affirm the linguistic richness that characterizes the continent. Its primary aim is to provide an accessible yet rigorous entry point for understanding the diverse language varieties spoken across the United States and Canada. Unlike comprehensive reference works or highly specialized monographs, this primer offers concise, focused introductions to a wide range of language varieties, emphasizing their distinctive features, historical development, status, and practical implications for various professional contexts.

The title reflects our dual commitment to linguistic knowledge and to practical utility. When we recognize the existing language diversity in North America and work to gain knowledge of that diversity, we position ourselves in opposition to the deficit perspectives used to characterize non-mainstream language varieties. At the same time, by identifying this work as a 'guide for practitioners', we signal our intention to move beyond abstract appreciation to concrete applications providing information that can inform and improve professional practice.

This volume addresses a diverse audience that spans both academia and applied professional contexts. It will serve researchers in linguistics, anthropology, education, and related fields who seek concise overviews of language varieties they may encounter in their work. It will support practitioners in speech-language pathology, education, healthcare, social work, and other human services who need to distinguish between language differences and language disorders, or who wish to provide more culturally and linguistically responsive services. It will benefit students preparing for careers in these fields, offering them foundational knowledge about linguistic diversity that many traditional curricula overlook. And it will assist language revitalizers, community advocates and policymakers who are working to support and strengthen diverse language communities.

The power of insider perspectives

A distinctive feature of this volume and one of its greatest strengths is its emphasis on insider perspectives. The contributors include not only scholars who have devoted their careers to studying language varieties but also practitioners who work directly with speakers of these varieties and, crucially, individuals who are themselves members of the linguistic communities they describe. This approach stands in contrast to the historical pattern in linguistics and anthropology, where researchers from dominant linguistic and cultural backgrounds have often studied minoritized language communities as outside observers.

The insider perspective offers multiple advantages. First, it brings to light nuances and contextual factors that might escape the notice of external researchers, however well-intentioned (Dwyer & Buckle, 2009; Suwankhong & Liamputtong, 2015). Community members possess what anthropologist Clifford Geertz called 'local knowledge' (Geertz, 1983), that is, intimate familiarity with the social meanings, pragmatic functions, and historical resonances of linguistic features. They understand when and why particular expressions are used, how speech patterns vary across different social contexts and how community members themselves perceive and evaluate linguistic variation (Eckert, 2000; Labov, 1972).

Second, the insider perspective helps correct misrepresentations and oversimplifications that have sometimes characterized academic accounts of non-mainstream language varieties. Too often, such varieties are described primarily in terms of how they differ from standardized forms, reinforcing notions of deficiency or deviation rather than recognizing their internal coherence and expressive power. Contributors who belong to the communities they describe can present these varieties on their own terms, highlighting their structural logic, aesthetic qualities, and communicative effectiveness.

Third, the inclusion of insider voices reflects a commitment to including all languages and all people as valuable in the production of human knowledge. This work recognizes that speakers of all language varieties are authorities on their own linguistic experience. By centering these voices, we challenge historical patterns of exclusion and marginalization in academic discourse. We acknowledge that expertise about language comes both from formal training in linguistics and from the lived experience of people within each language community.

The insider perspective bridges theory and practice in other ways. Contributors who work as speech-language pathologists, educators or other practitioners bring practical wisdom derived from applying linguistic knowledge in real-world contexts. They understand the challenges of distinguishing between language differences and language disorders, of supporting language development while respecting linguistic diversity and of navigating institutional systems that may not recognize or value non-mainstream varieties. Their insights help translate abstract linguistic principles into concrete professional applications.

The use of the insider perspective is shared to include the varied and diverse viewpoints about language use, maintenance, and change. The contributors to this volume are experts in their respective fields and are graciously offering a thoughtful and engaged account of their perspective on these topics. Many of the contributors occupy multiple positions as community members, researchers, active users of the language(s) under discussion and practitioners. These overlapping points of reference allow the contributors to integrate varied forms of knowledge, acquisition and perspective in to the information shared.

By privileging insider perspectives, the intent of this edited volume is to be academically sound, authentic, respectful, and directly relevant to the communities whose language varieties we describe. This approach will yield a richer, more nuanced understandings of language diversity and more effective guidance for those seeking to support it.

Bridging theory and practice: Applications for real-world impact

This volume is explicit in its emphasis on practical applications, particularly for educators and speech and language practitioners. The gap between linguistic research and professional practice has been noted by scholars and practitioners. This disconnection has profound consequences, especially for individuals from non-mainstream language backgrounds who interact with these systems.

Perhaps nowhere is this gap more consequential than in the assessment and treatment of speech and language disorders in children from linguistically diverse backgrounds. Without adequate knowledge of typical development patterns in different language varieties, practitioners may misinterpret features of African American English, Spanish-influenced English, or Indigenous language phonology as evidence of disorder rather than difference. Such misdiagnoses can lead to unnecessary intervention, wasted resources and potential psychological harm to children whose natural language development is pathologized. Conversely, practitioners unfamiliar with diverse language patterns may miss genuine disorders that require intervention when that practitioner attributes clinical markers of disorder to cultural difference.

This volume addresses these challenges by providing detailed information about typical phonetic, phonological, morphological, syntactic and pragmatic features of various language varieties. Contributors describe not only the features themselves but also their developmental trajectories when and how children typically acquire specific sounds or sound classes, grammatical structures, or discourse patterns within their language communities. This information will enable practitioners to establish appropriate benchmarks for assessment, distinguishing between developmental variations that reflect community norms and those that may indicate disorder.

The volume offers guidance for intervention and support of all multilingual learners. Contributors discuss culturally responsive approaches to speech and language therapy, educational strategies that build upon linguistic variation and frameworks for explaining language difference to families, educators, and other professionals. They address complex questions such as: How can therapists respect home language varieties while also helping children develop proficiency in standardized forms they may need for educational and professional advancement? How can educators distinguish between writing conventions that should be explicitly taught and those where variation should be accepted? How can healthcare providers ensure effective communication with patients from diverse linguistic backgrounds?

The volume also responds to recent calls within speech-language pathology, education, and related fields for more culturally and linguistically responsive practices. Professional organizations such as the American Speech-Language-Hearing Association (ASHA) and the International Association of Logopedics and Phoniatrics (IALP) have increasingly emphasized the importance of cultural competence in service delivery. Educational researchers have advocated for asset-based pedagogies that recognize and build upon students' linguistic resources. This volume provides concrete guidance for implementing these principles, moving beyond general statements about cultural sensitivity to specific information about language varieties.

By bridging theory and practice, this volume aims to have a real-world impact by improving assessment and intervention for individuals from multilingual language backgrounds, enhancing educational approaches that support linguistic diversity, informing policy decisions related to language in public institutions, and ultimately contributing to more equitable and effective services across North America.

Navigating the Linguistic Landscape: An Overview of the Book's Structure

This volume is organized into three main sections that systematically explore different dimensions of North America's linguistic diversity. This structure reflects both historical patterns of language development and contemporary sociolinguistic realities. It moves from established varieties with deep historical roots, through Indigenous languages that represent the continent's original linguistic heritage, to emerging varieties that display ongoing processes of language contact and evolution. Together, these sections offer a comprehensive portrait of North America's dynamic linguistic landscape.

Part 1: English, Spanish and Creole Varieties – Established Voices in the North American Chorus

The first part focuses on well-established language varieties that have shaped North American identity for generations yet often receive insufficient scholarly attention or institutional recognition. These include regional and social varieties of English, varieties of Spanish with long histories in specific regions and creole languages that emerged from complex histories of language contact. Though studied for decades, these varieties continue to evolve in response to social, demographic, and technological changes. Despite their historical significance and linguistic sophistication, speakers of these varieties frequently face linguistic discrimination, making accurate information about their features and development critical for professionals in education, healthcare, and speech-language pathology.

Contributors provide detailed analyses of phonetics, phonology, morphology, syntax, and pragmatics while tracing historical developments and describing contemporary usage patterns. They also address attitudes and ideologies surrounding these varieties and explore practical implications for professionals who serve speakers of these languages.

Among the varieties examined are African Diaspora Englishes and Creoles, which reflect the profound linguistic and cultural contributions of African-descended populations. African American English (AAE), Gullah Geechee and Jamaican Creole (as spoken in Canada, particularly Toronto) emerged through complex processes of language contact and adaptation under often oppressive conditions. These varieties feature distinctive phonological systems, grammatical structures and pragmatic conventions that have influenced broader patterns of North American English. Mills and Whitaker explore AAE's preverbal HAD construction in children's narratives, emphasizing its function as a past tense intensifier. For speech-language pathologists (SLPs), recognizing AAE as a legitimate linguistic system is crucial to preventing misdiagnosis, and narrative language sampling and recasting strategies offer valuable assessment tools. Likewise, Berry examines the historical development and resilience of Gullah Geechee language, stressing the need for nuanced assessments to avoid conflating linguistic differences with disorders. Peart and Washington investigate how Jamaican Creole shapes Canadian English, advocating for culturally responsive assessments to prevent misdiagnoses. Forrester further explores how Jamaican Creole influences Multiethnic Toronto English, underscoring the importance of inclusive diagnostic tools.

Regional Englishes, such as Appalachian English and Cajun English, demonstrate how geographical isolation, cultural distinctiveness, and settlement patterns shape linguistic development. Appalachian English, marked by monophthongization and nonstandard syntax, can be mischaracterized as an archaic 'Elizabethan dialect of English' rather than recognized as a modern dialect rich in cultural identity. Reed dispels this misconception, urging SLPs to recognize dialect features as accurate hallmarks of the language rather than pathologize them as indicative of speech or language errors. Similarly, Cajun English bears the imprint of French Acadian heritage and Louisiana Creole contact. Bennett, Weill and Rice discuss Cajun English's evolution and its role in cultural identity, emphasizing the need for appropriate assessment methods that distinguish dialect variation from speech and language disorder.

North American varieties emerging from Spanish English contact, including Blaxican Spanish and Texas Spanish/English, reflect the dynamic interaction between two of North America's most widely spoken languages and the cultural hybridity of borderland communities. Clemons' study of the Blaxican linguistic variety highlights the need to validate diverse linguistic practices and avoid pathologizing deviations from traditional norms in either Spanish or English.

Collectively, the discussions in this part challenge notions of linguistic purity or correctness, demonstrating that all language varieties evolve through contact and adaptation. They highlight the rich linguistic resources that speakers of these varieties possess, countering deficit perspectives that have often characterized institutional responses to linguistic diversity. Moreover, they provide essential information for practitioners seeking to distinguish between language difference and disorder while ensuring culturally and linguistically appropriate services for diverse communities.

Part 2: Indigenous Languages – Heritage, Vitality and Resilience

The second part turns to the Indigenous languages of North America – those spoken on the continent for thousands of years before European colonization and that continue to be vital elements of identity and sovereignty. These languages represent extraordinary diversity, belonging to dozens of language families with distinct historical origins, structural properties, and cultural associations. Some, like Diné (Navajo) and Inuktitut, have thousands of speakers and are used across multiple domains of community life. Other pre-colonial North American languages have experienced severe decline due to historical policies of enforced assimilation, child removal to English-only boarding schools, compulsory enrollment in English-only community schools and the devaluation of pre-colonial cultures in the colonial social economy. Currently, some Native North American languages live only in the speech of a few elders and individuals working on language revitalization both inside and outside the linguistic communities of practice. Yet even the most endangered languages remain a vital aspect of the cultural heritage and personhood of the communities and speakers shaped by those languages. It is our hope that this volume continues to honor the languages and the people that use them to name themselves and their homes.

This part highlights several interconnected themes central to understanding Native languages in contemporary North America. First is the importance of validating and supporting the everyday use of these languages. Contributors emphasize that Native languages are not merely historical artifacts or cultural curiosities but living communication systems that continue to evolve and adapt to changing circumstances. They describe current patterns of use in contexts ranging from traditional ceremonies to social media, highlighting both challenges and innovations. They discuss the emotional and psychological significance of language as a connection to ancestral knowledge and cultural identity, particularly for communities that have experienced historical trauma related to language loss.

A second key theme is the relationship between language and sovereignty. Contributors frame language maintenance and revitalization as an affirmation of the Native community's right to independently foster their cultural traditions. They describe the relationship of language reclamation to broader movements for political recognition, land rights, cultural preservation and self-determination, including international frameworks, such as the United Nations Declaration on the Rights of Indigenous Peoples, which affirm language rights as fundamental human rights.

A third theme concerns the practical challenges and strategies of language revitalization in contexts where Indigenous languages often exist alongside dominant languages like English, French, or Spanish. Contributors share approaches to language documentation, curriculum development, teacher training, and community engagement that have proven effective in various settings. They discuss innovations in language teaching methodology, multimedia resources and digital technologies that support language learning and use. They address the complexities of standardization, orthography development and terminology creation for languages that may have been primarily oral until recently. And they highlight the importance of creating new domains of use where Indigenous languages can fulfill contemporary communicative needs.

The specific languages covered in this section represent diverse geographic regions, linguistic families, and revitalization contexts. They include Diné, one of the most widely spoken Indigenous languages in the United States, with a rich tradition of literature and formal education. Studies conducted with Diné-speaking youth emphasize the need for culturally responsive assessments. These studies advocate for dynamic evaluation approaches that recognize Indigenous communication norms such as silence, indirect eye contact, and embedded humor; elements sometimes misinterpreted in mainstream assessment tools. The rigid use of standardized models without accounting for the linguistic variation that has always existed in North America advocates a prescriptive rather than descriptive view of language and dishonors Indigenous linguistic identities in educational and therapeutic settings.

The languages in the third section of the text include the following: Canadian Inuktitut, which encompasses a family of related Inuit languages spoken across the Canadian Arctic; Ishakkoy, an isolate language indigenous to the Gulf Coast that is undergoing revitalization after a period of dormancy; and Koasati, a Muskogean language spoken in

Louisiana and Texas. Koasati is being revitalized through an innovative community-driven language program. The practice of language revitalization is being used with multiple Indigenous languages of North America, including Samoan, which has developed distinctive patterns of use in diasporic contexts like California and Utah.

Allen and colleagues examine the Inuit languages spoken across Canada's Arctic regions, emphasizing the polysynthetic nature of Inuktut and its developmental progression in children. The authors caution against applying Eurocentric assessment methodologies to Inuktut speakers, advocating for community-driven language development strategies that support fluency while respecting Indigenous epistemologies.

Darensbourg and Badawy present approaches for learning and using Ishakkoy despite the absence of fluent speakers. They stress language revitalization as a decolonial act and encourage professionals to integrate Indigenous greetings and storytelling into their practice, fostering continuity even in contexts of dormancy.

Babatsouli and Sotiropoulou investigate Koasati, a Muskogean language spoken in Louisiana and Texas, alongside its accompanying English dialect. Their research, which includes a comparison with other Indigenous languages, stresses the need to distinguish between dialect differences and speech impairments when working with Indigenous populations to avoid misclassification of linguistic features as clinical disorders and in educational contexts.

Ballard and Fautua explore Samoan, an Indigenous language with a strong community presence in North America, particularly in California and Utah. Their work highlights distinctions between Samoan and English in phonology, morphology and syntax, advocating for bilingual assessments that differentiate between language differences and disorders while respecting cultural values emphasizing collectivism and nonverbal communication.

For each language, contributors provide information about phonological, grammatical, and discourse features that may be particularly relevant for practitioners. They describe typical patterns of language development for children acquiring these languages, either as monolingual speakers or in bilingual/multilingual contexts. They discuss common transfer effects that may appear when speakers of these languages use English or other majority languages. And they offer guidance to SLPs to help distinguish between language difference and language disorder. Identifying difference from disorder can be a particularly complex task in contexts where normative data may be limited.

Throughout this portion of the text, contributors emphasize the resilience of Indigenous languages and their speakers in the face of historical and ongoing hegemonic pressures for linguistic assimilation. The authors show the creativity and determination of communities engaged in linguistic revitalization work, often with limited resources but extraordinary commitment. They highlight the cultural, cognitive and ecological knowledge encoded in these languages, knowledge that represents an invaluable resource not only for Indigenous communities but for humanity. We must recognize that the loss of a language is not just the disappearance of words and grammar, but the loss of unique cultural perspectives and ways of knowing that have evolved over generations.

Part 3: Emerging Varieties – The Always Evolving Linguistic Frontier

The third part explores language varieties that are emerging in North America through the typical human processes of migration, language contact, and cultural exchange. These varieties represent the newest chapter in North America's linguistic story reflecting globalization on a micro-cultural scale. While some of these varieties have received scholarly attention, many are still in the early stages of documentation and analysis. Understanding them is crucial not only for tracking contemporary sociolinguistic trends but also for practitioners collaborating with newer immigrant communities and their children.

A central theme of this section is the process of language contact and adaptation. Contributors examine how languages change when they come into sustained contact with others, particularly in immigrant contexts where speakers must navigate between heritage languages and dominant societal languages. They describe phenomena such as code-switching (alternating between languages within a conversation or even within a single sentence), borrowing (incorporating elements from one language into another) and structural convergence (where grammatical patterns of different languages become more similar over time). They explore how speakers creatively blend linguistic resources to construct identities that reflect both their cultural heritage and their current social circumstances.

Another important theme concerns the emergence of distinctive language varieties within diasporic communities. Contributors investigate how languages like Korean, Vietnamese, Persian and Mandarin develop unique characteristics when spoken in North American contexts – features that distinguish them from the varieties spoken in their countries of origin. These diasporic varieties often incorporate English vocabulary, adopt new phonological patterns, develop innovative grammatical constructions, and establish norms of language mixing that reflect the bilingual realities of their speakers. The resulting varieties serve as powerful markers of hybrid or transnational identity, allowing speakers to express affiliation with both their heritage cultures and their North American homes.

Several researchers have contributed to the documentation and analysis of these emerging varieties. Carter examines Miami English, an ethno-regional variety shaped by Spanish English bilingualism in South Florida.

Its phonological and syntactic features reflect the influence of Spanish, forming a distinct linguistic identity within the region. Taghvafard and Babatsouli analyze Persian English bilingualism, highlighting phonological contrasts critical for speech assessment and emphasizing the importance of cultural sensitivity in clinical interactions. Choi explores Korean English bilingualism, identifying predictable patterns of phonological and grammatical transfer that speech-language pathologists must distinguish from speech disorders. Margetson and colleagues study Vietnamese English bilingualism, emphasizing the role of migration history in language maintenance and advocating for culturally responsive assessment approaches that account for dialectal variations and cross-linguistic influences.

Additional studies contribute to the broader understanding of bilingual adaptation. To and So describe Cantonese English bilingualism and examine transfer patterns in phonology, morphosyntax and vocabulary, recommending dynamic assessment methods to differentiate typical bilingual development from potential language impairments. An and Li discuss Mandarin English bilingualism, underscoring how Mandarin's distinct structures impact bilingual speech acquisition and addressing the lack of standardized assessments tailored to Mandarin-English speakers. Ning explores Mandarin-Catalan bilingualism, illustrating how prior language knowledge influences Catalan acquisition in Chinese multilingual adults and highlighting its relevance for professionals working with multilingual populations.

For practitioners collaborating with these communities, this section offers crucial guidance. Contributors discuss typical developmental patterns for children growing up with these language varieties, whether as simultaneous bilinguals from birth or as sequential bilinguals who acquire English after establishing a foundation in their heritage language. They address common transfer effects and cross-linguistic influences that may appear in children's speech and language development. They examine the impact of factors such as age of acquisition, language dominance, and patterns of language use within families and communities. And they offer strategies for assessment and intervention that respect the legitimacy of emergent bilingual varieties while supporting children's development across their full linguistic repertoire.

Throughout this section, contributors emphasize that the emergence of new language varieties is not a problem to be solved but a natural and creative response to changing social circumstances. They challenge deficit perspectives that frame language contact in terms of interference or contamination, instead highlighting the sophisticated metalinguistic awareness and communicative flexibility that bilingual speakers develop. They demonstrate how these emerging varieties enrich North America's linguistic landscape, introducing new sounds, structures, expressions and perspectives that may eventually influence mainstream varieties of English and other languages.

By documenting these emerging varieties, this section captures language evolution in progress, providing a snapshot of dynamic processes that continue to reshape North America's linguistic landscape. It reminds us that the story of language in North America is ongoing, with each new wave of migration contributing to the continent's extraordinary linguistic diversity.

The Journey Ahead

As we conclude this introduction, it is worth reiterating why *Linguistic Varieties in North America: A Guide for Speech and Language Practitioners* represents a timely and essential contribution to our understanding of language in contemporary society. First, it brings together scholarly rigor and practical application, addressing a gap that has too often separated academic research from professional practice. By providing accessible yet substantive information about diverse language varieties, it equips practitioners with knowledge that can directly improve service delivery to linguistically diverse populations. Second, it centers insider perspectives, amplifying the voices of community members, practitioners and scholar-activists who bring lived experience as well as academic expertise to their analyses. This approach yields richer, more nuanced understandings of language varieties than would be possible through external observation alone. Third, it encompasses an unusually broad range of language varieties from well-established Englishes to endangered Indigenous languages to emerging immigrant varieties, providing a comprehensive portrait of North America's linguistic landscape. Fourth, it consistently frames linguistic diversity not as a problem or challenge but as a useful resource to be recognized, supported and celebrated. This perspective runs counter to the deficit narratives that often dominate institutional responses to language difference.

The value for the reader

Different readers will use this volume for different purposes and evaluate the text based on their background, interests, needs, and professional context. Practitioners in speech-language pathology will gain specific information about the phonological, grammatical and pragmatic features of various language varieties, helping them distinguish between difference and disorder and develop culturally appropriate intervention strategies. Educators will find guidance for supporting students' language development while respecting their linguistic heritage, as well as approaches for teaching about language diversity as part of a comprehensive language arts curriculum. Researchers will discover both synthesized knowledge about well-studied varieties and preliminary descriptions of less-documented ones, potentially sparking new lines of inquiry. Students across multiple disciplines will gain foundational knowledge about linguistic diversity that will serve them throughout their academic and professional careers. Language activists and community members will find validation of their experiences and practical strategies for supporting language maintenance and revitalization. And general readers with an interest in language and culture will gain a deeper appreciation for the rich linguistic tapestry that characterizes North America.

A call to engagement

We invite readers to approach this volume not as a definitive statement but as an entry point, as a primer that introduces key concepts, varieties and issues while acknowledging the vast complexity that lies beyond these introductory discussions. The chapters that follow offer windows into different language communities, each with its own history, structural features, social dynamics, and future. We encourage readers to engage deeply with these chapters, to reflect on their implications for research and practice, and to continue exploring the language varieties that interest them most through further reading, direct engagement with language communities and through humble inquisitive application of this knowledge in their professional contexts.

We hope this volume will inspire readers to become advocates for linguistic diversity in their own spheres of influence. Whether as practitioners implementing more culturally responsive assessment procedures, as educators creating more inclusive classroom environments, as researchers pursuing community-engaged scholarship or as citizens supporting policies that protect language rights, each reader has opportunities to contribute to a society that values and sustains linguistic diversity. By deepening our understanding of language varieties and their significance, we can work toward a North America where all speakers have equitable access to education, healthcare and other essential services; where linguistic discrimination no longer limits individuals' opportunities; and where the continent's extraordinary linguistic heritage is preserved for future generations.

The journey toward full recognition and support for language diversity is ongoing, with both encouraging developments and persistent challenges. This volume represents one step in that journey, a contribution to the growing movement for recognizing the value of all people and all languages and an appreciation of language as a fundamental aspect of human dignity. We invite you to join us in celebrating and supporting the remarkable linguistic mosaic that is North America.

References

Boroditsky, L. (2001) Does language shape thought? Mandarin and English speakers' conceptions of time. *Cognitive Psychology* 43 (1), 1–22. https://doi.org/10.1006/cogp.2001.0748

Casasanto, D. (2008) Who's afraid of the big bad Whorf? Cross-linguistic differences in temporal language and thought. *Language Learning* 58 (s1), 63–79. https://doi.org/10.1111/j.1467-9922.2008.00462.x

Dwyer, S.C. and Buckle, J.L. (2009) The space between: On being an insider-outsider in qualitative research. *International Journal of Qualitative Methods* 8 (1), 54–63. https://doi.org/10.1177/160940690900800105

Eckert, P. (2000) *Linguistic Variation as Social Practice: The Linguistic Construction of Identity in Belten High*. Blackwell.

Evans, N. and Levinson, S.C. (2009) The myth of language universals: Language diversity and its importance for cognitive science. *Behavioral and Brain Sciences* 32 (5), 429–448. https://doi.org/10.1017/S0140525X0999094X

Geertz, C. (1983) *Local Knowledge: Further Essays in Interpretive Anthropology*. Basic Books.

Harrison, K.D. (2007) *When Languages Die: The Extinction of the World's Languages and the Erosion of Human Knowledge*. Oxford University Press.

Labov, W. (1972) *Language in the Inner City: Studies in the Black English Vernacular*. University of Pennsylvania Press.

Maffi, L. (2005) Linguistic, cultural, and biological diversity. *Annual Review of Anthropology* 34 (1), 599–617. https://doi.org/10.1146/annurev.anthro.34.081804.120437

Skutnabb-Kangas, T., Maffi, L. and Harmon, D. (2003) *Sharing a World of Difference: The Earth's Linguistic, Cultural, and Biological Diversity*. UNESCO.

Suwankhong, D. and Liamputtong, P. (2015) Cultural insiders and research fieldwork. *International Journal of Qualitative Methods* 14 (5), 1–7. https://doi.org/10.1177/1609406915621404

Wolff, P. and Holmes, K.J. (2011) Linguistic relativity. *Wiley Interdisciplinary Reviews: Cognitive Science* 2 (3), 253–265. https://doi.org/10.1002/wcs.104

2 African American English in the Personal Narratives of School-Age Children

An Exploration of Preverbal HAD

Monique T. Mills and Tynashia Whitaker

Introduction

Personal narration is as much an ordering of one's lived experience as it is an art form that grounds a past event into a social context such as casual conversation (Bauman, 1975; Ochs & Capps, 2009) or an elicited language assessment task (Mills *et al.*, 2013). We tell personal narratives to relive past events, share with others, communicate information about ourselves, make sense of our emotions connected to past events and solve cognitive puzzles (Engel, 1995: 84). Personal narratives are important clinically because they are a window into the sociolinguistic backgrounds of child narrators: through devices such as direct reported speech, [child] narrators tell of the language variation available to them (Bauman, 1975). Children produce 80 to 87% of personal narratives shared in working-class Black and White communities and in middle-class White communities (Blum-Kulka & Snow, 1992).

For Black children, personal narrative represents a relative strength, providing a context to express verve and linguistic creativity (Gardner-Neblett *et al.*, 2012; Mills *et al.*, 2017; Smitherman, 2000). Much of the work on African American English (AAE) in the communication sciences and disorders literature rests on dialect density measures developed to help clinicians identify features of child AAE and establish relative rate of AAE production in free play (Washington & Craig, 2002), picture description (Mills, 2015), and narrative (Mills *et al.*, 2013) elicitation tasks. To further illuminate the AAE linguistic system, noncontrastive alternatives exist to describe syntactic patterns within AAE (Green, 2011; Johnson & Koonce, 2018; Ross *et al.*, 2004). In an attempt to move beyond a feature list approach to describing AAE, we have conducted an in-depth exploration of preverbal HAD. We focus solely on the preverbal HAD construction in AAE, given the plethora of comprehensive descriptions of what

AAE is like in adults (Green, 2002; Lanehart, 2015; Mufwene *et al.*, 2022; Smitherman, 1986) and in children (Craig & Washington, 2006; Green, 2011; Oetting & Pruitt, 2005; Washington & Craig, 2002).

This chapter commences by situating AAE in a cultural and historical context. It then presents a study of preverbal HAD in child narration. Finally, the chapter provides clinical implications for researchers and for clinicians who examine, assess, and treat narrative language in school-age children.

Context and culture

African American English has a storied past. Sociolinguists have posited three main accounts of how AAE came to be: Anglicist Hypothesis (also known as Dialectologist), Creolist Hypothesis, and Divergence Hypothesis. For a comprehensive account of each theory, we urge the reader to review what sociolinguists and applied linguists have written about the sociohistorical context of AAE (Dillard, 1974; Lanehart, 2001; Redmond Taylor, 2016; Rickford & Rickford, 2000; Wolfram, 2005; Wolfram *et al.*, 1999). Here, we summarize each account of AAE's history in turn.

The Anglicist Hypothesis holds that, like other American English dialects, AAE is rooted in British English. As enslaved Blacks from West Africa interacted with White migrant workers and White slave owners, they learned to blend English into their linguistic repertoire, and AAE is the result of this linguistic union. Proponents of the Anglicist Hypothesis point to such phonological features as *r*-lessness (e.g. *cah* for *car*) that exist across many other American English dialects as evidence that AAE is indeed English.

In contrast, the Creolist Hypothesis holds that AAE is rooted in African languages. As Blacks traded goods with Europeans on the West Coast of Africa, they created a pidgin – a new and initially simple form of a language that arises out of language contact between two or more groups of people who do not share a common language (Swann *et al.*, 2004), such as Portuguese Pidgin. Combining Indo-European languages such as English, Portuguese, Spanish, Dutch and French with West African languages, Portuguese Pidgin was spoken in 'factories' on the West Coast of Africa and later adopted by enslaved persons transported to plantations in the Americas and the Caribbean (McGinnis, 1975). As Portuguese Pidgin was passed on to children on plantations across the Americas and Caribbean, a creole was formed. A creole is a new first language of a community that had previously communicated in a pidgin (Swann *et al.*, 2004). After the Great Emancipation of enslaved Blacks in the United States, the creole language underwent further modifications, becoming more similar to that of the local White population; AAE was formed.

Creolists hold firmly that even in its decreolized form, AAE retains an aspectual system that is rooted in African languages and similar in structure to those other African-based creoles such as Jamaican Creole, Haitian Creole and Liberian Settler English. For example, the remote past BIN (e.g. They *been* back from the store) and invariant BE (e.g. He *bees* bad) are grammatical structures not found in English. Moreover, Rickford (2022) demonstrated that copula absence patterns much the same way across African-based creoles and, critically, do not exist in White dialects of American English outside of the Atlantic South. He argues, 'decreolizing changes happen in a certain order, keyed to environment, and that the order of those changes could explain synchronic variability' (2022: 161). Yet, there is considerable contention among Creolist theorists regarding the extent of decreolization. For example, Winford (2015) argues that

> conditions were favorable for most Blacks to acquire relatively close approximations of the dialects spoken by White settlers throughout the Atlantic South, with creole formation restricted to the coastal areas of South Carolina, and later Georgia. (2015: 99)

Thus, the Gullah language (also known as Sea Island Creole) spoken off the coast of South Carolina presents an opportunity to test hypotheses about the formation of AAE. Because speakers of Gullah are geographically isolated by islands, their language structure may be more similar to African languages than is the AAE spoken on the mainland of the United States. We make this suggestion with caution, because, at the time of this writing, younger Gullah speakers are residing in speech communities across the United States, potentially creating a shift toward other American dialects. Learning more about child speakers of Gullah, AAE and African-based creoles in comparison to older speakers can lend support to the Creolist Hypothesis as well as best educational practices that Mainstream American English (MAE)-speaking language assessors might employ. In a recent clinical forum, Bazzocchi and colleagues (2025) presented a series of papers offering a comprehensive overview of how to formally assess language in multilingual child speakers of creole languages and varieties of AAE. They suggest language sampling, drawings, and nonword repetition tasks as culturally fair measures of language (Bazzocchi *et al.*, 2025; Washington, 2025).

Like the Creolist Hypothesis, the Divergence Hypothesis concedes that the aspectual system in AAE is unlike that of MAE. However, Divergence theorists suggest that AAE coexists with other American Dialects (Labov, 2013). In fact, the Divergence Hypothesis holds that AAE consists of a General English/MAE component and an African American component (Labov, 2013). According to this explanation, AAE's aspect system represents the African American, or decreolized, component while the tense system represents the MAE component, comprised of structures that are variably present (e.g. past tense -ed, plural -s).

Contemporary research on how children acquire AAE points to a roller-coaster trajectory, from ages four years to 20 years (Kohn *et al.*, 2021), with phonological and tense structures (/ŋ/ fronting, third person singular *-s* absence, copula absence) patterning differently than aspectual structures like invariant BE: invariant BE appears to have a later acquisition profile than do phonological and tense structures of AAE.

In the section that follows, we will briefly outline the major phonological and morphosyntactic structures of child AAE. Because we are interested in children's narrative language, we focus the remainder of the chapter on a structure of AAE that is linked with the language of storytelling: preverbal HAD.

Grammar of the Language

How phonology works in the child AAE system

The sound system of child AAE is an understudied area of inquiry. Yet, because the sound system of AAE is linked with language discrimination, which can negatively affect employability (Greer *et al.*, 2024) and housing opportunities (Baugh, 1996) in adults, and with negative test bias, which can negatively affect educational misplacement in children (Stockman, 1996; Wolfram, 1986), AAE phonology provides a promising space of investigation and advocacy.

Bailey and Thomas (2021) provide a framework for characterizing AAE phonology. They propose four types of phonological constructions in AAE: (1) processes that occur in all varieties of English but more frequently and in more varied contexts within AAE; (2) processes that occur in some other nonmainstream American English dialects, but not in MAE; (3) processes that co-occur in Southern American English, but are stigmatized outside of the Southern region of the United States; and finally (4) processes largely restricted to AAE. In Table 2.1, we provide a description of AAE phonological features within each of the four types of constructions. Drawing upon the scant but extant literature on child AAE phonology, we indicate features observed in child speech (Craig & Washington, 2004, 2006; Stockman, 1996). Craig and Washington indicate five important phonological patterns that persist between pre-kindergarten and Grade 5, yet are observed to decline in rate after Grade 1, as follows: 'g' dropping[1] (waiting → *waitin*); 'th' substitutions (birthday → *birfday*); consonant cluster reduction (world → *worl*); postvocalic reduction (mouth → *mouf*); and syllable deletion (became → *came*).

Over time, the AAE phonological system has changed in some respects and remained unchanged in others. In Table 2.2, we depict how AAE phonology has shifted since 1875, noting features observed in child AAE. For example, AAE has lost one phonological feature since 1875:

Table 2.1 Types of phonological patterns in AAE

Type of phonological construction	Linguistic term	Example	Observed in child AAE
Occur in most English dialects	Final consonant cluster reduction when stop consonant in final position of a word is preceded by a consonant of the same voicing	[lis] "least"	+
	Unstressed syllable deletion	[kem] "became"	+
	Haplology; reducing syllable in multisyllabic words with repeated similar sounds	[prali] "probably"	+
	Vocalization of postvocalic /l/ in unstressed syllable	[pi:pu] "people"	+
Occur in other NMAE dialects	r-lessness in medial and final positions of unstressed syllables and after postvocalic consonants	[mʌðə] "mother"	+
	Substitution of /f/ and /v/ for /θ/ and /ð/ in word-final or medial position; Labialization of interdental fricatives	[wrœf] "wrath" [tiv] "teethe"	+
	Stopping of syllable-initial fricatives (especially with voiced fricatives)	[dɪm] "them"	+
	Stopping of voiceless interdental fricative (especially contiguous to nasals)	[mənt] "month"	+

(Continued)

Table 2.1 (Continued)

Type of phonological construction	Linguistic term	Example	Observed in child AAE
Occur in Southern American English	Metathesis of final /s/+stop	[æks] "ask"	+
	Vocalization or loss of intersyllabic /r/	[wʌri] "worry"	NA
	Vocalization or stressed syllabic /r/	[θɛədi] "thirty"	NA
	Vocalization of unstressed syllabic /r/	[sɪstə] "sister"	+
	Glide reduction of /ai/ [ai → a] before voiced obstruents	[sad] "side"	+
	Glide reduction of /ɔɪ/ [ɔɪ → ɔə] before /l/	[bɔəl] "boil"	+
	Merger of /ɛ/ and /ɪ/ before nasals	[mɪn] "men"	+
	Merger of tense and lax front vowels before /l/	[dɪl] "deal"	NA
	Stopping of fricatives before nasals	[pæns] "pants"	NA
	Front stressing of initial syllables	[sɪstɚ] "sister"	+
Occurs only in AAE	Reduction of final nasal to vowel nasality	[mĩ] "mean"	+
	Final consonant deletion (especially affects nasals)	[goʊɪn] "going"	+
	Final stop devoicing (without shortening of preceding segment)	[bæɪ] "bag"	+
	Coarticulated glottal stop with devoiced final stop	[uʔp] "up"	NA
	Loss of /j/ after consonants	[nu] "knew"	+
	Substitution of /k/ for /t/ in /str/ clusters	[skrit] "street"	+

Note: NA = information not available.

Table 2.2 Phonological change in AAE vowel system

Feature	Pre 1875	1875–1900	After 1900	Example	Observed in child AAE
Monophthongal /e/ and /o/	+	+/–	–	[fes] "face" [sno] "snow"	NA
Central onsets of /au/	+	+	+	[əʊt] "out"	NA
'Back' back vowels	–	–/+	+	[daɔtɚ] "daughter"	NA
Raised /œ/	–	–/+	+	[bɛt] "bat"	NA
Glide-shortened /ai/ before voiced phoneme	–	–/+	+	[tam] "time"	+
Merger of /ɛ/ and /ɪ/ before nasals	–	–/+	+	[pɪn] "pen" and "pin"	+
Merger of tense/lax vowels before /l/	–	–/+	+	[dɪl] "dill" and "deal"	NA
Merger of /ɔ/ and /o/ before /r/	–	–/+	+	[hors] "horse" and "hoarse"	NA

Note: NA = information is not available.

monophthongal /e/ and /o/. AAE has two persistent phonological features since 1875: central onsets of /au/ and 'back' back vowels. Finally, AAE has gained five phonological features since 1875: raised /œ/; glide-shortened /ai/ before voiced consonants; merger of /ɛ/ and /ɪ/ before nasals; merger of tense/lax vowels before /l/; and merger of /ɔ/ and /o/ before /r/. Four of the five phonological features gained since 1875 are shared with Southern American English: raised /œ/ is additionally unique to AAE. According to Bailey and Thomas (2022: 116), the AAE vowel system 'suggests a history marked by unique origins, shared history, and independent development – the same kinds of things that characterize the histories of most languages'.

The AAE vowel system is complex and unique. According to Labov (1991), the AAE vowel system contains the same set of vowel phonemes that characterize Southern American English and other American dialects. However, AAE organizes its vowel space in a way that does not mirror that of other American dialects. Vowel differences are important because they provide many of the phonological cues that listeners use in ethnic identification (Bailey & Manor, 1989; Haley, 1990).

How morphosyntax works in the child AAE system

The aspect of AAE governing how words and sentences are structured is referred to as its morphosyntax. Morphemes – the smallest units of meaning – serve as the building blocks of sentences. Craig and Washington (2004, 2006) describe the features of morphosyntax that they observed in child AAE from pre-kindergarten to Grade 5 in a large sample of child speakers. Table 2.3 lists the major morphosyntactic features of child AAE, including examples. We refer the reader to Hamilton *et al.* (2018) for descriptions that are strengths-based.

Interestingly, five phonological patterns persist from pre-kindergarten to Grade 5 (zero copula, subject-verb agreement variation, zero article, zero preposition, appositive pronoun);[2] three are observed in pre-kindergarten and kindergarten but are dropped thereafter (zero past tense, zero plural, zero progressive *-ing*); and three others do not appear until Grade 2 or 3 (*fitna/sposeta/bouta*, indefinite article and existential *it*). Among the morphosyntactic features listed in Table 2.3, three are recognized as key components of the tense-aspect system in child AAE: zero copula, zero past tense and *fitna/sposeta/bouta* (Green, 2011). As we outline in the next section, preverbal HAD is also a notable feature of child AAE tense and aspect.

How preverbal HAD works in the child AAE system

To understand how preverbal HAD works, it helps to begin with an overview of the tense and aspect forms present in English (see Table 2.4). Preverbal HAD is an auxiliary that occurs with verbs in past contexts. As

Table 2.3 Types of morphosyntax patterns in child AAE

Type of morphosyntax construction	Linguistic term[3]	Example
Observed relatively early, but declines during elementary years.	Zero copula or auxiliary in present tense.	She (is) ready for bed. The frog (is) creeping out of the jar.
	Zero article.	He is running from (the) bees.
	Subject-verb agreement variations. Also referred to as zero verbal *-s*.	It don't (doesn't) go like that.
	Zero preposition. Prepositions are variably produced.	She was in the hospital (for) three days.
	Appositive pronoun.	Me and my friends *we* visit the library after school.
Variably present in elementary years.	Zero past tense. Regular past tense and irregular past tense may go unmarked on the verb when marked elsewhere in the sentence.	Yesterday we talk(ed) about the ocean.
	Zero plural. Plurality may not be marked on noun when marked elsewhere in the sentence.	He had a bunch of frog(s).
	Zero progressive *-ing*. Progressive *-ing* is unmarked in phonological contexts where 'gone' or 'gonna' would suffice.	She go(ing) be back.
Observed relatively late during elementary years.	*Fitna/sposeta/bouta* to indicate imminent action.	He *sposeta* be running for homecoming court.
	Indefinite article. Article *a* is used regardless of vowel context.	*A* owl is chasing the bees.
	Existential *it*. It is used regardless of referent.	*It*'s (There's) a gopher in the hole.

Note Features in parenthesis are not obligatory in AAE.

Table 2.4 Examples of tense and aspect forms of English

Present tense	
Simple	*escapes*
Perfect	*has escaped*
Progressive/Imperfect	*is escaping*
Past tense	
Simple	*escaped*
Perfect	*had escaped*
Progressive/Imperfect	*was escaping*

such, preverbal HAD is a complex verb form. Yet, preverbal HAD has been linked with ungrammaticality in children (see Berman & Slobin, 1994: 143), before the form was first described linguistically in children (Green, 2011; Ross *et al.*, 2004; Schachter & Craig, 2013). Preverbal HAD is identical in shape to past perfect, also known as pluperfect, (past before the past) sequences: preverbal HAD and past perfect are formed with HAD + verb (verb -ed) sequence. Yet, the two forms differ in meaning: past perfect refers to the past before the past (e.g. by the time the boy woke up, the frog *had escaped*), whereas preverbal HAD refers to the time before the present (e.g. the frog *had escaped* out of the jar during the night). Preverbal HAD may look like perfect aspect on the surface, but its goal is not a backwards temporal reference to events occurring relatively earlier in the past. Rather, preverbal HAD indicates time before the present, signaling that an event has culminated before the time of speaking. As such, sociolinguists consider preverbal HAD a *camouflage construction* – a form that looks similar to MAE but has different meanings (Rickford, 1999; Rickford & Rafal, 1996).

As a past tense auxiliary, preverbal HAD marks the completion of an event (*had looked*), but not the duration of an event (**had looking*): preverbal HAD is not observed in progressive or imperfect aspectual contexts in which events are ongoing. Further, preverbal HAD does not occur with emphatic forms (**DID/WILL had looked*) nor negative forms (**AIN'T/DON'T/WON'T had looked*). In AAE speakers across the lifespan, preverbal HAD precedes verbs that are irregular (*saw*) or regular (*searched*). However, in preschool-age AAE speakers, preverbal HAD may also precede verbs that are unmarked (*see, search*).

It appears that preverbal HAD (*had escaped*) is something more than its simple past counterpart (*escaped*). According to Green (2011):

> It is clear that HAD is compatible with past time marking, but it does not have the simple function of situating the event in the past or just marking it as past. The function of HAD is to indicate that an event has been achieved or accomplished. (2011: 82)

To determine the semantic meaning the child is aiming to convey, clinicians and clinical researchers must analyze verbs that occur in preverbal HAD constructions. Verbs in past tense express at least three situation types or aspectual properties, as outlined in Berman and Slobin (1994) and Smith (1997): activity – an event that does not have a final endpoint (e.g. *walk*, *play*, *ponder*); accomplishment – an event that has a final endpoint arrived at through a process (e.g. *wake up*, *make*, *manage to*); and achievement – an event that has a final endpoint that is reached relatively quickly (e.g. *fall*, *see*, *lock a door*). Because accomplishment and achievement situations have a final endpoint, they offer a perfective viewpoint. In contrast, the activity situation type, devoid of a final endpoint, offers an imperfective viewpoint of an event. Children developing AAE as well as other languages tend to first mark past tense in accomplishment and achievement contexts before they do so in an activity situation context. It appears easier for children to consider an event as past after it has been fully realize: thus, past perfect is acquired before past progressive/imperfect.

In addition to a marker of tense and aspect, preverbal HAD is also an intensifier in narrative discourse, signaling complicating actions within narratives of young school-age children (Ross *et al.*, 2004; Schachter & Craig, 2013), adolescents and adults (Rickford & Rafal, 1996). Green distinguishes preverbal and preterite HAD in Green (2011: 86) because young children do not use preverbal HAD in the same ways as adolescents and young adults. That is, young children use preverbal HAD with verbs that are overtly marked for past tense (e.g. *came, yelled*) as well as verbs that are bare (e.g. *come*, *yell*). At preschool, AAE speakers produce preverbal HAD more often with unmarked verbs than with verbs that are overtly marked morphologically. Finally, unlike older children and adults, preschoolers produce preverbal *had* in narration and in conversation (Green, 2011). Green notes that even when preverbal HAD is deployed in narratives of preschool AAE speakers, it is not necessary at the highpoint of the narrative. Young children appear to have more variability in their nascent linguistic systems than do adolescents and adults. Green (2011) argues that preverbal HAD may develop into preterite HAD with age: there may be a positive correlation between age and overt past tense marking on verbs in preverbal HAD construction present at narrative climax.

Examining preverbal HAD across narrative sampling contexts

Seventy-eight school-age African American children aged 7–11 years from central Illinois were included in this study. The mean age of the final group of participants was 8;7 years (range = 7;7–11;1). The children included in the final sample were typically developing, as represented by their performance on test batteries described below. The children included in this study were part of a larger study on language, literacy, and social capital in Black children (Mills & Fox, 2016). Following Peterson and McCabe (1983), we elicited personal narratives from a story prompt. Children then generated a personal narrative. Then they wrote the narrative. Finally, they read their narrative aloud. Using the Systematic Analysis of Language Transcripts (SALT) software, we extracted each utterance that included the word HAD. We coded each occurrence of preverbal HAD within two distinct situation types: achievement/accomplishment and activity, following Green (2011).

The results of our preliminary findings are displayed in Table 2.5 and Figure 2.1. We tallied 53 instances of preverbal HAD across all narrative conditions. As displayed in Table 2.5, school-age Black children in our pilot study produced preverbal HAD with more irregular verbs than regular verbs. Producing preverbal HAD with a greater number of irregular verbs than regular verbs may be a marker of language development, as preschool-age AAE speakers presented with the opposite profile. Although school-age AAE speakers tended to mark past tense overtly, there were a few cases in which verbs were bare. Again, overt past tense marking may be a sign of language development: preverbal HAD may be developing into preterite HAD. As Figure 2.1 illustrates, most preverbal HAD constructions occurred with achievement verbs (75%), rather than activity verbs (25%). During the school-age years, child AAE speakers continue to prefer past events that are complete, rather than ongoing. However, we did not analyze past progressive context directly, and this is a direction to take in the future.

Finally, with regard to narrative context, no child produced preverbal HAD in all three contexts. Two children produced preverbal HAD in more than one context: narrative generation and narrative writing. Across narrative context, narrative generation tended to include more instances of preverbal HAD than did narrative writing, which included more instances than narrative oral reading. The excerpts that follow are from a child ('Nadine') who is 11;5 and in Grade 5. We have selected sentences from her narrative generation and narrative writing that include preverbal HAD to illustrate her editing process:

Nadine's narrative generation sample

When we HAD went to Jamaica we went scuba diving.
It was funny because we HAD put on the mask and my dad jumped in.
And my mom HAD looked at her like 'no you didn't just say that'.

Nadine's narrative writing sample

We HAD went on a cruise, but my parents didn't tell us.
When we HAD got on the boat the first day we went swimming.

Table 2.5 Verbs within preverbal HAD constructions

HAD V-ed	HAD V-∅
Narrative generation	
walked	come
came	
left	
told	
found out	
slipped	
fell	
got	
forgot	
said	
made	
gotten	
woke up	
brung	
moved	
went	
locked	
put	
knew	
ate	
gave	
bought	
looked	
started	
saw	
jumped	
thought	
played	
Narrative writing	
started	walk
came	
called	
Narrative oral reading	
got	∅

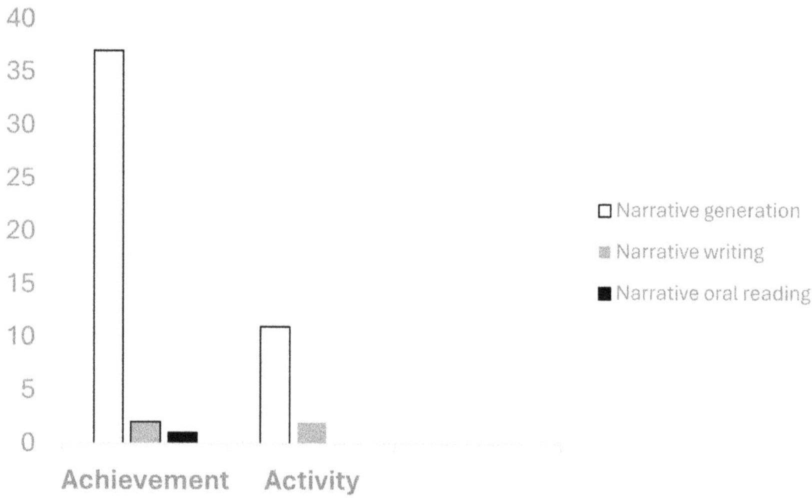

Figure 2.1 Preverbal HAD production within situation type and across narrative context

Children like Nadine may edit themselves across the tasks that moved from oral to literate. This movement may be explained by schooling. Children may have adopted school literacies that require more standardized grammatical forms in written language than in oral language. If children shift registers in this way – producing a more concise rendering of past events – it may be a sign of learning. Nadine's sentences display grammatical prowess, and she includes multiple clauses in each utterance and cohesive devices, such as coordinating conjunctions, whether narrating orally or in print. She includes narrative devices that assist with character development, such as direct reported speech. The narrative shared is of a past event that carried much joy and interest: her narrative generation was over eight minutes in length. Preverbal HAD is not just used to thicken the plot of the narrative; it is also deployed to initiate each narrative. Thus, school-age children like Nadine have room for improvement such that preverbal HAD develops into preterite HAD.

Clinical Implications for Researchers

Researchers interested in how children acquire AAE may think preverbal HAD an unimportant part of AAE grammar because it occurs so infrequently. However, based on the roller-coaster trajectory of AAE (Kohn *et al.*, 2021), we urge researchers to examine how preverbal HAD develops through adolescence and into emerging adulthood. Support for the Anglicist Hypothesis could be explored in future research by comparing preverbal HAD in child AAE speakers with auxiliary systems of children who speak other American dialects, such as Southern White English and Appalachian English. Does a comparable construction exist? If so, this may be evidence that preverbal HAD is part of the deep structure of English. Researchers with Creolist Hypothesis leanings may be interested in exploring narrative language in creoles spoken across the African diaspora to determine if children deploy similar auxiliary verb constructions. Such evidence may point to preverbal HAD as sharing in the deep structure of African languages. Those aligned with the Divergence Hypothesis may seek evidence in longitudinal studies suggesting that preverbal HAD is diverging from the auxiliaries that look similar on the surface, such as pluperfect in MAE, due to social segregation of Black and White speech communities. As Weldon (2021) suggests, such a study would also need to explore social stratification within race-based speech communities to examine how middle-class speakers deploy preverbal HAD.

Clinical Implications for Practitioners

Narrative language is critical in schools and in society. Most state educational standards include storytelling expectations. Children are expected to tell a story with a clear beginning, middle and end and with lots of descriptive detail. What happens when stories are presented in AAE? If child AAE narrators present their stories to an MAE-speaking audience in classrooms (Michaels, 1981), what is the likelihood that they will be understood? For example, studies have shown that court testimony presented in AAE is often misunderstood by court reporters (Eades, 2010; Green, 2002; Jones *et al.*, 2019; Rickford & King, 2016; Rickford & Rickford, 2000), threatening both linguistic justice (Baker-Bell, 2020) and justice. Jones and colleagues' findings indicated 'a court reporter may have heard and correctly transcribed stressed *been* or preterite *had*, but mistranscribed a different part of the utterance' (e234), suggesting that court reporters could accurately transcribe AAE constructions but the meanings of AAE constructions were often lost in translation. When MAE speakers listen to the preverbal HAD construction, do they imagine an event occurring in the near past or in the far past? If there is a cognitive cost to processing AAE, might this cost be exacerbated by pervasive ideologies of language standardization, leading to negative views of AAE and its speakers (see Greer *et al.*, 2024; Mills, 2024; Mills, 2025; Scrivner *et al.*, 2025)?

Language experts, particularly school-based speech-language pathologists (SLPs), play a critical role in advocating for AAE and its speakers (Gibson & Terrell Shockley, 2018). As frontline practitioners, SLPs and other educators have the power to shape inclusive learning environments by implementing best practices that support children's language development. One such approach involves recasting children's statements – preserving their intended meaning while modeling alternative language structures. By actively engaging with children's narratives, we foster deeper connections, encourage linguistic exploration and validate their cultural identity.

When children recount past events in AAE, we do more than simply listen – we empower. Through thoughtful questioning, we spark critical thinking, expand their expressive abilities and nurture linguistic security. The stories they share offer invaluable insights into their experiences and perspectives, reminding us of the profound humanity in their voices. In turn, we share stories that resonate with their realities, reinforcing a reciprocal learning process.

Conclusion

This chapter provides an in-depth analysis of preverbal HAD – a key narrative feature used by AAE speakers. SLPs and other school-based practitioners can add this chapter to their toolkit, advocating for language equity and cultural responsiveness in education. In conclusion, we aimed to demonstrate through this exploration of preverbal HAD the rich tense and aspect system that is inherent in AAE. Clinicians and clinical researchers might use this chapter to help them describe narrative language presented in AAE. With age, child AAE speakers are likely to increase the production of irregular verbs (this is also true for non-AAE speaking children). Likewise, over time, AAE-speaking children may reduce the number of past tense verbs that go unmarked. Finally, context matters: children are likely to produce a greater rate of AAE in contexts considered informal, such as speaking, than in formal contexts like writing and reading aloud.

Acknowledgments

We thank the parents who allowed their children to partake in our study. We are grateful to a grant that provided funds to collect and analyze data. We are forever thankful for members of the Child Language Ability Lab who transcribed and coded personal narratives. We appreciate sponsorship from the ASHFoundation, National Institutes of Health (1R21DC019997-01A1), and a Social and Behavioral Sciences Small Grant from The Ohio State University.

Notes

(1) ‘g’ dropping is the same phonological pattern as /ŋ/ fronting, which is described as having a ‘roller-coaster’ trajectory into emergent adulthood (Kohn *et al.*, 2021).
(2) Copula and subject-verb agreement variation have been described as having a ‘roller-coaster’ trajectory into emerging adulthood (Kohn *et al.*, 2021).
(3) For strengths-based descriptions of AAE rules, see Hamilton *et al.* (2018).

References

Bailey, G. and Maynor, N. (1989) The divergence controversy. *American Speech* 64 (1), 12–39. https://doi.org/10.2307/455110

Bailey, G. and Thomas, E. (2022) Some aspects of African-American vernacular English phonology. In S.S. Mufwene, J.R. Rickford, G. Bailey and J. Baugh (eds) *African-American English* (pp. 93–118). Routledge.

Baker-Bell, A. (2020) *Linguistic Justice: Black Language, Literacy, Identity, and Pedagogy*. NCTE.

Baugh, J. (2018) *Linguistics in Pursuit of Justice*. Cambridge University Press.

Bauman, R. (1975) Verbal art as performance 1. *American Anthropologist* 77 (2), 290–311.

Bazzocchi, N., Kokotek, L., Kathryn, C. and Washington, K. (2025) Beyond test scores: Using drawings and language samples to characterize multilingual children's language profiles. *Seminars in Speech and Language* (online) 46, 87–106. https://doi.org/10.1055/s-0044-1801814

Berman, R.A. and Slobin, D.I. (1994) *Relating Events in Narrative: A Crosslinguistic Developmental Study*. Psychology Press.

Blum-Kulka, S. and Snow, C.E. (1992) Developing autonomy for tellers, tales, and telling in family narrative events. *Journal of Narrative and Life History* 2 (3), 187–217. https://doi.org/10.1075/jnlh.2.3.02dev

Craig, H.K. and Washington, J. A. (2004) Grade-related changes in the production of African American English. *Journal of Speech, Language, and Hearing Research* 47 (2), 450–463. https://doi.org/10.1044/1092-4388(2004/036)

Craig, H.K. and Washington, J.A. (2006) *Malik Goes to School: Examining the Language Skills of African American Students from Preschool-5th Grade*. Psychology Press.

Dillard, J.L. (1974) *Black English: Its History and Usage in the United States*. Vintage.

Eades, D. (2010) *Sociolinguistics and the Legal Process*. Multilingual Matters.

Engel, S. (1995) *The Stories Children Tell: Making Sense of the Narratives of Childhood*. Macmillan.

Gardner-Neblett, N., Pungello, E.P. and Iruka, I.U. (2012) Oral narrative skills: Implications for the reading development of African American children. *Child Development Perspectives* 6 (3), 218–224.

Gibson, S. and Terrell Shockley, E. (2018) Walking the tightrope between advocacy and knowledge: An appeal from teacher educators to speech-language pathologists regarding African American English. *Perspectives of the ASHA Special Interest Groups* 3 (1), 147–158.

Green, L.J. (2002) *African American English: A Linguistic Introduction*. Cambridge University Press.

Green, L.J. (2011) *Language and the African American Child*. Cambridge University Press. https://doi.org/10.1017/cbo9780511975561

Greer, T.W., Mills, M.T. and Lapka, S. (2024) The influence of linguistic profiling on perceived employability: A new application of the systems theory framework of career development. *Career Development International* 29 (3), 352–366.

Haley, K. (1990) Some complexities in speech identification. *SECOL Review* 14, 101–113.

Hamilton, M.B., Mont, E.V. and McLain, C. (2018) Deletion, omission, reduction: Redefining the language we use to talk about African American English. *Perspectives of the ASHA Special Interest Groups* 3 (1), 107–117.

Johnson, V.E. and Koonce, N.M. (2018) Language sampling considerations for AAE speakers: A patterns- and systems-based approach. *Perspectives of the ASHA Special Interest Groups* 3 (1), 36–42.

Jones, T., Kalbfeld, J.R., Hancock, R. and Clark, R. (2019) Testifying while black: An experimental study of court reporter accuracy in transcription of African American English. *Language* 95 (2), e216–e252.

Kohn, M., Wolfram, W., Farrington, C., Renn, J. and Van Hofwegen, J. (2021) *African American Language: Language Development from Infancy to Adulthood*. Cambridge University Press.

Labov, W. (1991) The three dialects of English. In P. Eckert (ed.) *New Ways of Analyzung Sound Change* (pp. 1–44). Academic Press.

Labov, W. (2013) Co-existent systems in African–American vernacular English. In S.S. Mufwene, J.R. Rickford, G. Bailey and J. Baugh (eds) *African–American English: Structure, History, and Use* (pp. 119–168). Routledge.

Lanehart, S.J. (ed.) (2001) *Sociocultural and Historical Contexts of African American English*. John Benjamins.

Lanehart, S. (ed.) (2015) *The Oxford Handbook of African American Language*. Oxford University Press.

McCabe, A. and Peterson, C. (1984) What makes a good story. *Journal of Psycholinguistic Research* 13 (6), 457–480. https://doi.org/10.1007/BF01068179

McGinnis, J. (1975) Historical sketch of Black English. In R.L. Williams (ed.) *Ebonics: The True Language of Black Folks*. The Institute of Black Studies.

Michaels, S. (1981) Sharing time: Children's narrative styles and differential access to literacy. *Language in Society* 10 (3), 423–442. https://doi.org/10.1017/S0047404500008861

Mills, M.T. (2015) The effects of visual stimuli on the spoken narrative performance of school-age African American children. *Language, Speech, and Hearing Services in Schools* 46 (4), 337–351. https://doi.org/10.1044/2015_lshss-14-0070

Mills, M.T. (2024) *Language Ideology and Subtle Hate Speech*. Hate Speech Research Project, University of Houston. https://www.uh.edu/class/mcl/hate-speech-research-project/editorials/language-ideology-and-subtle-hate-speech/

Mills. M.T. (2025) Language, literacy, and identity: Clinical and educational perspectives on African American English in child development. *Seminars in Speech and Language* 46 (03), 159–161. https://doi.org/10.1055/a-2729-0763

Mills, M.T. and Fox, M. (2016) Language variation and theory of mind in typical development: An exploratory study of school-age African American narrators. *American Journal of Speech-Language Pathology* 25 (3), 426–440. https://doi.org/10.1044/2016_ajslp-15-0038

Mills, M.T., Watkins, R.V. and Washington, J.A. (2013) Structural and dialectal characteristics of the fictional and personal narratives of school-age African American children. *Language, Speech, and Hearing Services in Schools* 44 (2), 211–223. https://doi.org/10.1044/0161-1461(2012/12-0021

Mills, M.T., Mahurin-Smith, J. and Steele, S.C. (2017) Does rare vocabulary use distinguish giftedness from typical development? A study of school-age African American narrators. *American Journal of Speech-language Pathology* 26 (2), 511–523. https://doi.org/10.1044/2016_ajslp-15-0157

Mufwene, S.S., Rickford, J.R., Bailey, G. and Baugh, J. (2022) *African American English: Structure, History, and Use*. Routledge Linguistics Classics.

Ochs, E. and Capps, L. (2009) *Living Narrative: Creating Lives in Everyday Storytelling*. Harvard University Press. https://doi.org/10.2307/j.ctv2d7x4pr

Oetting, J.B. and Pruitt, S. (2005) Southern African–American English use across groups. *Journal of Multilingual Communication Disorders* 3 (2), 136–144.

Peterson, C. and McCabe, A. (1983) *Developmental Psycholinguistics: Three Ways of Looking at a Child's Narrative*. Plenum Press.

Redmond Taylor, L. (2016) *Introduction to Ebonics: The Reflexification of African Grammar with English and Other Indo-European Words*. Professional Publishing House, LLC.

Rickford, J.R. (1999) *African American Vernacular English: Features, Evolution, Educational Implications*. Blackwell.

Rickford, J.R. (2022) The creole origins of African-American vernacular English: Evidence from copula absence. In S.S. Mufwene, J.R. Rickford, G. Bailey and J. Baugh (eds) *African-American English: Structure, History, and Use* (pp. 169–220). Routledge.

Rickford, J.R. and King, S. (2016) Language and linguistics on trial: Hearing Rachel Jeantel (and other vernacular speakers) in the courtroom and beyond. *Language* 92 (4), 948–988.

Rickford, J.R. and Rafal, C.T. (1996) Preterite had+V-ed in the narratives of African-American preadolescents. *American Speech* 71 (3), 227–254. https://doi.org/10.1215/00031283-79-2-167

Rickford, J.R. and Rickford, R.J. (2000) *Spoken Soul: The Story of Black English.* Wiley.

Ross, S.H., Oetting, J.B. and Stapleton, B. (2004) Preterite had+ V-ed: A developmental narrative structure of African American English. *American Speech* 79 (2), 167–193. https://doi.org/10.1215/00031283-79-2-167

Schachter, R.E. and Craig, H.K. (2013) Students' production of narrative and AAE features during an emergent literacy task. *Language, Speech, and Hearing Services in Schools* 44, 227–238. https://doi.org/10.1044/0161-1461 (2013/12-0034)

Scrivner, S.A., Lee, G., Moore, L.C. and Mills, M.T. (2025) Teachers' beliefs about child AAE speakers' language and narratives: A qualitative exploration of language beliefs and informal narrative assessment. *Seminars in Speech and Language* 46 (4), 286–307. https://doi.org/10.1055/a-2763-3161

Smith, C. (1997) *The Parameter of Aspect* (2nd edn). Springer. https://doi.org/10.1007/978-94-011-5606-6

Smitherman, G. (1986) *Talkin and Testifyin: The Language of Black America.* Wayne State University Press.

Smitherman, G. (2000) *Talkin that Talk: Language, Culture, and Education in African America.* Routledge.

Stockman, I.J. (1996) Phonological development and disorders in African American children. In A.G. Kamhi, K.E. Pollock and J.L. Harris (eds) *Communication Development and Disorders in African American Children: Research, Assessment, and Intervention* (pp. 117–153). Paul H. Brookes Publishing Company.

Swann, J. (2019) *Dictionary of Sociolinguistics.* Edinburgh University Press.

Washington, J.A. and Craig, H.K. (2002) Morphosyntactic forms of African American English used by young children and their caregivers. *Applied Psycholinguistics* 23 (2), 209–231. https://doi.org/10.1017/s0142716402002035

Washington K.N. (2025) Creole languages and American Englishes: Multilingualism and pediatric speech-language pathology. *Seminars in Speech and Language*, 75–86.

Weldon, T.L. (2021) *Middle-Class African American English.* Cambridge University Press.

Winford, D. (2015) The origins of African American vernacular English. In S. Lanehart (ed.) *The Oxford Handbook of African American Language* (pp. 85–104). Oxford University Press.

Wolfram, W. (1986) Language variation in the United States. In O.L. Taylor (ed.) *Nature of Communication Disorders in Culturally and Linguistically Diverse Populations* (pp. 73–115). College-Hill Press.

Wolfram, W. (2005) African American English. In M.J. Ball (ed.) *Clinical Sociolinguistics* (pp. 87–100). Blackwell Publishing.

Wolfram, W., Adger, C.T. and Christian, D. (1999) *Language Variation in Schools and the Community.* Erlbaum.

3 Appalachian Englishes

Paul E. Reed

Introduction

The Appalachian region of the Southern and Eastern United States is a region that has experienced scrutiny from numerous disciplines, from geology to linguistics. And, for each discipline, a pervasive issue arises, best captured by a quote from John C. Campbell. He writes about Appalachia, 'there are more things known that are not true than of any region in the nation' (Campbell, 1921). As one can see from the date, this aphorism is now more than a century old, yet its truth remains. For speech-language clinicians working in Appalachia or working with clients from the region, it is very likely that certain beliefs and myths might be familiar, as well as a lacuna of knowledge regarding aspects of the language varieties spoken in the region. The present chapter hopes to address these.

There are numerous circulating myths regarding Appalachia and its language varieties. A careful reader will note that this chapter refers to Appalachian varieties, with care to emphasize the plural. I make this effort to help dispel the myth that there is but one variety spoken; the reality is many varieties are spoken. Much recent work in the region highlights intra-regional diversity, e.g. *Appalachian Englishes in the 21st Century* (Hazen, 2020). Another myth, well-known and oft repeated, is that Appalachian varieties are holdovers from earlier English forms, usually described as some type of Elizabethan or Chaucerian style. While false and debunked (Cramer, 2014; Montgomery, 1998), such a myth persists to help speakers fight the circulating stigmas about the region as a whole. Sadly, this myth is still believed by many both inside the region and outside it – I just recently heard it. But the fact that such mistruths persist suggests an overall lack of general understanding of the region and its culture. I hope to help inform readers regarding many of the linguistic aspects of the language varieties, focusing on those aspects that might present issues during a typical speech/language assessment. The chapter follows the following structure – first, I will address the fundamental and crucial question, where is Appalachia? While some might say this answer is obvious, it is more opaque than one might expect. Then, we will approach phonological variation, grammatical variation and I will briefly mention lexical variation.

Where Is Appalachia?

To begin our exploration of Appalachian Englishes, we must first establish where we are referring to – where is Appalachia? Such a question seems simple at first glance, but it is not as straightforward as one might think. Many people associate the region with the Appalachian Mountain range, which stretches from Georgia in the southeast to Maine in the northeast. Further, historically, many have assumed that there is some shared monolithic culture (and language variety) of the region. As a result, the massive area of the Appalachian Mountain range would be considered too broad. The official designation, which is not without discussion and controversy (see below), of Appalachia from the Appalachian Regional Commission (ARC), the governmental agency tasked with overseeing the region, labels 423 counties across 13 states – Mississippi, Alabama, Georgia, Tennessee, Kentucky, South Carolina, North Carolina, Ohio, Virginia, West Virginia, Maryland, Pennsylvania and New York – as Appalachian (see Figure 3.1 below). This massive area

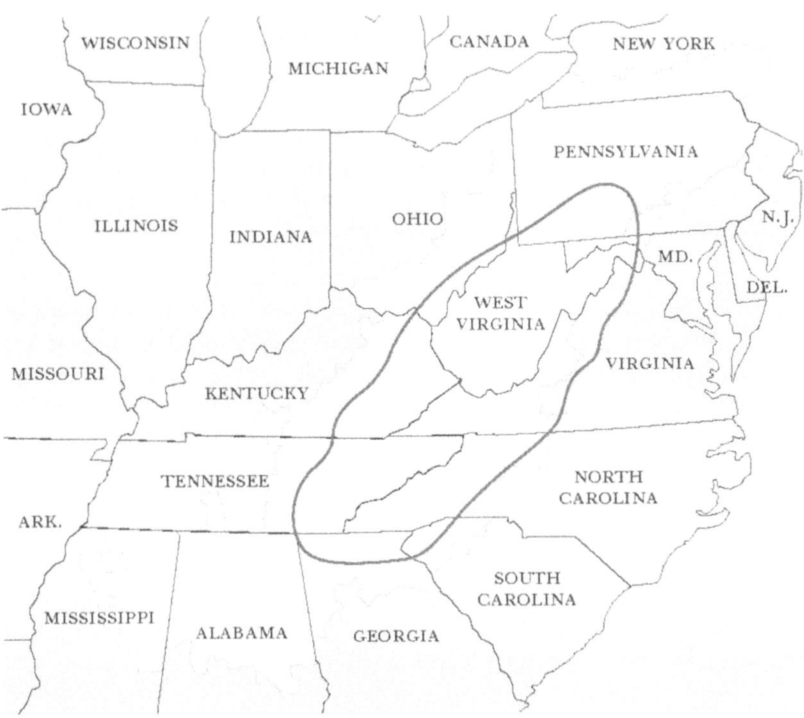

Figure 3.1 The Appalachian Region of the United States is outlined in white, with the core region encircled

encompasses urban areas, rural areas, suburban areas, different climate zones, etc. To arrive at this massive region, the ARC uses a combination of factors when assessing/assigning the label *Appalachian* for a county, using geographic factors, economic factors and transportation concerns. However, many folks are surprised at this expansive region, as both natives to the region and outsiders tend to have a much narrower conception of the region. By using economics and transportation, the ARC includes areas where both locals and non-locals do not (and we might say would not) consider themselves as Appalachian nor would they accept/embrace the label 'Appalachian'. However, as Puckett (2003) notes, 'both *Appalachia* and *Appalachian English* are therefore non-indigenous lexemes not recognized by community residents or, if recognized, used under systems of metapragmatic awareness and linguistic ideological construction that conform to the linguistic ideologies of their communities and networks...' (2003: 541; emphasis in original).

Thus, the term Appalachian Englishes should be understood best as a scholarly umbrella term to cover the numerous varieties spoken in this core area, which will have different local names (such as mountain, country, etc.). Perhaps a better definition includes where people, both inside and outside the region, *believe* Appalachia is (cf. the title of Batteau's (1990) book *The Invention of Appalachia*). In this vein, the seminal work is Ulack and Raitz (1981) that polled over 2000 insiders and outsiders to the region. They noted the areas where both insiders and outsiders agreed Appalachia was located. The area denoted in Figure 3.1 shows the core area wherein the overlap in agreement as to the location of Appalachia. This much more circumscribed area fits better with most folks' conception of where Appalachia is, and for the purposes of this chapter, where most of the linguistic features are concentrated.

Sub-regions

Within the expansive region, several sub-regions have been identified – Northern, Central and Southern (with smaller sub-sub-regions, see Figure 3.2). While each region has some similarities, linguistically, most of the features that tend to be recognized as regional and/or those that tend not to be used outside of the region are concentrated in Central and Southern Appalachia. However, there are ecological differences between and among these sub-regions. For example, in Central Appalachia, coal mining was a primary historic industry that is now waning. However, in Southern Appalachia, there was much less coal, and more forestry and timbering. They are united, however, in the fact that both industries fostered the creation of many small communities that were somewhat relatively isolated.

From a linguistic perspective, the Northern sub-regions tend to pattern more closely to varieties that are Midland and Mid-Atlantic

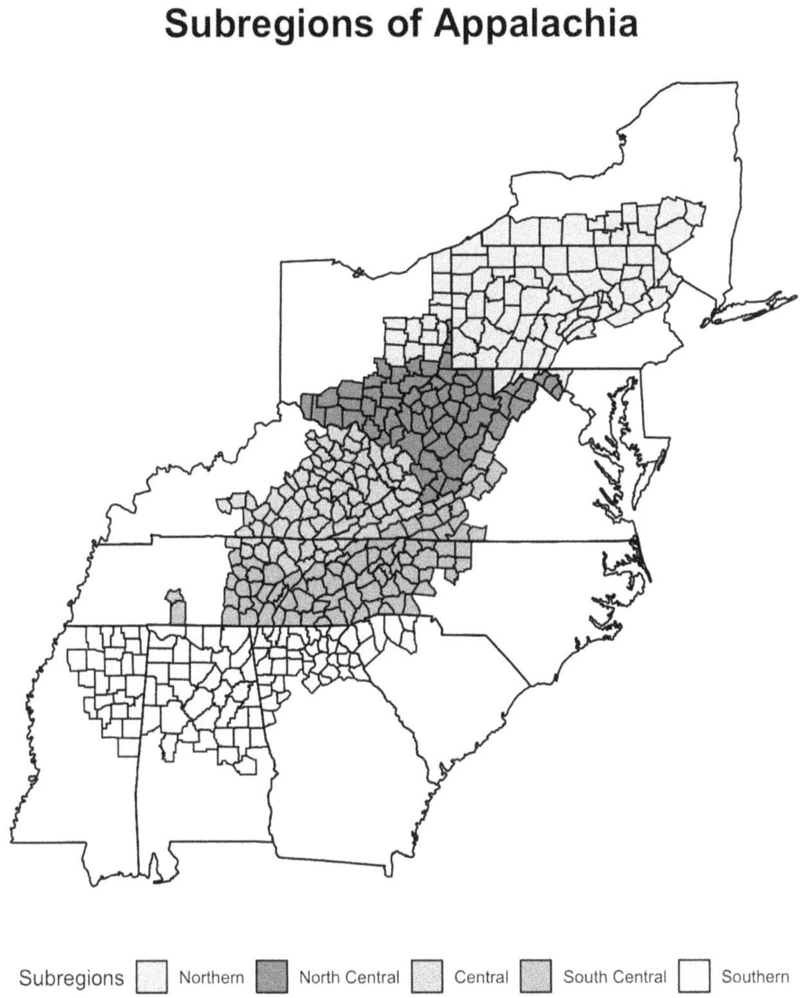

Figure 3.2 This figure shows the Appalachian sub-regions as defined by the Appalachian Regional Commission

(Hasty & Childs, 2021), depending on geography. Obviously, this is a bit of an overstatement, as any speech and language specialist or clinician should be cognizant of the potential for socially based variation. A note, many, if not most, of the features that have traditionally been considered Appalachian, and much of the published research has focused on the Southern half of the geographic Appalachian region, within the core region. Thus, for the remainder of this chapter, I will concentrate on the features associated with this part of Appalachia. Further, this area corresponds to the mental map of the core area mentioned above, which buttresses the rationale to focus primarily on it.

Rootedness

As referenced above, the region of Appalachia is routinely and pervasively stigmatized in the broader American society. The region is often ridiculed and denigrated, especially in popular media (see Billings *et al.*, 2000 or Harkins & McCarroll, 2019 for responses from Appalachian natives). Thus, many Appalachians are well aware of how they and their speech are viewed (Greene, 2010; Reed, 2014, 2016). However, Appalachians are also aware of how using the features and characteristics of the regional variety signal attachment to and orientation toward the region in the face of stigma. The language becomes a signal of home and belonging, what I have termed *rootedness*, a sense that Appalachia is important to the speaker's identity (Reed, 2016, 2020c). Like any disputed region (or group), some Appalachian speakers may have a stronger rootedness (i.e. a closer orientation to the region) and will use more of the features outlined below or will use them in a greater variety of interactions with more interlocutors. Others, in contrast, may have a weaker rootedness, and thus might not use as many of the features or will be more reticent to use the features with non-Appalachians. This avoidance might be due to the possible stigma associated with the features.

I want to emphasize that this chapter will describe many features that should best be considered as possibilities. Not every speaker will use all the features, although some very well might. Or a speaker might not use all the features with all conversational interlocutors, but they may use some of them. It will truly vary individually.

Appalachian English Features

Several linguistic features have been identified in most investigations of Appalachian English varieties (Wolfram & Christian, 1976). In this section, I highlight those that tend to differ from most other varieties of American English (although there will undoubtedly be overlap with many Southern American English varieties), with a particular emphasis on features that clinicians should be aware of as the discussed features can easily be misunderstood as 'errors' and/or might be scored as 'errors' on some diagnostic instruments. A note about overlap with other varieties – many of the following features correspond to both Southern American and African American varieties as well. And, for some features, there are differences with respect to ethnicity, i.e. some Black Appalachian speakers may use a feature more often. I will discuss some of those key features providing explanatory detail about the patterns found and, more importantly, about the ways in which they have been used as diagnostic indicators among regions and groups.

Pragmatics

One overarching characteristic of many speakers of Appalachian English varieties is a distinct focus on indirectness. In her seminal book on Appalachian pragmatics, Puckett notes that many of her participants and respondents assiduously avoided being direct. In fact, this linguistic aspect was so striking that she titled her book *Seldom Ask, Never Tell* to emphasize this (Puckett, 2000). During her fieldwork, she noted that speakers would use many indirect speech acts and indirect speech in general. Puckett elaborates on what she means as indirect in that Appalachian speakers tend to avoid statements that could be interpreted as imposing on the hearer, such as requests, commands and/or challenges. This avoidance of asking or telling helps to protect the independence and social standing of all persons involved (what some call *face* (Brown & Levinson, 1987)). Thus, to ask that someone do something requires much linguistic and social work to ensure that each person's face is maintained. To ensure face is maintained, the petitioner must be careful not to overly burden the petitionee. To move this discussion to current practitioners and other speech or language professionals, care must be taken when asking a person to do something, particularly before a very strong rapport has been built. Further forging strong rapport must be a high priority (as it would most likely be anyway), as to make an ask requires time and care. Thus, a clinician must be acquainted with this pragmatic focus. To give very direct instruction and/or very direct feedback could be interpreted as rude. Further, a client or someone affiliated with a client would most likely never directly ask questions, seek additional help or respond about difficulties, as such utterances might be understood as imposing on the clinician. Naturally, there is much individual and familial variation regarding this particular pragmatic aspect of language. So, a clinician must seek to build and foster rapport with the client and all those affiliated with the client, and any overt requests will need to be handled with care. And, when seeking feedback from a client or their family, several requests (appropriately made!) might be needed to receive it.

Lexical variation

Across the Appalachian region, and especially the Southern portions that are the focus of this chapter, there are many words, phrases and lexical items that are widespread within the region but are much lesser known outside it. However, a good number of them (if not the majority) are quite restricted to the speech of older residents, or at the very least tend to be used only among intimates. A full list of all the words and phrases goes beyond this chapter, but the most comprehensive resource is

Montgomery and Heinmiller (2021), a true magnum opus of Appalachian lexicography.

Two lexical items that are related to one another and are also quite common across the Appalachian region (and the South as a whole) are the second person plural *y'all* and *you'uns* (this is sometimes rendered *yinz* or *yunz* as the production of the vowel can vary) (Lipski, 1993). Most folks have heard *y'all* as it has greatly expanded its range beyond the American South. However, *you'uns* is much more restricted, but still common across parts of Appalachia (Hasty & Childs, 2021). Each of these arose due to the collapse of the singular second person pronoun series (*thou*, *thee*, *thine*) by around the year 1700. To address this loss, *you*, the formerly second person plural, began to be used in singular constructions. As a result, a gap emerged for second person plurals (Montgomery, 1989). Most varieties of English have created or adapted a second person plural (*you guys*, *youse*, *you all*), but *y'all* is the most common in the South and in Appalachia. But, in many areas, one will still hear *you'uns* as well.

Phonological features

Prosody

Prosody encompasses phonetic and phonological phenomena above the level of an individual phoneme, which can include aspects of speech such as speech rate, speech rhythm and intonation. Research into these phenomena is not quite as common or robust as research into vowels, consonants, syntax or grammatical differences. However, Appalachian Englishes are characterized by differences in both prosody and intonation. In fact, some investigators into the region and its language features have stated that the region's prosody might be what sets it apart most (Hall, 1942; Williams, 1992).

Intonation

Intonational variation in Appalachian varieties has received some recent scholarly attention. Several recent studies found that Appalachian intonation was distinct from that of other Southern varieties (Greene, 2006; Reed, 2020b) and from other American English varieties (Burdin *et al.*, 2018, 2022). These distinctions occur both in the relative frequency of pitch accents and in the phonetic realization of pitch accent contours. What this finding means is that Appalachian speakers use much more pitch variation than many other American English varieties. Speakers of Appalachian English varieties use a particular pitch contour (L+H*) that is often used as an emphatic or focus contour in many other varieties. To someone not familiar with these pitch contours, it can appear as if Appalachian speakers are being quite emphatic, or occasionally it can seem as if they have moved into a storytelling mode.

Prosodic rhythm

Prosodic rhythm, or how a language organizes the differences in strong and weak syllables, has produced fascinating research that has illuminated differences between languages, or, more important for the present chapter, differences between regional varieties of the same language. Languages or varieties with greater durational differences in adjacent syllables (i.e. specifically greater pairwise variability), such as English and German, were historically categorized as stress-timed. This means that a stressed syllable is much longer (and typically louder) than an unstressed syllable. Those languages with lesser differences in adjacent syllables (i.e. lesser pairwise variability), such as Spanish or Mandarin, were considered syllable-timed. This means there is not a large durational difference between stressed and unstressed syllables. Crucially, languages and varieties tend to fall on a continuum of more stress-timed (i.e. a greater difference in the duration of stressed to unstressed syllables) to less stress-timed (or more syllable-timed, i.e. more equal duration between stressed and unstressed syllables). In Reed (2020d), I compared a variety of Appalachian English to a variety of Southern American English (not from the mountains), and I found clear differences in prosodic rhythm using nPVI (Clopper & Smiljanic, 2015), which is a method of comparing the durations of adjacent syllables. The greater the nPVI the more stress-timed, and vice versa. The Appalachian variety had a greater nPVI than the Southern US variety, which indicates greater durational differences between adjacent syllables, i.e. more stress timing. Further, I found that more rooted Appalachian speakers had the greatest nPVI. What this means for clinicians is that Appalachian speakers can have very short, almost elided, unstressed syllables. Such productions are not errors, rather variable productions.

Consonants

Overall, the majority of consonants in Appalachia are in a very similar fashion to the consonants in other North American varieties. Within such a large geographic region, and with the social variation within the region, there will undoubtedly be much individual variation. However, in the aggregate, many of the consonants would follow other varieties. I note some of the exceptions below (most are derived from overviews such as Hall (1942) and Reed (2020a)), focusing primarily on those features that clinicians should be especially cognizant of.

/w/ and /ʍ/

Historically, many varieties of North American English had two labiovelar approximate sounds, the voiced /w/ and the voiceless /ʍ/, rendering *well* and *whale* as different, as well as other pairs such as *witch* and *which*. In many, if not most, modern North American English varieties, these two sounds have merged, leaving only one labiovelar approximate, the voiced /w/. The result of this merger is that *well/whale* and *witch/which* are now homophones. However, in many parts of Appalachia, the distinction of /w/ and /ʍ/ for some speakers is maintained, although it may be receding (Hazen *et al.*, 2016). Thus, clinicians should be aware that some speakers will have an additional phoneme, and they will need to adjust any scoring for an assessment to include the voiceless variant.

/l/ vocalization

Like many English varieties in North America, many Appalachian speakers have a very dark velarized /ɫ/ in syllable-final position. For many speakers, the syllable-final lateral will be realized as a vowel, with a resulting production of a vocalized /l/ that, depending upon the speaker, may be articulated more like /u/ or /ʊ/. Vocalization is very common across social boundaries and groups. However, akin to many features, /l/ vocalization may be receding across time (Dodsworth & Hazen, 2011). As stated above, clinicians will need to be very cognizant that some Appalachian speakers will not have a syllable-final /l/ – it will likely be produced as a vowel. Such productions are not the result of any deviant or delayed phonological pattern/process, rather a natural and grammatical production.

Devoicing of final /z/

A lesser known and yet fairly common consonantal feature of Appalachian Englishes is that of devoicing of word-final /z/, being realized very closely to /s/. Walker *et al.* (2017) found this in several Southern US varieties, but it was more common in Appalachian speakers. Such production renders words such as *cheese* /tʃiz/ as /tʃis/, or *keys* /kiz/ as /kis/. This production can mirror some phonological patterns/processes that would be labeled 'errors' or 'distortions' in certain assessments; however, they are not errors and should not be considered such.

Consonant reductions/deletions

Many Appalachian varieties permit the elision/deletions of consonants in certain phonological contexts (similar to most English varieties around the world). However, in contrast to other varieties, Appalachian varieties tend to have rates of deletions/elisions much higher than other varieties. For example, the voiced interdental fricative /ð/ in initial position, as in words like *this* or *there* (among other words) is often elided, where the phrase *in this* might sound as if the person produced *in is*, or the phrase *over there* might be produced as *over ere*. Further, the voiced labiovelar approximate /w/ in initial position, such as in the words *was* or *would* is routinely deleted if it occurs after pronouns, with the phrase *I was* being rendered *I'uz*. Contracting past tense *be* is relatively rare in other English varieties. Further, the phrase *I would* being rendered *I'ud*, again somewhat rare in some English varieties. Hazen (2011) found, however, that it appears to be spreading and becoming more common.

Clinicians must also be aware of the prevalence of coronal stop deletion in Appalachian varieties. This pattern is when a /t/ or /d/ is reduced/deleted in consonantal clusters that occur in final position. Deletion of the final /t/ or /d/ is a very common occurrence in Appalachian speech. Hazen (2011) found roughly 30% deletion pre-vocalically and 90% deletion in contexts before a non-alveolar consonant. Such high rates of deletion can easily be misinterpreted erroneously as 'errors', especially in the speech of Appalachian children. Clinicians must be aware and adjust their evaluations accordingly.

Vowels

Many of the varieties of Appalachian English found in the core area differ from many other English varieties with respect to the vocalic system. Several mergers and rotations exist, some of which are part of the Southern Vowel Shift (SVS) and are explained below. However, as with the consonant variation explored above, there will undoubtedly be much individual variation across the region.

The Southern Vowel Shift

In their seminal work on vowel variation across the United States, Labov *et al.* (1972) noted several vowel shifts happening across the nation. Using data from the Southern United States, they outlined systematic differences in the production of many vowels, what linguists term a chain shift, among many Southern speakers. The principal characteristic that they noticed in Southern US speakers was differences in the productions of the front vowels (along with other phenomena). The differences in production, when visualized with a plot of the first and second formants (an F1/F2 plot), showed a clockwise rotation in the nuclei of the front vowels, fronting of the back vowels and monophthongization of the diphthong /ay/ (see below for more detail regarding /ay/). Labov *et al.* (1972) termed these production differences the 'Southern Vowel Shift' (SVS). Figure 3.3, adapted from Reaser and Wolfram (2014), show these phenomena graphically. The SVS was found, to varying degrees, in the speech of Southerners across the South, and especially among Appalachian speakers. Naturally, there was much social and individual variation, with some groups having more of the features, or having more in certain speaking situations, while other speakers may not have many features at all, depending on the speaking situation (Labov *et al.*, 2005; Pederson *et al.*, 1986–1993). More recent scholarship has tended to find many of the features receding across the South, with fewer speakers having all the features and differences in social groups, with more rural

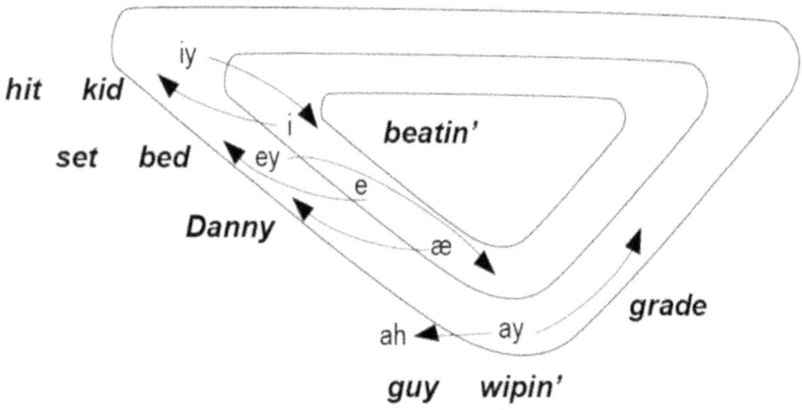

Figure 3.3 The Southern Vowel Shift, from Reaser and Wolfram (2014)

speakers having the most features and urban speakers showing fewer (Fridland, 2001). However, this recession has not occurred to the same degree in Appalachia. Irons (2007) found the SVS to actually be advancing across parts of Appalachian Kentucky. And I have found that the SVS has been maintained in Appalachian East Tennessee and Alabama (Reed, 2018b, 2022).

/ay/

Probably the most classic, and caricatured, linguistic feature of Southern and Appalachian speech is the production of /ay/. In fact, Feagin has said the 'most notable unchanging feature of Southern speech' is how Southerners produce /ay/ (2000: 342). Across the South and Appalachia, a process of glide weakening is widespread, across the social spectrum. In pre-voiced and open syllables, many speakers use a more monophthongal production of /ay/, approaching /a/ or /ɑ/ (Thomas, 2001, 2003). A more regionally restricted area, principally in Appalachia (although it is found in some other rural regions, and a smattering of other areas), takes this process of monophthongization further, with a more monophthongal and/or glide-weakened production in all phonetic contexts (Greene, 2010; Reed, 2016; Thomas, 2001).

PIN/PEN merger

Another widely described phonological feature of Appalachia (Hazen, 2005), and Southern speech more broadly, is the merger of /ɪ/ and /ɛ/ before nasal consonants – a phenomenon traditionally labeled the *PIN/PEN* merger. Speakers will tend to produce both as *pin* (Labov *et al.*, 2005; Montgomery & Eble, 2012). This merger is present across large swaths of the South, from the Atlantic Coast to the Gulf Coast, to the limits of the Southern dialect region. However, as with other features, there is a growing distinction between urban and rural speakers, where urban speakers are now producing distinct vowels in the pre-nasal position (Koops *et al.*, 2008).

Other vowel mergers

Other vowel mergers are present in the Appalachia; however, they are more regionally restricted. One such restricted merger is the pre-lateral merger of /i/ and /ɪ/ to /ɪ/, rendering *feel* and *fill* as near homophones as /fɪl/. The pre-lateral merger is widespread in the Upland South and can also be found in more rural regions across the Lower South (Thomas, 2004).

A more recent merger, similar to what is occurring across the United States, is the low back vowel merger, often titled the *COT/CAUGHT* merger, where /ɑ/ and /ɔ/ are merged (or near merged) to /ɑ/, where *cot* and *caught* are produced similarly, something near /kɑt/ (Thomas, 2001). However, this merger is not present everywhere. Parts of Appalachia maintain a distinction, with *caught* produced as an upgliding diphthong.

Word stress

Another widespread phonological feature of Appalachian Englishes (and other Southern US varieties) is strong initial stress on many words. This phenomenon is often commented upon when folks travel. Many Appalachian speakers will produce the primary stress on the first syllable of words like *umbrella*, *insurance*, *guitar*, *police*, *cement*. Speakers from most other varieties of American English produce these words with stress on the second syllable (Thomas, 2004). Thomas discusses how producing these words, especially *insurance* and *umbrella*, with strong initial stress is more indicative of a Southern identity, and I would also note Appalachian identity. See above for a discussion about *rootedness*.

Grammatical Variation

Grammatical, morphosyntactic and lexical variables have also received a good deal of attention in studies of Appalachian English. As mentioned above, several patterns might be misconstrued as 'errors'. Clinicians should be aware of these patterns, especially as they tend to differ from many standardized varieties of American English. These differences tend to be quite salient to the hearer, especially when one is not aware of them.

Double modals

One of the most interesting syntactic variables found in the Southern United States, and especially in Appalachia, is double modals, occasionally called multiple modals (Montgomery, 1998; Reed & Montgomery, 2023). Double modals are where a modal verb (typically *might* or *may*) occurs in the same verb phrase as another modal verb (e.g. *might could*, *may can*, etc.). These are quite interesting in part because of their saliency. Many users of double modals are unaware that other English speakers do not use them. Over the years, research on double modals has shown that the structure is quite common across the Southern United States and is found from Texas and Oklahoma to the Atlantic and Gulf Coasts, and as far north as the Mid-Atlantic. However, there is a concentration of use within the Appalachian region, particularly the core region. Further, investigators have identified preferred double modal forms (i.e. *might could*, *might should*), which are very common across the region and across social groups within the region. Double modals are common in the speech of both young and old speakers, urban and rural, Black and White, and there does not appear to be any social stigma regarding their use within the region. However, there does appear to be a small shift in their use across generations, with younger speakers not using as many double modals and using a smaller number of the possible combinations of modals. It is notable that outside of the South and Appalachia, double modals are practically absent. Clinicians who are unfamiliar with double modals will need to be aware of their presence and their frequent use within the region.

A-prefixing

The use of the *a*- prefix on present participle verbs (*a-huntin'*) is a highly salient feature of Appalachian English varieties (Montgomery, 2009; Wolfram, 1980). With both syntactic and phonological constraints on its occurrence, the origins of this variable have been traced to Southern England (Montgomery, 2009). Work on *a*-prefixing has shown that while the linguistic constraints remain the same across Appalachia (Wolfram, 1988), some locally based variations have been found (Montgomery, 2009). This feature is not as common in the speech of younger Appalachians.

Completive done

Completive *done*, sometimes called perfective done or preverbal done, is the use of *done* as a verbal auxiliary to indicate and/or emphasize that an action has been completed, as in the sentence 'I done told him three times'. In this sentence, *done* conveys that the action occurred in the past and was completed, but also connotes that the speaker is emphasizing that the person was told the information multiple times. This feature can be found across the South and in Appalachia and is used by both White and Black speakers (Mallinson & Childs, 2004).

Other grammatical variables

In addition to the grammatical features above, Appalachian speakers may also produce variation in reflexive pronouns (e.g. *hisself*), use multiple negation (e.g. *you can't see nothing*) and have variations in the *be* verbal paradigms (e.g. leveled *was* as in *we was there too*) (see Wolfram, 2003 or Hazen's chapter in Hazen, 2020 for overviews). While these features might be present, they are not unique nor exclusive to Appalachia and Appalachian varieties; rather, they are common to non-mainstream varieties in general and thus go beyond the scope of the present chapter.

Conclusion

In this chapter, I have outlined several linguistic features of Appalachian English varieties, from pragmatic concerns to lexicon to phonology and grammar. I have centered my discussion on those aspects of the language varieties that might have clinical impact, i.e. that might be scored as 'errors' on a language or phonological assessment. Through covering so many different aspects of language, a clinically oriented reader can clearly see that a good number of the features of Appalachian varieties have the potential to be mislabeled as errors. While no short overview can be comprehensive, my hope with this overview is that it aids clinicians in understanding the systematicity of Appalachian varieties while also conveying their beauty and how much language can mean to speakers.

References

Appalachian Regional Commission. (2021) *Subregions in Appalachia*. https://www.arc.gov/map/subregions-in-appalachia/

Batteau, A.W. (1990) *The Invention of Appalachia*. The University of Arizona Press.

Burdin, R.S., Holliday, N., Reed, P. (2018) Rising Above the Standard: Variation in L+H* contour use across 5 varieties of American English. Proceedings Speech Prosody 2018, 354–358. https://doi.org/10.21437/SpeechProsody.2018-72

Billings, D., Norman, G. and Ledford, K. (2000) *Back Talk from Appalachia: Confronting Stereotypes*. University of Kentucky Press.

Brown, P. and Levinson, S. (1987) *Politeness: Some Universals in Language Usage*. Cambridge University Press.

Burdin, R.S., Holliday, N.R. and Reed, P.E. (2022) American English pitch accents in variation: Pushing the boundaries of Mainstream American English ToBI conventions. *Journal of Phonetics* 94, 101163.

Campbell, J.C. (1921) *The Southern Highlander and his Homeland*. The Russell Sage Foundation.

Clopper, C.G. and Smiljanic, R. (2015) Regional variation in temporal organization in American English. *Journal of Phonetics* 39, 237–245.

Cramer, J. (2014) Is Shakespeare still in the holler? The death of a language myth. *Southern Journal of Linguistics* 38 (1), 95–207.

Dodsworth, R. and Hazen, K. (2011) Following L over hill and dale: Changes in l-vocalization through space, time, and methods. Paper presented at *New Ways of Analyzing Variation 40*, Georgetown University, Washington, DC, October 2011.

Feagin, C. (2000) Sound change in the South. *American Speech* 75 (4), 342–344.

Fridland, V. (2001) The social dimension of the Southern vowel shift: Gender, age, and class. *Journal of Sociolinguistics* 5, 233–253.
Greene, R. (2006) Pitch accents in Appalachian English. Unpublished Qualifying Paper. Stanford University.
Greene, R. (2010) Language, ideology, and identity in rural Eastern Kentucky. Stanford University Dissertation. See https://purl.stanford.edu/fh361zh5489.
Hall, J. S. (1942) The phonetics of Great Smoky Mountain Speech. *American Speech*, 17 (2), 1–110. https://doi.org/10.2307/487132
Harkins, A. and McCarroll, M. (2019) *Appalachian Reckoning: A Region Responds to Hillbilly Elegy*. West Virginia University Press.
Hasty, J.D. and Childs, B. (2021) Investigating Appalachian Englishes: Subregional variation in the new Appalachia. *Journal of Appalachian Studies* 27 (1), 69–88.
Hazen, K. (2005) Mergers in the mountains. *English World-Wide* 26 (2), 199–221.
Hazen, K. (2011) Flying high above the social radar: Coronal stop deletion in modern Appalachia. *Language Variation and Change* 23 (1), 105–137.
Hazen, K. (ed.) (2020) *Appalachian Englishes in the Twenty-First Century*. West Virginia University Press.
Hazen, K., Lovejoy, J., Daugherty, J. and Vandevender, M. (2016) Continuity and change of English consonants in Appalachia. In W. Schumann and R. Adkins Fletcher (eds) *Appalachia Revisited: New Perspectives on Place, Tradition, and Progress* (pp. 119–138). University Press of Kentucky.
Irons, T. (2007) On the Southern shift in Appalachia. *University of Pennsylvania Working Papers in Linguistics* 13 (2), 121–134.
Koops, C., Gentry, E. and Pantos, A. (2008) The effect of perceived speaker age on the perception of PIN and PEN vowels in Houston, Texas. *University of Pennsylvania Working Papers in Linguistics* 14 (2).
Labov, W., Yaeger, M. and Steiner, R. (1972) *A Quantitative Study of Sound Change in Progress, Volumes 1 and 2*. Report on National Science Foundation Contract NSF-GS-3287.
Labov, W., Ash, S. and Boberg, C. (2005) *The Atlas of North American English: Phonetics, Phonology and Sound Change*. De Gruyter Mouton. https://doi.org/10.1515/9783110167467
Labov, W., Ash, S. and Boberg, C. (2006) *Atlas of North American English*. Mouton de Gruyter.
Lipski, J.M. (1993) Y'all in American English: From Black to White, from phrase to pronoun. *English World-wide* 14 (1), 23–56.
Mallinson, C. and Childs, B. (2004) The intersection of regional and ethnic identity: African American English in Appalachia. *Journal of Appalachian Studies* 10 (1/2), 129–142.
Montgomery, M. (1989) A note on y'all. *American Speech* 64 (3), 273–275.
Montgomery, M. (1998) In the Appalachians they talk like Shakespeare. In L. Bauer and P. Trudgill (eds) *Language Myths* (pp. 66–76). Penguin.
Montgomery, M. (2009) Historical and comparative perspectives on a-prefixing in the English of Appalachia. *American Speech* 84 (1), 5–26.
Montgomery, M. and Eble, C. (2012) Historical perspectives on the pen/pin merger in Southern American English. In A. Curzan and K. Emmons (eds) *Studies in the History of the English Language II* (pp. 415–434). De Gruyter Mouton.
Montgomery, M. and Heinmiller, J. (2021) *The Dictionary of Southern Appalachian English*. The University of North Carolina Press.
Pederson, L., McDaniel, S.L. and Adams, C.M. (eds) (1986–93) *Linguistic Atlas of the Gulf States* (7 vols). University of Georgia Press.
Puckett, A. (2000) *Seldom Ask, Never Tell: Labor and Discourse in Appalachia*. Oxford University Press.

Puckett, A. (2003) The "value" of dialect as object: The case of Appalachian English. *Pragmatics* 13 (4), 539–549.
Reaser, J. and Wolfram, W. (2014) *Talkin' Tar Heel*. University of North Carolina Press.
Reed, P.E. (2014) Inter- and intra-generational monophthongization and Southern Appalachian Identity. *Southern Journal of Linguistics* 38 (1), 159–193.
Reed, P.E. (2016) Sounding Appalachian: /ai/ monophthongization, rising pitch accents, and rootedness. University of South Carolina dissertation.
Reed, P.E. (2018a) The importance of Appalachian identity: A case study in rootedness. *American Speech* 93 (3–4), 409–424.
Reed, P.E. (2018b) Rootedness and the Southern vowel shift in Appalachia. Paper presented at the *American Dialect Society (ADS) Annual Meeting*. Salt Lake City, UT, 4–7 January.
Reed, P.E. (2020a) Phonological possibilities in Appalachian Englishes. In K. Hazen (ed.) *Appalachian Englishes in the Twenty-First Century* (pp. 20–35). WVU Press.
Reed, P.E. (2020b) Inter- and intra-regional variation in intonation: An analysis of rising pitch accents and rootedness. *Journal of the Acoustical Society of America* 147 (1), 616–626.
Reed, P.E. (2020c) Place and language: Links between speech, region, and connection to place. *WIREs Cognitive Science* 11 (60).
Reed, P.E. (2020d) Prosodic variation and rootedness in Appalachian English. *Penn Working Papers in Linguistics* 25 (2).
Reed, P.E. (Jan. 2022) The Southern Vowel Shift and meaningful places: how attachment to place affects vowel production among college students. Paper presented at the American Dialect Society (ADS) Annual Meeting. Virtual meeting.
Reed, P. and Montgomery, M. (2023) Multimo. See https://artsandsciences.sc.edu/multimo/welcome
Thomas, E.R. (2001) *An Acoustic Analysis of Vowel Variation in New World English*. Publication of the American Dialect Society 85. Duke University Press.
Thomas, E.R. (2003) Secrets revealed by Southern vowel shifting. *American Speech* 78 (2), 150–170.
Thomas, E.R. (2004) Rural white Southern accents. In B. Kortmann, E.W. Schneider, K. Burridge, R. Meshthrie and C. Upton (eds) *A Handbook of Varieties of English: A Multimedia Reference Tool* (pp. 300–324). Mouton de Gruyter.
Ulack, R. and Raitz, K. (1981) Appalachia: A comparison of the cognitive and Appalachian commission regions. *Southeastern Geographer* 21 (1), 40–53.
Walker, A., Southall, A. and Hargrave, R. (2017) An acoustic and phonological description of /z/-devoicing in Southern American English. *The Journal of the Acoustical Society of America* 142 (4), 2678–2678.
Williams, C.D. (1992) *Southern Mountain Speech*. Berea College Press.
Wolfram, W. (1980) "A"-prefixing in Appalachian English. In W. Labov (ed.) *Locating Language in Time and Space* (pp. 107–142). Academic Press.
Wolfram, W. (1988) Reconsidering the semantics of *a*-prefixing . *American Speech* 63, 247–253.
Wolfram, W. (2003) Language variation in the American South: An introduction. *American Speech* 78 (2), 123–129.
Wolfram, W. and Christian, D. (1976) *Appalachian Speech*. Center for Applied Linguistics.

4 Cajun English

Wilbur V. Bennett III, Christine P. Weill
and Claiborne Rice

Introduction

Cajun English (CE) is a dialect of English influenced by the many varieties of Louisiana French (LF) spoken in Southern Louisiana. While Cajun English, narrowly defined, may be an ethnolect indexing Cajun ethnicity, we will use the term to refer more broadly to any variety of French-influenced English spoken in the Southern Louisiana region (exclusive of New Orleans) (Carmichael, 2019; Dubois & Melançon, 1997; Eble, 1993; Rubrecht, 1971; Scott, 1992; Walton, 1994). What little research has been done specifically on non-Cajun versions of this dialect will be mentioned when relevant. Originally an L2 variety of English for native speakers of LF, CE gradually emerged as a marker of ethnic and cultural identity as French waned in importance through the course of the 20th century. This chapter provides a brief history of the speech community, describes the unique features of the dialect, discusses the clinical implications and calls for more research into a language that may not exist in a generation.

The CE Speech Community

Cajuns are predominantly a white ethnic group living in Acadiana, a region of Southern Louisiana composed of 22 parishes with Lafayette at its heart (Figure 4.1). Cajuns trace their ancestry back to Acadia (today Nova Scotia, Canada). Acadia was founded in 1603 and remained isolated for nearly 150 years, and the Acadians developed a strong identity with a shared culture focused on the Catholic religion and distinct French dialect (Ancelet *et al.*, 2009; Brasseaux, 1987). Around 1755, the British attempted to violently force the Acadians to convert to the Anglican Church, adopt the English language and pledge loyalty to the crown. This led to the expulsion of Acadians between 1763 and 1776. After several years of travel, thousands of Acadians accepted an offer from Spain to settle west of New Orleans in Louisiana since this allowed them to reestablish their community and maintain their culture and language.

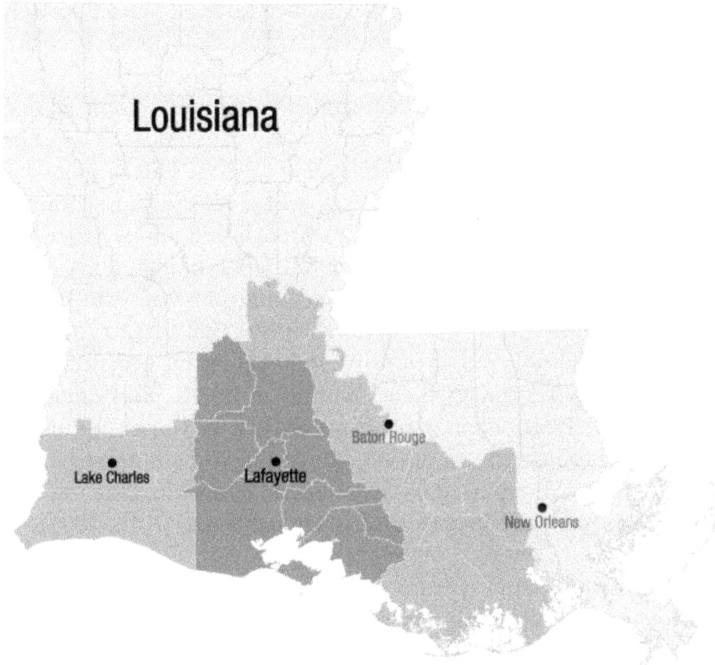

Figure 4.1 Parishes of Acadiana in Louisiana (note: Darker areas are Acadiana Heartland) Map adapted from Wikimedia commons: QuartierLatin, 1968

The Acadians remained relatively isolated until after the Louisiana Purchase in 1803 and statehood in 1813 (Brasseaux, 1987; Rubrecht, 1971). With statehood and the innovations in travel, Anglo and Germanic immigrants began settling in the region and shifting Louisiana away from French culture and language in an effort to Americanize (Ancelet *et al.*, 2009; Brasseaux, 1987; Estaville, 1987). During this time, many French and Spanish Louisianians began to identify themselves as Creole to separate themselves from Anglo-Americans (Kein, 2000). Estaville (1987) and Ancelet (2009) argue that the decline of French in Louisiana began before the American Civil War, with the English-speaking families already outnumbering the French. The breaking point for Louisiana French was the 1921 constitution requiring English-only instruction in public classrooms (*CODOFIL | Council for the Development of French in Louisiana*, 2014; Ward, 1997). Subjected to institutional discrimination and hostility, Cajuns underwent a second 'expulsion', selling their lands and moving to more rural areas. Rubrecht (1971) categorizes the French-speaking population at this time into three groups: the wealthy French Creoles and Cajuns who lived in cities, primarily spoke English, and welcomed the adoption of American values and traditions; Cajuns who worked on large farms, spoke French and English, and were indifferent to but influenced by American culture; and Cajuns who lived in small communities in rural or isolated locations in the bayous, only spoke French, and actively resisted Americanization.

As population demographics continued to change, Cajuns were denigrated as coarse ruffians who preferred sinful pursuits such as dancing, drinking, hunting and fighting (Ancelet *et al.*, 2009). This, along with the wealth and increased prestige held by the English-speaking community, led subsequent generations to disregard French and adopt English. This pressure increased during WWI and WWII when bilingual Cajuns were mobilized for the war. Many French-speaking parents, who desired to protect their children from the harsh discipline that often resulted from using French at school, and to improve their economic prospects as well, stopped speaking French to their children at home. This erasure continued until the 1960s when a renewed interest in Cajun culture led to the provision requiring English-only education to be removed from the constitution in 1973, replaced by a statement acknowledging the right of people to preserve their culture and language (CODOFIL, 2014; Ward, 1997).

The revival of Cajun culture and language, sometimes billed as the Cajun Renaissance (Bernard, 2003), helped bring Cajun music, food and some traditions (like The Courir de Mardi Gras) to the nation. With the harshest criticism softened, CE has become 'enregistered' (Johnstone, 2016) as a recognizable dialect of English by Acadiana residents wishing to reinforce their Cajun identity. Because many typical Cajun-identified activities, like music performance or crawfish boiling, have historically been the province of men, younger male speakers tend to use features of CE more frequently than female speakers do (Dubois & Horvath, 2000).

Phonological Features Distinct from Mainstream American English (MAE)

Consonants and vowels

Cajun English phonetic inventory is similar to both Southern American English (SAE) and Black English (BE) with a few differences. The Appendix provides a table with the consonants of CE (Tables 4.1A and B) and a table comparing the vowels of MAE, SAE, BE and CE (Table 4.2C). The information for the tables was compiled from Kretzschmar, Jr (2004), Thomas (2004), Edwards (2004), Dubois and Horvath (2004) and Hannegan and Shport (2024).

Monophthongization of tense vowels and diphthongs

A prominent feature of CE is the reduction or absence of glides in tense vowels (/i, e, o, u/) (Carmichael, 2019; Dubois & Horvath, 2004; Glain, 2021; Rubrecht, 1971; Walton, 1994). Tense vowels are produced as monophthongs ([iː], [eː], [oː], and [uː]) with slightly longer durations than lax vowels [ɪ, ʊ], [eː] and [oː] appear more frequently than [iː] and [uː]. This feature has increased in frequency with younger generations as Cajun culture has gained prestige. Also, like SAE, the diphthongs /ɑɪ, ɑʊ, ɔɪ/ are monophthongized as [aː], [ɑː] and [ɔː]. The monophthongization of /ɑɪ, ɑʊ, ɔɪ/ is more frequent and produced with a much shorter duration when followed by an approximant (especially [l] and [ɹ]). Words like *night*, *pow* and *oil* sound like 'not', 'pa' and 'all'.

Deletion of final consonants

Another prominent feature is the deletion of final consonants and consonant clusters (Dubois & Horvath, 2004; Glain, 2021). This feature is also prevalent in Louisiana French. Some examples cataloged have been [leː] for *late*, [skuː] for *school* or [boː] for *both*. Older CE speakers frequently delete the third person singular present tense marker (*-s*) and the past tense marker (*-ed*), while younger CE speakers have a much lower frequency of deletion (Dubois & Horvath, 2003). Similar to BE and SAE, CE speakers drop the *-s* and *-ed* endings from verbs though at a higher frequency (Dubois & Horvath, 2003).

CARD/CORD merger

Another feature distinguishing Cajun English from MAE, SAE and BE is the merger of the vowels in CORD and CARD ([ɔɹ] and [aɹ]). This merger has been reported for English varieties in Utah, Delaware and central and east Texas (Bowie, 2003, 2008), while Duncan (2022) states that the merger has reversed in the St. Louis area, where it had been a well-known feature of the local dialect. Research is needed to determine the precise parameters of this merger for CE, whether the CORD vowel has lowered into the CARD space, or has simply unrounded, or something else. This merger can be heard in CE with the distinctive pronunciations of, for example, *important* as 'impartant' and *horse* as 'harse'. The merger appears more often in the formal speech of CE speakers.

Nasalization

CE speakers also produce vowels (and some intervocalic consonants) with heavy nasalization (Carmichael, 2019; Coyne, 2008; Dubois & Horvath, 2004; Glain, 2021). This feature is more common in older speakers (who are usually bilingual).

Aspiration and voice onset time (VOT) of plosives

Older CE speakers frequently produce voiceless stops (/p, t, k/) without aspiration especially in word-initial positions before a stressed vowel or [ɹ, l, w, j] (Carmichael, 2013, 2019; Dubois & Horvath, 2004;

Glain, 2021; Rubrecht, 1971; Walton, 1994). Bennett (2025) found that monolingual CE speakers produce plosives similar to European French speakers with lead voicing and short lag VOT, but CE speakers also produce voiceless stops with aspiration. The lead voicing and short lag VOT appear to be a transfer feature from Louisiana French (LF) that continues with monolingual speakers.

/h/ dropping

CE speakers also frequently drop /h/ in word-initial positions, so *hair* is pronounced like 'air' (Carmichael, 2013, 2019; Dubois & Horvath, 2004; Rubrecht, 1971; Walton, 1994).

Stopping of interdentals

The stopping of interdental fricatives /θ, ð/ as [t, d] is a feature of CE that connects to the community and Louisiana as a whole (Carmichael, 2019; Coyne, 2008; Dubois & Horvath, 2004; Glain, 2021; Rubrecht, 1971). This feature is shared by BE speakers in the region and many New Orleanians. This highly stigmatized feature has gained prestige at sporting events where fans chant, 'Who dat going to beat X?' in support of their teams. CE has also been informally called 'dat' speak. Carmichael (2013) found that this feature acts as a marker for Cajun identity and is commonly used by joke tellers to signify a Cajun speaker.

Trilled /r/ and deletion of /l/

CE speakers produce the sound /ɹ/ in a variety of forms (Carmichael, 2019; Coyne, 2008; Dubois & Horvath, 2004; Glain, 2021; Walton, 1994). Many older CE speakers only produce [ɹ] in the pre-vocalic position. CE speakers also produce /ɹ/ as a flap [ɾ] or trill [r] in word-initial consonant clusters [tɹ, dɹ, fɹ]. There are also instances of the /ɹ/ being produced as a uvular fricative [ʁ] especially with traditional French vocabulary, i.e. *traiteur* [tʁeːtø] (Rubrecht, 1971). The lateral approximant /l/ is frequently dropped in intervocalic and preconsonantal positions in words such as *celery* as [sɛri], *help* as [hɛp] and *alright* as [ɑːit].

Prosody

CE speech is often described as 'flat speech' (Walton, 1994). Glain (2021) argues that the syllable stress and intonation patterns of CE resemble LF (syllable-timed language) more than MAE (stress-timed language). Stressed syllables in LF and CE are shorter than those of MAE, and CE speakers (similar to LF) usually produce the tonic syllable on the final words in the clause (Walton, 1994). Rubrecht (1971) noted the lack of difference between stressed and unstressed syllables in CE. Scott

(1992) remarked that CE had a 'clipped, staccato sound' and emphasized the end of the sentence. Glain (2021) analyzed several audios collected by Carmichael (2013) and found that CE speakers shifted to a more syllable-timed rhythm when telling jokes about Cajuns. This shows that CE speakers are changing their stress and intonation pattern as a marker for Cajun identity.

Other phonological features

CE, SAE and BE speakers are noted to pronounce *ask* as [æks] (Cheramie, 1998; Glain, 2021). Hannegan and Shport (2024) reported that CE speakers often front back vowels (/u, ʊ, o/), producing them with a higher F2 in comparison to /ʌ/.

Grammatical Features

Reduplicated adjectives

CE speakers frequently repeat adjectives to intensify the meaning. For example, 'he likes the gumbo thick, thick'. Rubrecht (1971) gives an example of a St Francisville informant using 'bumpy bumpy' meaning 'very bumpy'.

Left and right dislocation of pronouns

Another feature that can be traced back to LF is the dislocation of pronouns or emphatic repetition of pronouns (Carmichael, 2013; Cheramie, 1998). Dislocation occurs when an extra pronoun is produced either at the beginning or end of the clause. For example, 'I don't trust him, me', or 'Him, he caused trouble'.

Right dislocation of markers 'yes' and 'no'

CE speakers will also emphasize the positive or negative polarity of a clause by adding *yes* or *no* at the end, as in 'You shouldn't go there, no'. CE speakers usually avoid placing emphatic stress inside the clause, so the two types of dislocation help achieve the emphatic sense (Cheramie, 1998; Scott, 1992).

Absence of subject auxiliary inversion

CE speakers often form questions without subject auxiliary inversion, the process where the subject swaps position with the auxiliary verb or auxiliary DO is inserted before the subject if no auxiliary is present. The following table lists example interrogatives in MAE and CE. This lack of inversion is influenced by Louisiana French syntax (Table 4.1).

Table 4.1 Example interrogatives in Cajun English (CE) and Mainstream American English (MAE)

CE	MAE
"what that is?" (Scott, 1992)	"what is that?"
"How she writes dat?"(Marshall, 1982)	"how did she write that?"
"how long it took you?" (Glain, 2021)	"how long did it take you?"
"how much it is?" (Glain, 2021)	"how much is it?"

Tag questions

Tag questions are shortened questions used at the end of declarative statements to confirm information or indicate surprise. These questions are commonly produced in MAE as 'you are going to the store, aren't you?' In CE, older bilingual speakers use /æ̃/ (nasalized ash vowel) usually spelled as 'hein' (Scott, 1992) or 'anh' (Sothern, 2001) as a marker for surprise or not understanding. For an older CE speaker, the above statement would be 'you are going to the store, hein?'

Y'all as possessive

CE shares with SAE and BE the widespread use of *y'all* as a second person plural pronoun. While the possessive form of this pronoun for SAE is *y'all's*, both BE (Wolfram, 2004: 125) and CE speakers (Cheramie & Gill, 1992) favor the unmarked *y'all*, as in 'what are y'all thoughts?' (Rice, 2014).

Grammatical features shared with other dialects

CE shares many grammatical features with other local dialects of SAE and BE. For example, CE speakers frequently use negative concord (or multiple negation) to emphasize the negative, 'They didn't want no schooling' (Rubrecht, 1971). Older French CE speakers use *was* leveling ('He was happy', 'They was happy'), similar to SAE and BE speakers, but at a much lower frequency (Dubois & Horvath, 2002, 2003). Copula deletion ('He ugly', 'Where we going?') is a feature shared among CE, BE and SAE speakers. CE speakers drop both *is* and *are* more frequently than SAE speakers, while only *is* deletion occurs at a higher frequency than BE speakers (Dubois & Horvath, 2003). These verb features are still prevalent with monolingual CE speakers.

Semantic calques and vocabulary

There are numerous verb phrases that are unique to CE due to its contact with Louisiana French speakers. The most common phrases brought over to CE from LF are: *come see*, cf. *viens voir* or *viens voir ici*, meaning come here, 'Come see. I have something to show' (Cheramie & Gill, 1992); *get down*, cf. *descendre*, meaning to visit with someone or enter a location ('Are you going to get down?'); *pass by*, cf. French *passe chez,* similar meaning to *get down* though usually indicates a shorter visit, 'No, I can only pass by' (Carmichael, 2019); *save* X meaning to put away or store something, 'It's time to save your toys'; or *make*, cf. *faire*, with a number meaning to become an age, 'He made ten last summer', or usually with the noun *groceries* to mean 'buying groceries' – 'I make groceries on the Weekends' (Cheramie & Gill, 1992).

CE speakers also borrow words from LF. Most common words are *cher* meaning 'loved one', *mais* meaning 'well then', *frisson* meaning 'a chill', *lagniappe* meaning 'something extra', and others focused on food (e.g. *roux*, *boudin*, *jambalaya*).

Language Sample

The following sample is from an interview with a 70-year-old male who identifies as Cajun. He was asked to read the Rainbow Passage as part of a project to gather language samples of CE. Instances of CE features are highlighted with bold words and transcription. The speaker produces *take*, *shape*, *gold*, *no* and *people* with longer durations without a glide. He drops the /t/ in light and stops the interdental /ð/ in *there* but produced other examples of these phonemes according to MAE (see first line of passage).

When	*the*	*sunlight*	*strikes*	*raindrops*	*in*	*the*	*air,*	*they*	*act*	*as*
wɛn	ðə	sʌnlaɪt	stɹaɪks	ɹeɪndɹaps	ɪn	ði	ɛɹ,	ðeɪ	ækt	æz

a	*prism*	*and*	*form*	*a*	*rainbow.*	*The*	*rainbow*	*is*	*a*	*division*
ə	pɹɪzəm	ænd	fɔɹm	ə	ɹeɪnboʊ.	ðə	ɹeɪnboʊ	ɪz	ə	dɪvɪʒən

of	*white*	***light***	*into*	*many*	***beautiful***	*colors.*	*These*	***take***
ʌv	waɪt	**laɪ**	ɪntu	mɛni	**bjʉ:təfʌl**	kʌləɹz.	ðiz	**te:k**

the	***shape***	*of*	*a*	*long*	*round*	*arch,*	*with*	*its*	*path*	*high*	*above,*
ði	**ʃe:p**	ʌv	ə	lɔŋ	ɹa:nd	aɹk,	wɪð	ɪts	pæθ	haɪ	əbʌv,

and	*its*	*two*	*ends*	*apparently*	*beyond*	*the*	*horizon.*
ænd	ɪts	tu	ɛndz	əpɛɹəntli	bɪand	ðə	həɹaɪzən.

There	*is,*	*according*	*to*	*legend,*	*a*	*boiling*	*pot*	*of*	***gold***
dɛɹ	ɪz,	əkɔɹdɪŋ	tu	lɛʤənd,	ə	bɔɪlɪŋ	pat	ʌv	**go:ld**

at	*one*	*end.*	***People***	*look,*	*but*	***no***	*one*	*ever*	*finds*	*it.*
æt	wʌn	ɛnd.	**pi:pəl**	lʊk,	bʌt	**no:**	wʌn	ɛvəɹ	faɪndz	ɪt.

Excerpt from 'The Rainbow Passage' (Fairbanks, 1960)

Community Efforts Supporting CE in Acadiana

Individuals throughout the southern parishes of Louisiana maintain a general familiarity with CE thanks to the efforts of such organizations as the Council for the Development of French in Louisiana (CODIFIL), the Lafayette Parish School System French Immersion programs and the University of Louisiana at Lafayette (UL Lafayette). UL Lafayette further supports the increased study of the sociolinguistic characteristics and culture of CE through efforts such as the Cajun and Creole Music Collection, doctorate programming in Francophone Studies and Communicative Disorders, The Center for Louisiana Studies and the housing of Southwest Louisiana's National Public Radio Station affiliate KRVS Radio Acadie since 1963. KRVS Radio Acadie's mission to be '…the source of spoken and sung Louisiana Cajun French and Creole' (KRVS, 2024) has immersed generations in the melody of these dialects, making them a linguistic marker of home.

Clinical Implications for Researchers

Little research has been conducted specifically on CE dialects and speech-language-hearing disorders. Those researchers who are immersed in this area cite the complexity of identifying impairment within dialect (Hendricks & Adlof, 2017; Oetting *et al.*, 2013; Oetting & Garrity, 2006); an assertion shared by practitioners in the field. Essentially, like all dialects, CE is not a monolith but instead a continuum of dialectical adjustments coalescing with other local dialects of SAE (i.e. Southern Black English and Southern White English) to create distinctive geographical and cultural norms (Oetting & Garrity, 2006; Rivière *et al.*, 2018).

Further research into CE dialect should investigate the changing characteristics of CE and how those same characteristics differ by geographic location. Research on CE should be expanded to include characteristics present during the period of emerging development of both speech-language and literacy skills, including the use of CE characteristics as cultural markers and elements of distinctive voice within the home, community and larger society. See emerging work as part of the 'UL Lullaby' project at the University of Louisiana at Lafayette (e.g. Babatsouli *et al.*, 2025; Leal *et al.*, 2026). Additional investigations into regional narratives and CE narrative structures would contribute to our current understanding of the linguistic characteristics of CE and how these characteristics carry over to the development of literacy skills for school-age children. Significantly, the prevalence of speech-language and literacy disorders in CE dialect speakers has not been thoroughly investigated. Additional research in this area may help to illuminate educational practices to best support the development of literacy and academic skills for children in the Acadiana area (Puranik *et al.*, 2020; Washington *et al.*, 2018).

As the region experiences the negative effects of climate change on the lower-lying communities of Acadiana, the movements of CE dialect speakers to different areas of the state and country will offer opportunities to view dialectal shifts and the effects of those shifts on this culture. Advances in the use of artificial intelligence (AI) and language models on the sounds and rhythms of written language (and the voices they represent) offer an interesting line of research on the value of dialects and dialectal storytelling traditions. These two trends result in a growing critical importance in the study of CE and the position of this dialect in the future.

Clinical Implications for Practitioners

Outside the specific realm of the CE dialect, the field of speech-language pathology (SLP) continues to grow its research base on culturally responsive and collaborative practices for the assessment of speech, language and cognitive disorders in individuals who speak an ever-growing variety of Non-Mainstream American English (NMAE) dialects (Babatsouli, 2021, 2023, 2024; Damico *et al.*, 1996; Hamayan & Damico, 1991; Hendricks & Adolf, 2017; McLeod, Verdon, & *The International Expert Panel on Multilingual Children's Speech* (*IEPMCS*), 2017; Reid *et al.*, 1993; Velleman & Zurer Pearson, 2010; Verdon *et al.*, 2016; Washington *et al.*, 2018, 2023). Practice has grown considerably from our disappointing past of SLPs teaching standard English dialects to speakers of NMAE dialects (Adler, 1977). While SLPs have reported an increased awareness of dialectal considerations (Vafadar & Utt, 1992) practitioners may still demonstrate errors in clinical judgment when working with individuals with dialects different from their own (Easton & Verdon, 2021; Hendricks *et al.*, 2021; Robinson & Stockman, 2009). This 'linguistic subordination' can result in either the refusal of services or the overidentification of speakers of NMAE dialects on the already bursting caseloads of American SLPs (Forrest & Wolfram, 2019). To the knowledge of this researcher, the prevalence of overidentification of speech and language disorders in CE dialect speakers has not been studied to date.

Theoretically sound assessment practices

What is documented by the SLP community, regarding CE speakers in Louisiana, points to a diverse group of individuals who share a variety of characteristics with other dialect speakers (Oetting & Garrity, 2006; Rivière *et al.*, 2018). Research has shown the inconsistent nature of dialect characteristics in CE depending on the location, age, gender and contextual variables for communication (Dubois & Horvath, 1998). For this reason, SLPs should begin any assessment or screening process with theoretically sound methods that reflect collaborative practice and cultural humility. The following discussion will detail several practices that have specific application to the CE dialectal community.

Assessment as advocacy

In line with ethnographic methods of inquiry (McCurdy *et al.*, 2004; Spradley, 1980) is the assessment approach known as the bi-level analysis paradigm (Damico, 1991). In this assessment paradigm, systematic techniques are selected by the SLP to determine where communication breakdowns occur and the contribution of both extrinsic and intrinsic factors to those breakdowns. The evaluator is then left to function as an advocate for the client in the context of interest (Damico, 1991) using multiple tools, techniques and informant perspectives (e.g. caregiver, teacher, peers) around authentic social phenomena to determine how best to facilitate successful development of speech, language or academic skills. No one tool, perspective or observation carries all information needed to determine the presence of an intrinsic disorder. Instead, the evaluator seeks to understand the interaction between the communicator and the multiple environments of interest. While this chapter is not intended to be a tutorial on this form of assessment, several techniques used in this paradigm will be highlighted here to expand the discussion of CE.

Use of informants

The use of caregivers and other community members has been established as a best practice for the assessment of multilingual and NMAE dialect speakers (Babatsouli, 2024; Damico & Hamayan, 1992; McLeod *et al.*, 2017; Westby, 1990). Several studies detail the use of informants as part of culturally responsive screening and assessment of multilingual individuals (Babatsouli, 2023, 2024; Damico, 1991; Damico & Hamayan, 1992; Oetting *et al.*, 2016; Washington *et al.*, 2023). The *Intelligibility in Context Scale* (ICS; McLeod *et al.*, 2012) is one tool that has been used as an effective starting point when creating a sense of the presence or magnitude of a speech disorder in a child's developing communication abilities. This seven-item scale can be provided for several members of the extended family or community as a starting point for discussing the impact of the communication difficulty from the perspective of the caregivers. Use of informants in this matter demonstrates respect for the role of the extended family in the care of a child within a CE speaking community while also contextualizing the scope of the concern for the SLP. For example, a child who is developing speech in an environment with multiple generations speaking multiple dialects and/or varieties of CE and LF (not to mention the environmental sounds of Cajun dialects and languages present on the radio and television systems in Acadiana) may have differing levels of intelligibility to different members of their daily care teams. In rural and suburban communities in Acadiana, extended family are frequently the daily caregivers of children as the main caregivers work to support the larger family. Conversely, given the close family units often seen in the Acadiana communities, children play an important role in caring for elderly members of the extended family/community alongside their main caregivers and siblings. This cultural norm leads to a child's possible interactions with multiple dialects of CE and LF as well as multilingual/multicultural experiences within the Cajun communities of Louisiana. Readers are directed to McLeod, Verdon and IEPMCS (2017) for an in-depth discussion on the complexity of assessing the speech of multilingual children and to Babatsouli (2023) for the ecosystemic approach and Action Plan to assessing linguistic diversity. Although the above-mentioned work does not specifically address the needs of CE dialect users, the methods discussed are certainly applicable to CE dialects. The American Speech-Language-Hearing Association (ASHA) also provides resources and further information on several recorded dialects at the following website (https://www.asha.org/practice/multicultural/phono/) although CE is not included currently.

Informants provide for the SLP a view of a certain dialect, language or culture from the perspective of the users. Informants can be interpreters who are not only proficient in the language or dialect but also familiar with the cultural traditions and viewpoints shared by the client. An informant may be the caregiver, family members or members of the community for the individual being assessed. One such member of the community that might be included as an informant for a member of a Cajun community is the *traiteur* (pronounced commonly as /tʁeːtø/). These faith or folk healers are said to have gifts as an intermediary between the community and a higher power (Daigle, 1991). Traiteurs can provide important developmental history and cultural perspectives on the lived experience of some Cajun community members. A partnership here demonstrates an SLP's cultural humility and willingness to share in the assessment and treatment of a whole person within a whole culture (Westby & Washington, 2017).

One example from this researcher's clinical practice is the case of a nine-year-old male from a rural Acadiana parish who presented at our university clinic with an undiagnosed severe childhood apraxia of speech (CAS) and expressive language disorder. The caregiver's primary concern was delayed literacy development, which she noted in her daily interactions as the homeschool teacher for their extended family of 12 children ages 5 through 16. The primary language used in the home was LF, with exposure to LF and CE within the larger community circles. Both the classroom and the community had adapted their communication styles with this child to be a visual style of communication using gestures, pointing and pantomime as the child's primary mode of communication in connection with nasalized, open-vowel single-syllable verbalizations. Assessment and treatment sessions were conducted in a group setting with four of the siblings, the primary caregiver and the community traiteur present to maintain culturally responsive and collaborative practices. Intervention was conducted in a collaborative environment using SAE, CE and LF to maximize carryover into the child's community. For this child, the traiteur served as an informant, teacher and conduit between the SLP and the family as a whole. Respectful collaboration with this family took the form of a coaching methodology (Greenspan *et al.*, 1998) with careful consideration of the family and traiteur as the primary teachers of the child. The SLP appropriately and humbly took the role of only a facilitator, a tertiary collaborator, whose suggestions and observations were offered to assist the larger community in incorporating the needs and goals of the child as part of that community. This collaboration lasted for a consistent duration of two years (semester system with fall, spring and summer) and continues with periodic meetings to facilitate adjustments as the caregiver sees a need. While not representative of the majority of Cajun community experiences, this example does provide a sample of how culturally responsive practices can facilitate collaboration for SLPs and their clientele.

For additional guidelines on the use of informants as collaborators in clinical practice, the reader is directed to Damico and Hamayan (1992) for a detailed tutorial.

Use of authentic and functional contexts

The result of the bilevel analysis paradigm is a rich description and explication of complex social phenomena focusing on a pragmatic (or use-based) approach to speech and language assessment (Smith & Damico, 1992). This pragmatic approach to the communication of minority dialect speakers starts with a functional assessment of communication in authentic settings (e.g. home, school, work). The use of descriptive measures to examine the effects of context, namely communicative context and the effect that has on the person's ability to function, allows the SLP to not only locate breakdowns or barriers to successful environments but situate those breakdowns in either extrinsic or intrinsic factors that lead to answers for more successful interactions.

Recent movements to assert dialect use as a characteristic of all language users have helped to highlight the importance of considering the effects of dialect on the assessment of speech-language disorders (Oetting *et al.*, 2016). Assessment techniques should allow for explication of the effects of the bias of the examiners' language/dialect, the bias of any testing instruments' language/dialect use, as well as the possible ignorance on the part of the examiner regarding the client's language/dialect (Babatsouli, 2021, 2023, 2024; Damico *et al.*, 1996; Hamayan & Damico, 1991; McLeod *et al.*, 2017; Velleman & Zurer Pearson, 2010; Washington *et al.*, 2023). The complexity of this process is best represented when multiple levels of assessment are considered, including assessment in authentic and functional contexts of interest. Particularly when given the goal of assessment, which is the careful design of strategies to address the potential barriers to successful learning, growing and participating in life events (Brinton *et al.*, 2021; Reid *et al.*, 1993).

One context of communication, which must be included in the assessment of a suspected speech-language disorder is literacy development. The effects of a mismatch in language or dialect are a perfect example of where the NMAE dialect user may be considered intrinsically disordered by an inexperienced evaluator (Easton & Verdon, 2021). The use of descriptive assessment measures during literacy activities with culturally appropriate or culturally inspiring texts and partners familiar to the child can provide a wealth of speech and language information when determining the presence of an intrinsic disorder versus a possible mismatch. In an article published in (2018), Holt describes the effect of culturally inclusive writers on the interactional styles and demonstrations of competency for BE dialect users during shared reading activities. The author describes the use of 'dialect inspired poetry and verse' for effective intervention with users of BE dialects. This same context can assist clinicians in describing strengths and areas for growth in literacy development more readily than the use of a traditional or standardized assessment tool alone.

Thankfully, researchers will continue to develop language and/or dialect-specific assessments to aid in the clinical decisions of SLPs and to expand the knowledge base of the profession. These researchers have provided additional tools and techniques for SLPs to assess the growing variety of NMAE dialects. SLPs' integration of dialect or language-specific assessments, along with dynamic and descriptive assessment practices, will ensure better outcomes for the whole child situated within their various communities.

Conclusion

The careful and intentional study of dialect extends beyond simple speech sounds and the linguistic attributes of a particular region. In the Acadiana parishes of Louisiana, the CE dialect calls back to old traditions and a sense of community that is experiencing many of the changes of a modern society. In this chapter, the authors provide some historical context for the complexity of the Acadiana area, and they highlight the characteristics of CE that make it both distinctive and familiar among other regional dialects. The field of speech-language pathology has evidence-informed tools and procedures ready to serve and collaborate with CE dialect speakers in all aspects of communicative care. Additional research will enhance our understanding of the dialectal voice within our modern society and assist in the preservation of these ways of being in the world.

References

Adler, S. (1977) Dialectal differences: Professional and clinical implications. *Journal of Speech and Hearing Disorders* XXXVI (1), 90–100.

Ancelet, B.J., Edwards, J. and Pitre, G. (2009) *Cajun Country*. University Press of Mississippi.

Babatsouli, E. (2021) Diversity considerations in speech and language disorders: A focus on training. In *The Handbook of Language and Speech Disorders* (2nd edn, pp. 33–52). Wiley Blackwell.

Babatsouli, E. (2023) Ecosystemic clinical assessment of linguistic diversity: Greek-dominant speech. *Perspectives of the ASHA Special Interest Groups* 9 (3), 692–714.

Babatsouli, E. (2024) Phonological disorders in child bilingualism. In M. Amengual (ed.) *The Cambridge Handbook of Bilingual Phonetics and Phonology* (pp. 309–337). Cambridge University Press.

Babatsouli, E., Dore, E., Durand, C., Glaeser, C., Johnson, M., Leal, A. and Savant, E. (2025) Piloting the UL Lullaby Project: First Data. Poster presented at the *5th International Symposium on Monolingual and Bilingual Speech (ISMBS) 2025*. 16–19 June 2025. Chania, Greece.

Bennett III, W. (2025, June 16–19) Voice Onset Time of Cajun English speakers. Oral Paper presentation at the *International Symposium on Monolingual and Bilingual Speech (ISMBS) 2025*. 16–19 June, Chania, Greece.

Bernard, S.K. (2003) *The Cajuns: Americanization of a People*. University Press of Mississippi.

Bowie, D. (2003) Early development of the CARD-CORD merger in Utah. *American Speech* 78, 31–51. https://doi.org/10.1215/00031283-78-1-31

Bowie, D. (2008) Acoustic characteristics of Utah's CARD-CORD merger. *American Speech* 83 (1), 35–61. https://doi.org/10.1215/00031283-2008-002

Brasseaux, C.A. (1987) *The Founding of New Acadia: The Beginnings of Acadian Life in Louisiana, 1765–1803*. LSU Press.

Brinton, B., Fujiki, M. and Brinton Fujiki, R. (2021) Principles of assessment and intervention. In *The Handbook of Language and Speech Disorders* (2nd edn, pp. 110–128). Wiley Blackwell.

Carmichael, K. (2013) The performance of Cajun English in Boudreaux and Thibodeaux jokes. *American Speech* 88 (4), 377–412. https://doi.org/10.1215/00031283-2691415

Carmichael, K. (2019) Cajun English: A linguistic and cultural profile. In N. Dajko and S. Walton (eds) *Language in Louisiana* (pp. 159–172). University Press of Mississippi; JSTOR. https://doi.org/10.2307/j.ctvkwnnm1.19

Cheramie, D.M. (1998) Cajun Vernacular English and the influence of vernacular on student writing in South Louisiana. Ph.D., University of Southwestern Louisiana. See https://www.proquest.com/docview/304466027/abstract/E2533474B1FD4B85PQ/1

Cheramie, D.M. and Gill, D.A. (1992) Lexical choice in Cajun Vernacular English. In A.M. Scott (ed.) *Cajun Vernacular English: Informal English in French Louisiana*. Technical Writing Laboratory, Department of English, University of Southwestern Louisiana.

CODOFIL | Council for the Development of French in Louisiana, 29 May. (2014) [Page]. OCD-Division-Homepage. See https://DCRT-MAIN/cultural-development/codofil/index

Coyne, A.L. (2008) Intergenerational patterns of phonological features and linguistic attitudes of Cajun English speakers. M.A., Southern Illinois University at Carbondale. See https://www.proquest.com/docview/304463361/abstract/4C797C49F1AB48F8PQ/1

Daigle, E. (1991) Traiteurs and their power of healing: The story of Doris Bergeron. *Louisiana Folklore Miscellany* 6 (4), 43–48.

Damico, J. and Hamayan, E.V. (1992) *Multicultural Language Intervention: Addressing Cultural and Linguistic Diversity*. EDUCOM.

Damico, J.S. (1991) Descriptive assessment of communicative ability in limited English proficient students. In *Limiting Bias in the Assessment of Bilingual Students* (pp. 157–217). Pro-Ed. See https://scholar.google.com/scholar?cluster=8858866582260394788&hl=en&oi=scholarr

Damico, J.S., Smith, M. and Augustine, LLoyd E. (1996) Multicultural populations and language disorders. In W.H. Perkins (ed.) *Childhood Language Disorders* (pp. 272–299). Thieme Publishing.

Dubois, S. and Horvath, B.M. (1998) From accent to marker in Cajun English: A study of dialect formation in progress. *English World-Wide* 19 (2), 161–188. https://doi.org/10.1075/eww.19.2.02dub

Dubois, S. and Horvath, B.M. (2000) When the music changes, you change too: Gender and language change in Cajun English. *Language Variation and Change* 11, 287–313.

Dubois, S. and Horvath, B.M. (2002) Sounding Cajun: The rhetorical use of dialect in speech and writing. *American Speech* 77 (3), 264–287. https://doi.org/10.1215/00031283-77-3-264

Dubois, S. and Horvath, B.M. (2003) Verbal morphology in Cajun Vernacular English: A comparison with other varieties of Southern English. *Journal of English Linguistics* 31 (1), 34–59. https://doi.org/10.1177/0075424202250296

Dubois, S. and Horvath, B.M. (2004) Cajun vernacular English: Phonology. In *The Americas and the Caribbean* (Vol. 2, pp. 407–416). De Gruyter Mouton. https://www.degruyter.com/view/title/30937

Dubois, S. and Melançon, M. (1997) Cajun is dead-long live Cajun: Shifting from a linguistic to a cultural community. *Journal of Sociolinguistics* 1 (1), 63–93. https://doi.org/10.1111/1467-9481.00004

Duncan, D. (2022) Merger reversal in St. Louis: Implementation and implications. *Journal of English Linguistics* 50 (1), 72–105. https://doi.org/10.1177/00754242221083648

Easton, C. and Verdon, S. (2021) The influence of linguistic bias upon speech-language pathologists' attitudes toward clinical scenarios involving nonstandard dialects of English. *American Journal of Speech-Language Pathology* 30, 1973–1989.

Eble, C. (1993) Prolegomenon to the study of Cajun English. *SECOL Review* 17 (2), 165–177.

Edwards, W.F. (2004) African American vernacular English: Phonology. In E.W. Schneider and B. Kortmann (eds) *A Handbook Varieties of English, Volume 1 Phonology* (Vol. 1). Mouton de Gruyter.

Estaville, L.E. (1987) Changeless Cajuns: Nineteenth-century reality or myth? *Louisiana History: The Journal of the Louisiana Historical Association* 28 (2), 117–140.

Fairbanks, G. (1960) The rainbow passage. In *Voice and Articulation Drillbook* (2nd edn, pp. 124–139). Harper & Row.

Forrest, J. and Wolfram, W. (2019) The status of (ing) in African American Language: A quantitative analysis of social factors and internal constraints. *American Speech: A Quarterly of Linguistic Usage* 94 (1), 72–90

Glain, O. (2021) The Cajun renaissance and Cajun English. The social, the linguistic, the imaginary. *Anglophonia. French Journal of English Linguistics* 32, Article 32. https://doi.org/10.4000/anglophonia.4049

Greenspan, S., Wieder, S. and Simons, R. (1998) *The Child with Special Needs: Encouraging Intellectual and Emotional Growth*. Perseus Books.

Hamayan, E.V. and Damico, J.S. (1991) *Limiting Bias in the Assessment of Bilingual Students*. https://cir.nii.ac.jp/crid/1130000795184827392

Hannegan, J. and Shport, I. (2024) *Examining Back-Vowel Fronting in Cajun English*. 2024 LAVIS Conference: The Changing South, Athens, GA. https://www.linguistics.uga.edu/lavis

Hendricks, A.E., Watson-Wales, M. and Reed, P.E. (2021) Perceptions of African American English by students in speech-language pathology programs. *American Journal of Speech-Language Pathology* 30 (5), 1962–1972.

Hendricks, A. and Adolf, S. (2017) Language assessment with children who speak nonmainstream dialects: Examining the effects of scoring modifications in norm-referenced assessment. *Language, Speech, and Hearing Services in Schools* 48, 168–182.

Holt, Y. (2018) Using African American literature in the therapy setting. *eHearsay: Electronic Journal of the Ohio Speech-Language Hearing Association* 8 (1), 43–50.

Johnstone, B. (2016) Enregisterment: How linguistic items become linked with ways of speaking: Enregisterment. *Language and Linguistics Compass* 10, 632–643. https://doi.org/10.1111/lnc3.12210

Kein, S. (ed.) (2000) *Creole: The History and Legacy of Louisiana's Free People of Color*. Louisiana State University Press.

Kretzschmar, Jr., W.A. (2004) Standard American English pronunciation. In E.W. Schneider and B. Kortmann (eds) *A Handbook Varieties of English, Volume 1 Phonology* (Vol. 1). Mouton de Gruyter.

KRVS. (2024) *KRVS*. KRVS Radio Acadie. See https://www.krvs.org/

Leal, A., Dore, E., Durand, C., Glaeser, C., Savant, E. and Babatsouli, E. (2026) Capturing dialectal and hierarchical representations for the evaluation of English developmental speech. Poster presented at the *National Conference on Undergraduate Research (NCUR) 2026*. Richmond, VA.

Marshall, M.M. (1982) Bilingualism in Southern Louisiana: A sociolinguistic analysis. *Anthropological Linguistics* 24 (3), 308–324.

McCurdy, D., Spradley, J. and Shandy, D. (2004) *The Cultural Experience: Ethnography in Complex Society* (2nd edn). Waveland Press.

McLeod, S., Harrison, L.J. and McCormack, J. (2012) The intelligibility in context scale: Validity and reliability of a subjective rating measure. *Journal of Speech, Language, and Hearing Research: JSLHR* 55 (2), 648–656. https://doi.org/10.1044/1092-4388(2011/10-0130)

McLeod, S., Verdon, S. and The International Expert Panel on Multilingual Children's Speech. (2017) Tutorial: Speech assessment for multilingual children who do not speak the same language(s) as the speech-language pathologist. *American Journal of Speech-Language Pathology* 26, 691–708.

Oetting, J.B., Gregory, K.D. and Riviere, A. (2016) Changing how speech-language pathologists think and talk about dialect variation. *Perspectives of the ASHA Special Interest Groups* 1 (16), 28–37. https://doi.org/10.1044/persp1.SIG16.28

Oetting, J. and Garrity, A.W. (2006) Variation within dialects: A case of Cajun/Creole influence with child SAAE and SWE. *Journal of Speech, Language, and Hearing Research* 49 (1), 16–26. https://doi.org/10.1044/1092-4388(2006/002)

Oetting, J., Lee, R. and Porter, K. (2013) Evaluating the grammars of children who speak mainstream dialects of English. *Topics in Language Disorders* 33, 140–151.

Puranik, C., Branum-Martin, L. and Washington, J.A. (2020) The relation between dialect density and the codevelopment of writing and reading in African American children. *Child Development* 91 (4), e866–e882. https://doi.org/10.1111/cdev.13318

Reid, B.M., Secord, W.A. and Damico, J.S. (1993) Strategies for the integration of collaborative theory into practice. *National Student Speech Language and Hearing Association Journal* 20, 32–42.

Rice, C. (2014) Bare possessive yall: Documentation and exploration. Southeastern Conference on Linguistics Annual Conference, Myrtle Beach, NC.

Rivière, A.M., Oetting, J.B. and Roy, J. (2018) Effects of specific language impairment on a contrastive dialect structure: The case of infinitival to across various nonmainstream dialects of English. *Journal of Speech, Language, and Hearing Research* 61 (8), 1989–2001. https://doi.org/10.1044/2018_JSLHR-L-17-0209

Robinson, G.C. and Stockman, I.J. (2009) Cross-dialectal perceptual experiences of speech-language pathologists in predominantly Caucasian American school districts. *Language, Speech, and Hearing Services in Schools* 40 (2), 138–149.

Rubrecht, A.W. (1971) Regional phonological variants in louisiana speech [Doctoral]. University of Florida.

Scott, A.M. (1992) *Cajun Vernacular English: Informal English in French Louisiana.* Technical Writing Laboratory, Department of English, University of Southwestern Louisiana.

Smith, M. and Damico, J.S. (1992) *Childhood Language Disorders.* Thieme.

Sothern, J.M. (with Charpentier, J.). (2001) *Cajun Dictionary: A Collection of Some Commonly Used Words & Phrases by the People of South Louisiana* (2nd edn). Bayou Printing & Graphics, Inc.

Spradley, J. (1980) *Participant Observation.* Holt, Rinehart and Winston.

Thomas, E.R. (2004) Rural Southern white accents. In E.W. Schneider and B. Kortmann (eds) *A Handbook Varieties of English, Volume 1 Phonology* (Vol. 1). Mouton de Gruyter.

Vafadar, A.C. and Utt, H. (1992) A Survey of speech-language pathologists' attitudes about, self-perceived knowledge of, and competency in dealing with social dialects: Language differences versus language disorders. *NSSLHA Journal* (20), 65–72.

Velleman, S. and Zurer Pearson, B. (2010) Differentiating speech sound disorders from phonological dialect differences: Implications for assessment and intervention. *Topics in Language Disorders* 30 (3), 176–188.

Verdon, S., Blake, H.L., Hopf, S.C., Phạm, B. and McLeod, S. (2016) Cultural and linguistic diversity in speech-language pathology. *International Journal of Speech-Language Pathology* 18 (2), 109–110.

Walton, S.L. (1994) Flat speech and Cajun ethnic identity in Terrebonne parish, Louisiana. Ph.D., Tulane University. See https://www.proquest.com/docview/304127894/abstract/76764B9FDF724F51PQ/1

Ward, R.K. (1997) The French language in Louisiana law and legal education: A requiem. *Louisiana Law Review* 57 (4), 1283–1324.

Washington, J.A., Branum-Martin, L., Sun, C. and Lee-James, R. (2018) The impact of dialect density on the growth of language and reading in African American children. *Language, Speech, and Hearing Services in Schools* 49 (2), 232–247. https://doi.org/10.1044/2018_LSHSS-17-0063

Washington, K.N., Wright Karem, R., Kokotek, L. and Leon, M. (2023) Supporting culturally responsive assessment practices with preschoolers: Guidance from methods in the Jamaican context. *Journal of Speech, Language, and Hearing Research* 66, 4716–4738.

Westby, C. (1990) Ethnographic interviewing: Asking the right questions to the right people in the right ways. *Communication Disorders Quarterly* 13, 101–111. https://doi.org/10.1177/152574019001300111

Westby, C. and Washington, K. (2017) Using the international classification of functioning, disability and health in assessment and intervention of school-aged children with language impairments. *Language, Speech, and Hearing Services in Schools* 48 (3), 137–152.

Wolfram, W. (2004) The grammar of urban African American Vernacular English. In B. Kortmann and E.W. Schneider (eds) *A Handbook of Varieties of English* (pp. 111–132). Mouton de Gruyter.

Appendix

Table 4.1A Consonants of Cajun English

	Bilabial		Labio dental		Labial-velar		Dental		Alveolar	
Plosive (stop)	p	b							t	d
Nasal		m								n
Trill										r*
Tap or Flap										ɾ
Fricative			f	v			θ	ð	s	z
Affricate										
Approximant						w				ɹ
Lateral approximant										l

*only produced in Cajun French vocabulary.

Table 4.2B Consonants of Cajun English

	Post-alveolar		Palatal		Velar		Uvular		Glottal	
Plosive (stop)					k	g			ʔ	
Nasal						ŋ				
Trill										
Tap or Flap										
Fricative	ʃ	ʒ						ʁ*	h	
Affricate	ʧ	dʒ								
Approximant				j						
Lateral approximant										

*only produced in Cajun French vocabulary.

Table 4.3C Vowels of Mainstream American English, Southern American English, African American English and Cajun English

Target word	MAE	SAE	BE	CE
KIT	ɪ	ɪ~iə	iə,iɪ	ɪ, i
DRESS	ɛ	ɛ~eə	ɛɪ	ɛ, æ
TRAP	æ	æ	æɛ	æ
LOT	ɑ	ɑ	ɑ	ɑ, a
STRUT	ʌ	ɜ	ʌ	ʌ
FOOT	ʊ	Y	ʊ	ʊ, ʉ
BATH	æ	æ	æɛ	æ
DANCE	æ	eə		æ̃, æ
CLOTH	ɔ, ɑ	ɑɒ	ɑ	a
NURSE	ɚ	ɚ>eɚ	ɣ,əɹ	ʌɹ, ʌɘ
FLEECE	i	ʝi~ɪi	ɪɪ	i:
FACE	eɪ	ɛi~æ̞i	eɪ	e:
PALM	ɑ	ɑ~ɒO	æ	ɑ
THOUGHT	ɔ, ɑ	ɑɒ	ɔʊ	a
GOAT	Oʊ	ɜy~ɜu>æ̞u	O	O:
GOAL	Oʊ	ɔ̞u~ɒ̞u	O	O:
GOOSE	u	ʉ̞ų~yʉ̞~ʉ̞y~yy	u	U:
PRICE	ɑɪ	ai~a:æ~a:	ɑ:	ai, ɑ:
PRIZE	ɑɪ	a:ɛ~a:æ~a:	ɑ:	ai, ɑ:
CHOICE	ɔɪ	oi	Oɪ	ɔi, ɔ:
MOUTH	aʊ	æɔ~æɒ~aɒ	æə	au, a:
LOUD	aʊ	æɔ~æɒ~aɒ		au, a:
NEAR	iɚ,ɪɚ	iɚ	iɣ,ɪəɹ	i:
SQUARE	ɛɚ	e̞ɚ	æə	ɛ, æ
MARRY	ɛ	e̞		ɛ, æ
MERRY	ɛ	e̞		ɛ
MARY	ɛ	e̞		ɛ
START	ɑɚ	ɒɚ>ɑɚ	ɑ:	ɑ, a
NORTH	ɔɚ	Oɚ	ɔə	ɔɹ, ɔɘ
FORCE	ɔɚ	Oɚ	ɔə	ɔɹ, ɔɘ
ORANGE	ɔ	ɑ~ɒ~O		ɔɹ, ɑ
CURE	jʊɚ	uɚ~ɚ	uə	ʊə
FIRE	aiɚ	aæɚ~a:ɚ		ai, ɑ:
POWER		aɔɚ		au, ɑ:
happY	i	i		ɪ, i
lettER	ɚ	ɚ		əɹ, ə

(Continued)

Table 4.3C (Continued)

Target word	MAE	SAE	BE	CE
horsES	ə, i	ɪ~ï		ɪ,ɪ̃
commA	ə	ə		ə
HAND		eə		æ, æ̃
PIN	ɪ	ɪ~iə		ɪ,ɪ̃
PEN	ɛ	ɪ~iə		ɪ,ɪ̃
THINK		ɪ~ɪi		i,ɪ̃
LENGTH		ɪ~ɪi		i,ɪ̃
GOING		ɔ̹u~ɒ̹u		ɔi,ɔ
POOL		ʊ̹~u		u:
PULL		ʊ̹~u		ʊ, ʉ
FEEL		ɪ~iə~ji		i:
FILL		ɪ~iə~ï		
FAIL		ei~ɛ		ei, e:
FELL		ɛ		ɛ
MIRROR		ɪ̞		i:, ɪ
NEARER		ɪ̞		i:, ɪ
TOMORROW		ɑ~ɒ		a, ɑ

5 Gullah Geechee

Jessica R. Berry

Introduction

Gullah Geechee context and culture

Gullah, Geechee, Gullah-Geechee, Gullah/Geechee and Gullah Geechee are among the many representations used to identify a unique group of indigenous African American people who primarily live on the southeastern coast of the United States. Some controversy has been noted among local scholars and advocates about the appropriate way to write the name of the language, with some entities opting for the use of the '/', i.e. Gullah/Geechee, while others opting not to use the slash, Gullah Geechee. To avoid presenting any separation between the two terms Gullah and Geechee, for the remainder of this chapter, Gullah Geechee will be used to reference the language, culture and people in recognition of their unity as one.

Gullah Geechee people have made significant contributions to the fabric of the United States, specifically to Southern American history. Gullah Geechee people are descendants of enslaved Africans who were kidnapped and brought to the United States during the transatlantic slave trade. Many of the enslaved were brought from West African countries like Sierra Leone, Angola, Benin, Senegal and The Gambia, while many were also brought from Afro-Caribbean countries like Jamaica, Guyana and Barbados to work at the behest of cruel owners with a singular focus on building wealth for their families. The origins of the Gullah Geechee language and people are deeply rooted in African traditions, language and the history of slavery in the southeastern United States.

Gullah Geechee ancestors were brought to the United States for exploitation of their ability to plant, harvest, birth and care for their owners, the land and their families. The enslaved were primarily responsible for the creation, maintenance and harvesting of major southern cash crops including Carolina Gold rice, cotton and indigo (Cooper, 2017; Eltis, 2000). Their unique knowledge of rice cultivation and harvesting, learned on the West African coast, was integral in creating the wealth that remains in Charleston and other low-country regions of South Carolina today.

Gullah Geechee constructed identity

The construction of Gullah Geechee identity has been debated and reshaped by scholars including anthropologists, historians, folklorists, journalists, tourists and the Gullah Geechee community itself over time (Cooper, 2017). Given the nature of Gullah Geechee people's existence as property and not people, they were not able to leave a written record of the origins of their identity. In recent years, Gullah Geechee have begun to use their language on social media platforms as a way to demonstrate their pride in being identified as Gullah Geechee. Within these instances of written Gullah Geechee use, the variation in the written form of the language has been evident. A group of Gullah Geechee community members and linguists collaborated to translate the New Testament of the Bible into Gullah Geechee. To date, this remains the most comprehensive written translation of the language that many used as a guide to standardize the written Gullah Geechee language. Currently, Gullah Geechee does not have a standardized written version; therefore, variations in the spelling of words occur based on speaker preference.

It has been left to descendants and historians to preserve and interpret the intricate nuances involved in the creation of this culture and language. Like other languages and cultures, Gullah Geechee is dynamic and resilient in the face of constant, often unsolicited change within and around their families and communities. The existence of modern Gullah Geechee culture, language and history is a testament to Gullah Geechee ancestral resilience in the face of unprecedented circumstances.

Gullah Geechee geography

During the transatlantic slave trade, South Carolina received more slaves than any of the other colonies. Scholars document that over 40% of the Africans kidnapped from Africa disembarked at Gadsden's Wharf in Charleston, South Carolina, from the late 1760s to 1801 and were subsequently dispersed along the Southeastern coast. Today, Gadsden's Wharf is home to the International African American Museum, which is a raised design that does not sit on the ground in honor of the many lives lost and forever changed during the journey to American soil ('Preservation Society of Charleston', 2024; 'IAAM'). In 1996 the US Congress officially established The Gullah Geechee Cultural Heritage Corridor (GGCHC) as a National Heritage Area to preserve cultural and natural resources associated with the Gullah Geechee culture and heritage. Additionally, the GGCHC was created to recognize the unique culture of the Gullah Geechee people who live along the sea islands and up to 30 miles inland on the coastal areas of North Carolina, South Carolina, Georgia and Florida (Figure 5.1).

Although Gullah Geechee people have traditionally resided in these areas, the great migration of the 1960s and 70s contributed to many Gullah Geechee people moving north to Chicago, Maryland, Detroit, Pennsylvania, New Jersey and New York in search of work and economic and social advancement opportunities ('National Archives: The Great Migration'). Therefore, the imprint of Gullah Geechee culture and language can be heard and felt in African American communities beyond the confines of the GGCHC areas. Gullah Geechee people have special

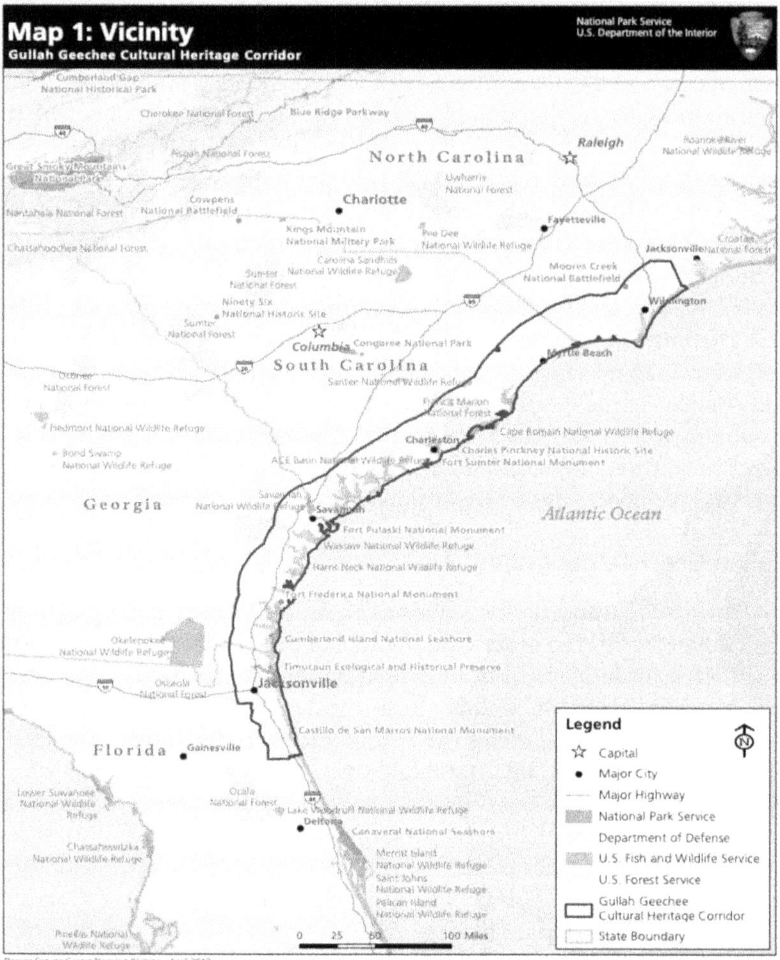

Figure 5.1 Gullah Geechee Cultural Heritage Corridor Image Credit: Gullah Geechee Cultural Heritage Corridor Management Plan [https://gullahgeecheecorridor.org/management-plan/].

names for the identity of those who reside along the corridor. Those who are born Gullah Geechee, speak the language and practice the culture are referred to as *Been ya* or *Bin ya* which means 'been here' or native. Many Gullah Geechee will refer to themselves as Been yas to distinguish themselves from those who are not Gullah Geechee. Those who are not native are considered *Come yas*. Those whose families moved away from the Gullah Geechee regions but have relocated to reclaim their Gullah Geechee properties are considered *Come back yas* as they have come back to reclaim their place on the land.

The development of Gullah Geechee

Vestiges of African culture can still be seen through the Gullah Geechee cultural and spiritual practices, crafts, religion and spirituality, cuisine and music (Berry, 2020; Crawford, 2020a; Jones-Jackson, 1987b). The development of the Gullah Geechee is attributed to the social and geographical isolation of enslaved Africans on sea islands and rural low-country plantations. In the book *Gullah Days: Hilton Head Islanders before the Bridge 1861–1956,* Emory Campbell *et al.* (2019) provide a detailed account of the traditions and resilience of the Gullah people on Hilton Head Island, South Carolina, from the Civil War era to the construction of the bridge in 1956 that connected the island to the mainland. This isolation provided the opportunity for the enslaved Africans to retain traditional African practices. Moreover, given that many of the enslaved were not members of the same African tribes, they did not speak the same languages. The isolation on these islands was an incubator for the creation of a pidgin language variety. A pidgin language is a simplified form of communication that develops between two or more groups of people who do not share a common language. It arises when speakers of different native languages need to communicate for trade, work or other purposes but have no shared language. Pidgins are often temporary and pragmatic but can evolve into fully developed languages, known as creoles, if they become the first language of a community. In the case of Gullah Geechee, the pidgin variety created out of the isolation of pre-bridge rural sea islands and forced labor on Southern plantations became the first language with each new generation of children and creolized to form the Gullah Geechee language discussed, studied and preserved today.

The isolation that Gullah Geechee people endured was fertile ground for the retention of African ways. Unlike other enslaved Africans who were dispersed across the developing United States, Gullah Geechee remained together, preserving and practicing many traditional African crafts, cuisine, medicinal practices and religious customs.

In an overview of the Gullah Geechee culture and language, Campbell (1997) highlights the various traditions central to Gullah Geechee culture. Basket weaving is one of the most distinguishable cultural practices of the Gullah Geechee culture. The weaving of sweetgrass baskets is one of the Gullah Geechee crafts directly tied to African culture. The baskets are made from natural materials like sweetgrass, bulrush and pine straw. Local basket makers forage via coastal forests and wetlands to harvest items needed to complete their baskets. The tradition of sweetgrass baskets is closely tied to basket weaving, documented as being done in Sierra Leone Africa (Opala, 1987). Although baskets now are largely collected and used as decor, their original designs were functional, used to separate rice, carry items, and fruits and vegetables.

African connection and retention

African retentions are present throughout Gullah Geechee culture in various facets like names, arts, crafts, music, folklore, cuisine and culture. Turner (1949), one of the early scholars to formally study the Gullah Geechee language, noted the use of 'basket names' (e.g. *Cudda*, *Tittuh*) among Gullah Geechee people. These were additional names given to a child at birth that typically reflected their appearance or something about their personality.

Mufwene (1997) places Gullah Geechee within the broader framework of creole formation, which occurs when speakers of different languages come into contact, typically under conditions of forced migration, such as the transatlantic slave trade. English, as the dominant colonial language, provided the lexical base, but many African grammatical structures were retained. The formation of Gullah Geechee was thus a result of this creolization process, where African languages influenced English, creating a distinct creole language.

Crawford (2020b) describes the significant role of spirituals in Gullah Geechee culture and African Americans' protests for freedom. The sound of Africa can be heard through Gullah Geechee spirituals. These spirituals feature rich musical traditions and lyrical content that reflect the struggles, hopes and resilience of the Gullah Geechee community. The spirituals draw heavily on African musical elements, incorporating call-and-response patterns, improvisation and rhythmic complexity. Gullah Geechee musical traditions include a distinct double, polyrhythmic clap used in the early praise houses on the sea islands and remain prevalently used in modern Gullah Geechee churches across the corridor. Many spirituals contained coded messages, providing communication among enslaved individuals regarding escape routes, uprisings or plans for freedom. Songs like 'Wade in the Water' represent dual meanings – both as expressions of faith and as metaphors for navigating the dangers of escape. The ring shout is a spiritual and musical expression retained from African practices within the Gullah Geechee culture. The ring shout includes singing using call and response, clapping and percussive movements in a counterclockwise circle. This practice is traced back to West and Central African religious practices and communal rituals, where music, dance and spirituality are interconnected (Crawford, 2020a). In celebration of Emancipation on 31 December 1862, Gullah Geechee people gathered at the praise house to celebrate their freedom from enslavement. The Watch Night service has remained a cultural practice of Gullah Geechee still practiced in many churches today. At Watch Night services, Gullah Geechee people sing classic spirituals, dance and praise God in preparation, celebration and thanksgiving for the new year approaching. Additionally, they discuss the significance of Gullah storytelling, spirituals and communal traditions, such as 'shouts' in worship services, all of which reflect the blend of African and American elements in Gullah Geechee culture (Campbell, 1997; Campbell *et al.*, 2019; Campbell, 2020). The construction of the first bridge to Hilton Head Island in 1956 marked the end of an era of isolation and the beginning of rapid modernization (Campbell, 1997; Campbell *et al.*, 2019).

Cooking the Gullah Geechee way is a testament to the African dishes that were retained by those stolen and to the creativity of the enslaved in the use of locally available resources for sustenance and survival. Gullah Geechee cuisine features locally sourced ingredients such as seafood, rice and vegetables. The recipes are practical and rooted in the history of the community, with dishes like fried fish, okra soup, crab rice, Frogmore stew, oysters, blue crabs, sweet potato pie and in' john (i.e. peas and rice) (Meggett, 2022; Robinson, 2005). Gullah Geechee cuisine is not typically cooked by recipe but by traditions passed down through generations. Young Gullah Geechee women are brought alongside the elder women to learn how to cook by intuition and touch using the available ingredients from local and familial farms (Smart-Grosvenor, 2011).

Through cultural practices, storytelling and folklore, many African retentions remain prevalent within the Gullah Geechee language and community through cultural practices like storytelling and folklore. Each of these oral cultural practices contributes to the continuance of Gullah Geechee as an oral language with no written standard variety. Within the folklore are stories of voodoo healers and witchcraft practitioners like Dr Buzzard. Gullah Geechee people paint the ceiling of their porches blue to ward off spirits, and many yards are lined with blue bottle trees, which are meant to capture spirits that may come to their property and symbolize good luck.

Gullah Geechee culture was created and is sustained by the water. The movement of the enslaved across the Atlantic Ocean, then being held hostage on foreign soil, forced them to recreate their lives. Therefore, the Gullah Geechee people relied on their hunter-gatherer skills of crabbing, fishing, harvesting oysters and creating fishing cast nets for survival. In modern times, Gullah Geechee people are fighting to retain the rights to the land that their ancestors occupied by force and after emancipation by sharecropping to modern heirs' property ownership. In 2023, South Carolina was considered the fastest-growing state, according to US Census Bureau Data (2023). As a result, rapid gentrification of traditional Gullah Geechee communities threatens the retention of the Gullah Geechee people, culture and language.

Gullah Geechee Language

In 1949, Dr Lorenzo Dow Turner was the first African American linguist to introduce the world to the Gullah Geechee language and document its connections to Africa through his seminal book titled *Africanisms in the Gullah Dialect* (Turner, 1949). His work elevated Gullah Geechee's status as a language by providing phonetic transcriptions that demonstrated the grammatical, phonological, morphological, semantic and syntactical patterns and uniqueness of the language and cultural traditions of the people. These phonetic transcriptions created a platform for future scholars in various fields to examine and document Gullah Geechee's grammar rules and structures. Since this publication, Gullah Geechee has been recognized as an English-based creole language by scholars across fields of study like African American Studies, linguistics (Turner, 1949; Winford, 1992; Wolfram, 1973), sociolinguistics (Weldon, 2003) and communication sciences and disorders academics (Berry & Oetting, 2017). Moreover, Gullah Geechee is revered as the only English-based creole still alive in the United States.

Turner is revered as the father of Gullah Geechee studies (Wade-Lewis, 2007). His publication provided evidence of significant cultural and linguistic retentions of African cultures among the Gullah Geechee people. Turner's father was born free, but his mother was born enslaved. He earned his PhD in English from the University of Chicago in 1926 and was a second-generation college student at a time when most African Americans were only receiving up to a fourth-grade education. Although Turner was not of Gullah Geechee descent, his ethnographic research approach centered on time spent immersed living in the community to observe and understand the daily practices, beliefs and interactions. This time allowed him to build relationships with the Gullah Geechee community, which was necessary for the ultimate success of the work. Turner's work identified more than 4000 words in the Gullah Geechee language that trace lexical descent from several languages in West, Central Africa and Niger-Congo language families like Mende, Kissi, Kikongo, Ewe, Yoruba, Igbo, Mandinka and Wolof (Mufwene, 1997). Turner phonetically transcribed narratives from residents of low country on James Island and Wadmalaw Island. From these transcriptions, he identified specific connections to several African languages that had not been documented. Turner's work created a pathway for scholars to study and document the nuances of the Gullah Geechee language.

Table 5.1 Gullah Geechee phonological features

Phonological feature	Example
Consonant cluster simplification	*cold* → *cole*, *left* → *lef*, *test* → *tes*
Voicing assimilation	*car* → *cah*
Unstressed syllable reduction or deletion	*because* → *cause*
Variable pronunciation of <th> sounds	*this* → *dis*, *think* → *tink*

Gullah Geechee phonology

The Gullah Geechee sound system reflects its creole heritage and African influences while exhibiting features common to other African American English (AAE) varieties. Gullah Geechee evolved as a practical means of communication among enslaved Africans from different language backgrounds, leading to a phonological system that is streamlined yet dynamic.

The simplifications in its phonology, such as consonant cluster reduction or vowel centralization, reflect processes common in creole languages where multiple linguistic influences converge (Weldon, 1998a, 2003). Weldon (1998b) situates Gullah Geechee within the broader context of creole phonology, comparing it with other English-based creoles like Jamaican Patois or Bahamian Creole. Gullah Geechee has a five-vowel system but with variations in pronunciation, especially in the tense-lax vowel pairs, which differ from Mainstream American English (MAE) pronunciation. Though less pronounced than African tonal languages, Gullah Geechee shows traces of African intonation and emphasis patterns (Jones-Jackson, 1987a; Mufwene, 1997; Turner, 1949; Weldon, 1998b, 2003). Gullah Geechee has less use of complex consonant clusters by simplifying word-final consonants, a pattern consistent with African phonological systems. Gullah Geechee favors open syllables (consonant-vowel, CV). This contrasts with MAE's tolerance for complex consonant clusters (Weldon, 1998b). Table 5.1 provides examples of Gullah Geechee's phonological features.

Gullah Geechee morphology

The Gullah Geechee morphological system is described as simple compared to the complex nature of the morphological system of other language varieties (Jones-Jackson, 1987a; Mufwene, 1997, 2001; Weldon, 1998b, 2003). Mufwene (2001) highlights how Gullah Geechee has simple rather than complex inflectional morphology (changes to word forms based on tense, number or case). Gullah Geechee and AAE exhibit copula variability, however. Mufwene describes copula variability as a hallmark feature of the language. Weldon (1998b) specifies how the copula (such as *is*, *are* or *be*) is often omitted or variably used depending on the context.

Table 5.2 Gullah Geechee morphology

Morphological feature	Example
Zero copula: the form *to be* (*is*, *are*, *was*, *were*, *am*)	She is tall → She tall They are ready → They ready I am happy → I happy
Lack of inflection of tense: does not inflect verbs for tense or number, using context and auxiliary verbs instead	He goes or He is going → He go
Regularized plural: indicated using context rather than explicit morphological markers	Two men → Two man
Zero plural marking: no *-s* suffix to mark plural forms	He runs home → He run home
Habitual BE	He's always running → He be running
Negative concord: double negatives	I don't have any money → I een got no money
Tense, mood, aspect markers (TMA): these markers help express when an action occurs, the speaker's attitude toward it, and its completion or repetition	He walked home → E walk home yestaday or Yestaday e walk home
• *Done* is used to mark completed actions • *Bin* marks past actions • Progressive marking: *da*	I have eaten already → I done eat I did it already → I bin did dat He is running → He da run

One of the central questions in Weldon's (1998b) study is what grammatical factors influence the presence or absence of the copula in Gullah Geechee. She analyzes various factors, such as tense, aspect and sentence structure that affect how the copula is used, finding that copula omission occurs more frequently in the present tense, before adjectives or in habitual contexts, much like in AAE. Via the patterns of copula variability, the findings underscore that Gullah Geechee is rule-governed and not random. Table 5.2 provides examples of Gullah Geechee morphological features as examined and described by various scholars (Jones-Jackson, 1987a; Mufwene, 1997, 2001; Weldon, 1998b).

Gullah Geechee syntax

Gullah Geechee's pronoun system and subject-verb agreement are simplified compared to MAE with less variation between subject and object forms. Berry (2020) describes the pronouns *he*, *she* and *it to* make distinctions between masculine (i.e. *he*), feminine (i.e. *she*) and neutral (i.e. *it*) gender pronouns in MAE. However, Gullah Geechee uses the 'universal' creole pronoun, *E* (also written as *ee*/*Ee*), which does not distinguish between gender pronouns. For example, the MAE phrase *He/she was here yesterday* in Gullah Geechee would be *E been ya yestaday*. The term *universal pronoun* is not an official term used in linguistics but represents how Gullah Geechee people use this creole form.

Other unique pronominal features of Gullah Geechee include the first-person pronoun *us* realized as *we*. For example, in Gullah Geechee

They'n ga do um fa we is *They aren't going to do it for us*, while the second person pronoun *you/your* is represented by a different word *Hunnuh*, e.g. *How hunnuh fa do?* for *How are you doing?*

Gullah Geechee follows a subject-auxiliary-verb (SAV) order, where auxiliary verbs precede main verbs. In Gullah Geechee, as in other languages, auxiliary verbs are crucial in expressing complex verb tenses and grammatical relations (Mufwene, 1997). For example, in the sentence *He done gone*, *done* is the auxiliary indicating the completed action. This structure contrasts with MAE, which often employs subject-verb-object (SVO) order (Mufwene, 1986).

Mufwene (2001) also notes that flexible word order is observed in the Gullah Geechee language, which is influenced by various African languages. For example, Gullah Geechee speakers use topicalization to move an element to the front of a sentence for emphasis: *Dis boy ya, I know him* for *I know this boy*. Gullah Geechee does not mark agreement with the subject; for example, *He talk* and *They talk* are both grammatically correct in Gullah Geechee without the requirement of adding an *-s* to talk for marking third-person plural subjects or the *-ed* for past tense marking. Question formation in Gullah Geechee is distinct and uses question words (i.e. *who, what, where*) but may not invert the subject and verb, e.g. *Wha e say?* instead of *What did he say?* (Jones Jackson, 1987b). In Gullah Geechee, actions are often expressed with emphasis on aspect markers rather than tense. Tense in MAE is often indicated through adverbs, like *yesterday*, or particles like *done* for past actions or *go* for future actions. Gullah Geechee's tense/aspect system mirrors the structure of many African languages (Mufwene, 1986). This construct is shown through *bin* to indicate past actions, *da* to indicate present progressive actions and *done* to indicate completed actions. Examples of these constructs include the following:

bin (used to indicate past actions): *He bin run* means He had run or He ran.
da (used to indicate present continuous actions): *He da run* means He is running.
done (used for completed actions): *He done run* means He has run.

Gullah Geechee pragmatics

The pragmatic elements of the Gullah Geechee language reflect the solidarity and communal nature of the people, historical roots and strategy for maintaining cultural and communal identity. Key pragmatic elements of the language include expressive language and expressive non-verbal communication, call and response patterns, use of proverbs, stories, indirect communications, in-group communications, honorifics and respect patterns.

In Gullah Geechee, strong emphasis is placed on the use of nonverbal cues such as gestures, body language and tone. Gullah Geechee speakers often use unique intonation, rhythm and pacing features to facilitate communication that can convey layers of meaning, adding emphasis, emotion or humor.

Given that Gullah Geechee is used most often during in-group settings (i.e. community events, family gatherings, religious gatherings), many speakers employ code-switching as a pragmatic strategy when interacting with outsiders. Code-switching to MAE allows Gullah Geechee speakers to align themselves with different social identities and norms based on the audience and setting. However, Gullah Geechee speakers often use their language to establish and reinforce social bonds within the community. Certain phrases, slang or grammatical constructions may signal in-group membership and shared cultural identity. Pragmatically, this serves to create a sense of solidarity, belonging and mutual understanding. Young (2009) critiques the educational practice of code-switching, particularly its application to speakers of AAE. He contends that promoting code-switching reinforces linguistic segregation and perpetuates racial biases. Conversely, switching to MAE or avoiding Gullah Geechee could signal distance or formality. As an alternative, scholars recommend 'code-meshing', which encourages the blending of dialects and languages in both speech and writing. This approach aims to validate diverse linguistic identities and promote inclusivity (Lee, 2014; Young *et al.*, 2014). Regrettably, the negative stereotypes that have been associated with being Gullah Geechee have forced many speakers to code-switch more frequently and subsequently abandon the use of the language. Many are not fully aware of the strengths that are associated with the ability to code-switch. In a 2020 study, Kuzyk *et al.*'s findings support the idea that bilingualism, including the practice of code-switching, is associated with cognitive advantages such as improved problem-solving skills and better task-switching abilities. This may be due to the constant mental management of multiple linguistic systems. This ability to code-switch, even under less-than-ideal circumstances, demonstrates a sophisticated understanding of linguistic structures and contexts, which may indicate advanced cognitive abilities (Hughes *et al.*, 2006).

Complex ideas and values of the Gullah Geechee people are shared through storytelling via proverbs, folktales and idiomatic expressions. These stories typically teach a lesson and give advice in an indirect but culturally meaningful way. Indirect communication is a pragmatic practice of the Gullah Geechee people that is used to maintain respect and politeness, especially when discussing sensitive topics or when engaging in conversations with community elders. In Gullah Geechee, ideals and values are often conveyed using fewer words but manipulating tone, intonation and pitch to convey rich and deep meaning. For example, in

MAE one may say, *Get out of here now before you get in trouble* while in Gullah Geechee a simplified *Gone nah!* in a deep serious tone conveys the same message employing an economy of words.

Important to the Gullah Geechee are pragmatic choices related to politeness and respect. Language use varies depending on the age, social status or familiarity between speakers. Elders are addressed with more deference and respect, as shown through the use of respectful greetings or pleasantries that convey respect. Call-and-response patterns are typically seen in religious settings and music within the Gullah Geechee culture. However, this pattern of back-and-forth communication style is common during communicative exchanges and serves as a way to establish rapport, maintain group cohesion and facilitate understanding. This call-and-response pattern often results in overlapping speech, nonverbal cues and communal references.

These pragmatic practices within the Gullah Geechee culture are most frequently used in communal settings like church events, family reunions and festivals. These gatherings provide space for elders to pass down stories, songs and folklore, reinforcing moral values, community history and collective memory. Gullah Geechee people use these pragmatic elements as a strategy to maintain the close-knit nature of the community identity and solidarity as the landscape of the community changes.

Gullah Geechee semantics

The Gullah Geechee people use many phrases to communicate that are not heard within MAE or AAE varieties. Visitors to the Charleston area can hear some Gullah Geechee phrases during the Gullah tour with Alphonso Brown. Brown (2008) captures insights into Charleston's Gullah Geechee history, offering a guide that highlights significant sites and stories related to the Gullah Geechee people. Table 5.3 provides some common Gullah Geechee phrases used across the corridor (Berry, 2020; Brown, 2008; Lee, 2010).

Gullah Geechee people have common phrases and words associated with people, animals, lifestyles and traditions among many others. Table 5.4 summarizes some of these variations as they are currently used (Berry, 2020).

Table 5.3 Common phrases and words I

Gullah Geechee phrase	MAE gloss
Unrabble e mout'	Talked a lot
E long eye	He/she wants too much
Krak teet	To talk
Mek so?	Why?
Day clean	In the morning

Table 5.4 Common phrases and words II

Gullah Geechee phrases	MAE gloss
Bin ya or Been ya	Native Gullah Geechee; been here
Come ya	Non-native Gullah Geechee
Buckruh	Caucasian person
Churn or chillen	Children
Hunnah or Oona	You
Cudda	Turtle
Fush	Fish
Innit or inny	Right?
Yeddi	To hear
Dareckly	In a moment or soon
Up da winda	Put the window up
Beenga	Was going to

Implications for researchers

Weldon (2003) places Gullah within a broader 'African American linguistic continuum', arguing that Gullah is historically and linguistically significant to understanding the development of AAE and its dialectal variations. Social factors, such as class, education and regional differences, affect the linguistic continuum. Gullah is most commonly spoken among older generations and those living in more rural or isolated areas (Weldon, 2003). As the awareness and interest in studying and documenting the Gullah Geechee people, culture and language increases, researchers should be reminded of the in-group nature of the culture. Due to the historical context in which Gullah Geechee was created and continues to exist, non-Gullah Geechee scholars may find it difficult to identify individuals or families willing to self-identify or participate in research studies. Like Turner in 1949, spending time within the community to establish relationships and trust will be essential to conducting research within the Gullah Geechee community.

Gullah Geechee's self-identity is deeply rooted in a history of Geechee being used as a derogatory term. Those who speak the language are encouraged to codeswitch to MAE seeking economic and social mobility. However, modern generations of Gullah Geechee speakers are reenergizing the conversation, research and scholarship of Gullah Geechee. Therefore, future research should consider examining past, present and future Gullah Geechee identity and the impact that it may have on the existence of the language.

Unlike AAE, which has been thoroughly examined for decades, Gullah Geechee language within the field of speech-language pathology has not been extensively studied. Therefore, researchers should consider studies that provide normative data to provide data-driven normative resources for use in clinical practice.

Implications for practitioners

A lot has changed in the landscape of Gullah Geechee as people have migrated to the coastal regions for its warm temperatures and access to many beaches. As a result, Gullah Geechee communities have begun to shrink over time. The integration of schools in many Gullah Geechee-only communities has allowed access to education and different language varieties that were not always available to the Gullah Geechee people. This new access has had an impact on the density of the Gullah Geechee language that is heard throughout the corridor as seen through a gradual shift away from Gullah towards more standardized forms of MAE, including AAE and MAE, particularly among younger generations of Gullah speakers. This shift is partly due to increased contact with the mainland, changes in education and economic pressures. However, Weldon (2003) highlights efforts to preserve Gullah Geechee, particularly through cultural revitalization programs, educational initiatives and the documentation of the language.

When assessing Gullah Geechee speakers, clinicians should consider that many people who speak the language do not self-identify as Gullah Geechee. The lingering effect of the negative stereotypes associated with the Gullah Geechee language has left a mark on the families that reside along the corridor. Specifically, when asking caregivers to identify if their student speaks Gullah Geechee, the clinician may need to give some examples of the common phrases and grammatical structures used within the language to help the family recognize the language. An additional consideration is that even if the family does self-identify as Gullah Geechee, they may not want the name of the language placed in their formal educational records. Clinicians should be prepared to provide information to caregivers about how the identification of the child's complete linguistic profile and culture will support efforts to improve their communication skills over time. Furthermore, clinicians can explain to parents the professional perspective that being bilingual is considered a strength. They can emphasize that all languages, including Gullah Geechee, are to be respected and included. Additionally, clinicians should use assessments that have been normed with speakers of non-mainstream English when available (i.e. Diagnostic Evaluation of Language Variation (DELV_NR), Seymour *et al.*, 2005). However, given that Gullah Geechee speakers have not been included in the samples of existing norm-referenced assessments, clinicians should use criterion-referenced assessments, dynamic assessments and language samples as best practices for assessment. The use of the DELV-S screening tool may be useful in determining dialect density and risk for language impairment that can inform the need for further assessment measures (Seymour *et. al.*, 2003).

Beyond assessment, clinicians should use culturally relevant materials within clinical practice, including the use of books that represent the Gullah Geechee and African diaspora. Research has shown that students respond to culturally relevant education efforts. A unique aspect of the Gullah Geechee culture that may be observed if the clinician is working with children is that children are taught to not talk back to their elders; therefore, some children may be slower to respond to clinicians out of a demonstration of respect for the person that they view as an elder to them. Similarly, if a clinician is working with an adult client, they should recognize that older clients may bring their children with them to help assist in their understanding of the information that is being shared.

Conclusion

The Gullah Geechee language is a living testament to the blending of African and English linguistic traditions, shaped by the unique circumstances of slavery in the American South. The language's origins lie in the need for communication among enslaved Africans from various ethnic backgrounds and between Africans and English-speaking colonists. This blending process, combined with the isolation of the Gullah Geechee people in the coastal regions, helped create a distinctive Creole language that has preserved many African linguistic elements to this day.

References

Berry, J.R. and Oetting, J.B. (2017) Dialect variation of copula and auxiliary verb BE: African American English-speaking children with and without Gullah/Geechee Heritage. *Journal of Speech, Language, and Hearing Research: JSLHR* 60 (9), 2557–2568. https://doi.org/10.1044/2017_JSLHR-L-16-0120

Berry, J. (2020) *The Little Gullah Geechee Book: A Guide for the Come Ya.* J. Berry Collective.

Brown, A. (2008) *A Gullah Guide to Charleston: Walking through Black history.* The History Press.

Campbell, E.S. (1997) *Gullah Cultural Legacies: A Synopsis of Gullah Traditions, Customary Beliefs, Art Forms and Speech on Hilton Head Island and Vicinal Sea Islands in South Carolina and Georgia.* Gullah Heritage Society.

Campbell, E.S. (2020) *Gullah Cultural Legacies, Second Edition: A Synopsis of Gullah Traditions, Customary Beliefs, Artforms and Speech on Hilton Head Island and Vicinal Sea Islands in South Carolina and Georgia.* Gullah Heritage Society.

Campbell, T.E., Campbell, L.G. and Grant, E.W. (2019) *Gullah Days: Hilton Head Islanders before the Bridge 1861–1956.* Lydia Ingram Keith & Teal Enterprises.

Cooper, M. (2017) *Making Gullah: A History of Sapelo Island, Georgia's African American Community.* University of Georgia Press.

Crawford, E. (2020a) *Gullah Culture in America.* University of South Carolina Press.

Crawford, E. (2020b) *The Sound of Freedom and Protest in the South Carolina Sea Islands.* University of South Carolina Press.

Eltis, D. (2000) The transatlantic slave trade: A review of the evidence. *Social Science History* 24 (4), 557–579. https://doi.org/10.1017/S0145553200013065

Gullah Geechee Cultural Heritage Corridor Commission. (2012) *Gullah Geechee Cultural Heritage Corridor Management Plan*. Prepared and published by the National Park Service, Denver Service Center.

Hughes, C.E., Shaunessy, E.S., Brice, A.R., Ratliff, M.A. and McHatton, P.A. (2006) Code switching among bilingual and limited English proficient students: Possible indicators of giftedness. *Journal for the Education of the Gifted* 30 (1), 7–28.

International African American Museum (2025) See https://iaamuseum.org/about/

Jones-Jackson, P. (1987a) *Contemporary Gullah Speech: Some Persistent Linguistic Features*. University of Georgia Press.

Jones-Jackson, P. (1987b) *When Roots Die: Endangered Traditions on the Sea Islands*. University of Georgia Press.

Kuzyk, K.G., Friend, M. and Keown, L.J. (2020) Are there cognitive benefits of code-switching in bilingual children? A longitudinal study. *Developmental Science* 23 (6), e12947. https://doi.org/10.1111/desc.12947

Lee, M.A. (2010) *Krak Teet*. CreateSpace Independent Publishing Platform.

Lee, M.E. (2014) Shifting to the world Englishes paradigm by way of the translingual approach: Code-meshing as a necessary means of transforming composition pedagogy. *TESOL Journal* 5 (2), 312–329. https://doi.org/10.1002/tesj.121

Meggett, E. (2022) *Gullah Geechee Home Cooking: Recipes from the Matriarch of Edisto Island*. Abrams Books.

Mufwene, S.S. (1986) On the status of auxiliary verbs in Gullah. In M. Montgomery and P. Eckstein (eds) *The Emergence of Black English: Texts and Commentary* (pp. 243–263). University of Michigan Press.

Mufwene, S.S. (1997) How African is Gullah, and why? In S. Mufwene (ed.) *African-American English: Structure, History, and Use* (pp. 129–154). Routledge.

Mufwene, S.S. (2001) Morphology and syntax. In N.J. Smelser and P.B. Baltes (eds) *International Encyclopedia of the Social & Behavioral Sciences* (pp. 9823–9829). Elsevier.

National Archives. June 28, 2021. See https://www.archives.gov/research/african-americans/migrations/great-migration

Opala, J.A. (1987) *The Gullah: Rice, Slavery and the Sierra Leone-American Connection*. USIS.

Preservation Society of Charleston (2024) See https://www.preservationsociety.org/locations/gadsdens-wharf/.

Robinson, S.A. (2005) *Cooking the Gullah Way, Morning, Noon, and Night*. University of North Carolina Press.

Seymour, H.N., Roeper, T. and de Villiers, P.A. (2003) *Diagnostic Evaluation of Language Variation: Screening (DELV-S)*. Psychological Corporation.

Seymour, H.N., Roeper, T. and de Villiers, P.A. (2005) *Diagnostic Evaluation of Language Variation: Norm-referenced (DELV-NR)*. Psychological Corporation.

Smart-Grosvenor, V. (2011) *Vibration Cooking: Or, the Travel Notes of a Geechee Girl*. University of Georgia Press. (Original work published 1970).

Turner, L.D. (1949) *Africanisms in the Gullah Dialect*. Arno Press. (Original work published 1949)

US Census Bureau (2023) https://www.census.gov/newsroom/press-releases/2023/population-trends-return-to-pre-pandemic

Wade-Lewis, M. (2007) *Lorenzo Dow Turner: Father of Gullah Studies*. University of South Carolina Press.

Weldon, T.L. (1998a) Copula variability in Gullah. In S. Mufwene, J. Rickford, G. Bailey and J. Baugh (eds) *African–American English: Structure, History, and Use* (pp. 191–210). Routledge.

Weldon, T.L. (1998b) Gullah phonology. In S. Mufwene, J. Rickford, G. Bailey and J. Baugh (eds) *African-American English: Structure, History, and Use* (pp. 35–51). Routledge.

Weldon, T.L. (2003) The place of Gullah in the African American linguistic continuum. In S.J. Nagle and S.L. Sanders (eds) *English in the Southern United States* (pp. 21–48). Cambridge University Press.

Winford, D. (1992) The BEV/Creole connection revisited. *Language Variation and Change* 4, 311–357.

Wolfram, W. (1973) [Review of *Black English: Its History and Usage in the United States*, by J.L. Dillard]. *Language* 49 (3), 670–679. https://doi.org/10.2307/412356

Young, V.A. (2009) "Nah, We Straight": An argument against code switching. *JAC* 29 (1–2), 49–76. https://www.jstor.org/stable/20866886

Young, V.A., Barrett, R., Young-Rivera, Y. and Lovejoy, K.B. (2014) *Other People's English: Code-Meshing, Code-Switching, and African American Literacy*. Teachers College Press.

6 Jamaican Creole in Canada

Shamara A. Peart and Karla N. Washington

Introduction

Context and culture

Jamaican culture in Canada and Black Canadian English are discussed in this chapter. In doing so, this chapter aims to educate researchers and practitioners on Jamaican Creole (i.e. Patwa or JamC) in Canadian diaspora populations. Some speakers also use Patois, although all three terms are interchangeable. The Black community is not a monolith but a group of people who speak languages unique to their ancestry. The content of this chapter offers a cross-linguistic examination of JamC use in Canada; specifically, the place of the language in the Greater Toronto Area and the role it plays in conversations about Canadian English (CanE). The history and cultural context of JamC, the grammar and clinical implications are discussed. The goal is to broaden the field of research about how JamC has evolved into Toronto's metropolitan vocabulary and ensure that there are culturally responsive practices and analyses unique to JamC moving forward. This will limit the number of misdiagnoses that Jamaican Canadian speakers encounter, since linguistic variation has been viewed as speech disorders or educational deficits.

Jamaican heritage has played a pivotal role in the multicultural population of Toronto since the immigration of many to the city in the 1980s; today, the country remains the largest source of Caribbean immigrants to Canada, followed closely by occupants from Haiti, Trinidad and Tobago, and Cuba (Statistics Canada, 2022). In 2022, the Government of Canada reported that 249,070 Canadians had Jamaican ancestry (Statistics Canada, 2022). Among these, over 80% of Jamaican Canadians were living in Ontario (Statistics Canada, 2022). Today, the total population is expected to be higher. Jamaican Creole is an informal oral language, so it is most often used in social or familial settings. Recent studies have found that North American teachers are not trained to deal with the linguistic structures of English-based creoles, since they misplace children who speak English varieties in English as a Second Language classes (Clachar, 2005). There are limited studies that highlight the complexity of JamC amidst screening tools such as the Intelligibility in Context Scale (ICS; McLeod *et al.*, 2012a) and ICS-Jamaican Creole (ICS-JC; McLeod *et al.*, 2012b). The distinction between those in Black populations of Jamaican ancestry with poor speech intelligibility and those who simply speak differently than Canada's White monolingual majority is restricted (León *et al.*, 2023).

A pidgin is created when two distinct languages interact for the first time. The result is a simplified communication system that borrows vocabulary from both languages; however, the dominant group contributes more words (Decamp, 1977). There are a few methods to determine whether a pidgin has evolved into a creole. Two examples are whether the language has native speakers (Decamp, 1977), or whether it has its own grammatical systems (Tucker & Murphy, 2023). JamC has British English as its lexifier, with a combination of borrowed words from Twi and Ewe, as well as Spanish and Portuguese (Cassidy & Page, 2002; Tucker & Murphy, 2023) among others. As such, there is parentage across English and West African languages. This crossover was the result of slaves who were brought to Jamaica. They created a *lingua franca* to communicate when living and working alongside others from different countries. Over many generations, their pidgin evolved into a complex creole. Today, the language is subjected to regional differences across the island and in its larger diaspora populations abroad, such as in Canada, the UK, the United States and Costa Rica (MFAFT – Jamaica, n.d.).

Cross-linguistic influence is characterized by transformations across various levels, including phonology, lexicon, morphosyntax and pragmatics (Malcolm, 2021). While the previous sociolinguistic factors created JamC, currently the language's livelihood relies on the motivation and attitudes of its speakers worldwide. There is growing research about Patwa's influence on international English varieties, as many Jamaicans understand both an L1 (JamC) and an L2 (an English variety). Some consider JamC and Jamaican English as part of the same language continuum (Bailey, 1966), while others view the languages as part of separate language systems (Holm, 1988; Winford, 1988). Diaspora populations with a different dialect (in this case, CanE) are not excluded from cross-linguistic changes either. The variability between how JamC and Canadian English manifests in mesolectal speakers as well as whether this difference is something that researchers and practitioners should consider moving forward is unclear.

Jamaican Creole Grammar

Vowels and consonants

Cassidy LePage and David Decamp were some of the first linguists to propose that creoles operate on a continuum in the Caribbean (Bickerton, 1973). LePage initially proposed the Cassidy System to document a phonemic/written version of the language. The system has since been updated by the University of the West Indies into the Cassidy-Jamaican Language Unit writing system (Farquharson, 2013). The continuum has been applied to other creoles in the Caribbean, being studied by linguists such as Beryl Bailey, Mervyn Alleyne and Richard Allsopp. Creolists have also expanded the term to 'post-creole continuum' to include intermediate varieties (Bickerton, 1975). Although there is ongoing research about JamC as the basilect and Jamaican English as the corresponding acrolect, scholarship is working to determine which traits most affect intermediate varieties. While this paper focuses on a mesolect, many scholars find it important to distinguish whether their work focuses on acrolectal, mesolectal or basilectal varieties due to phonological differences such as rhoticity (Beckford-Wassink, 1999; Harry, 2006; Irvine, 2004).

Otelemate Harry (2006) described JamC as having 12 vowel phonemes: 5 short vowels, 3 long vowels and 4 diphthongs (see Table 6.1). While the number of complex vowels and diphthongs varies based on vowel harmony (peripheral and back), a system containing at least 12 vowels is widely accepted. One proposed reason for the discrepancy is that JamC seems to follow the phonological structures of its substrate languages while loosely following the grammatical structure of its signifier. Vowel quality is used to distinguish at least some vowels, and down gliding occurs in /e:/ and /o:/ sounds (Beckford-Wassink, 2001). Harry notes that in JamC, back harmony is restricted to high vowels since primarily sequences of back vowels can be heard (e.g. /i/, /u:/ and /a:/) (2006).

Devonish and Harry (2004) compared the phonology of Patwa and Jamaican English, acknowledging that JamC's diphthongs cover a range of sounds of the allophone /a/; in their study, the range the diphthongs cover includes: /ia/ covers [iɛ] ~ [ie] ~ [ia] (e.g. *face*, *near* and *square* become [fies], [niɛr] and [skwiɛr]), /ua/ covers [uo] ~ [ua] (e.g. *goat* and *force* become [guot] and [fuos]), the sound of /ai/ is still [ai] (e.g. *price* sounds like [p^hrais]), and /au/ covers [aʊ] ~ [θʊ] (e.g. *mouth* is pronounced [maut]) (2004: 260). One resource that linguists and speech-language researchers have returned to in order to help determine which sounds dialects use is vowel length (Coy & Watson, 2020). León *et al.* (2023) conducted a cross-sectional study to examine if there are differences in acoustic duration between bilingual preschoolers and adults. Collected in both Kingston, Jamaica and New York City, the study compared audio

Table 6.1 Vowel inventory of Jamaican Creole

Simple vowels	/ɪ,u,e,o,a/
Long vowels	/i:, u:, a:/
Diphthongs	/ɪa, ai, ua, au/

Adapted from source: Harry, 2006: 127–128.

recordings from both age groups so that researchers could determine voice onset time (VOT), vowel duration, whole-word duration and the proportion of vowel to whole-word duration. Moreover, they questioned whether personal factors (i.e. age, sex, percentage of language use) played a role in linguistic differences. The results indicated that the preschoolers were in the process of developing speech-motor skills as their durational patterns differed from the adults (León *et al.*, 2023). However, VOT, vowel duration and whole-word duration were similar across JamC and US English speakers (León *et al.*, 2023). The findings indicate that there are similar acoustic characteristics between JamC and English, a result that could be due to the communities circulating use of both languages. While US English draws on duration and vowel quality equally, speech sounds in JamC are differentiated further through vowel quality (high front, low and high back) and harmony. Findings such as these strengthen the field of research on JamC in its diaspora populations and are a stepping stone to conversations about Canada's Jamaican population since Canadian English has consistent phonology with US English.

The vowel system of CanE has phonemes to represent short and long vowels, in addition to digraphs and r-controlled sounds. One prominent feature is the Canadian Vowel shift, where the pronunciation of the front vowels /ɪ/ (kit), /ɛ/ (dress), /æ/ (trap) is changing. Later, Roeder and Jarmasz (2010) conducted a study with Toronto natives that confirmed the lowering of /ɪ/, /ɛ/, /æ/ but showed little retraction. Ongoing studies debate the details of which vowels are shifting and in what direction, as the claims appear contradictory at times. Whether /ɪ/ is said to be moving at all, /ɛ/ is moving down or inward (or on occasion, both), and /æ/ is moving down and back, sound changes are occurring in CanE that have regional differences (Sadlier-Brown & Tamminga, 2008). As a result, the Canadian Vowel shift is one of the most widely described phonetic features of Canadian English (Boberg, 2008; Hoffman, 2010). Another similarity between CanE and JamC lies in the /a/ allophones. In CanE, this sound change occurs when [a], in a low front position, is pronounced as [ɒ], a low back rounded vowel (Hall-Lew, 2009). This vowel can take on a variety of forms depending on the speakers, even changing from [ɑ] to [ɔ] (Bigham, 2010). JamC has already begun to see this. Beckford-Wassink's (2001) study only had one vowel pair with complete spectral and temporal overlap for several Jamaican speakers, /a/ and /ɔ/. This data suggests that the phonemes are on their way to a similar merger. Patwa and CanE overlap regarding vowel quality and mergers.

A few other CanE features include Canadian raising, the long vowel /e/ and /o/ being pronounced with tense, and [aʊ] being pronounced in a relatively back position (Boberg, 2008). Charles Boberg worked on *The Atlas of North American English* in 2006, the first national view of CanE phonetics that identified the countries' broad sound changes (2008). Updated data suggests that the primary dialect divisions in Canada exist at the phonetic level between six regions: the West, Ontario, Quebec, the Maritimes, Newfoundland and a secondary division in 'the West' between British Columbia and the Prairies (Boberg, 2008). He continued this study and identified several features that further established Canadian speech into regional divisions. The inhabitants of Toronto are applicable to three of them. The first is the Canadian Shift; the second is the merger of /e/ and /æ/ before /r/ (e.g. *marry* and *merry*); and the last is the allophonic distribution of /æ/ (Boberg, 2008). Boberg acknowledges the limitations of his study, noting that sound changes in North American English involve consonants (-r), (-ng), (-t), (-d), (th), whereas regional variation involves vocalic variables (Boberg, 2008).

One process that relates to adjacent consonants in CanE is Canadian raising, where the starting sound of /aʊ/ and /aɪ/ is raised before voiceless consonants; another is the pronunciation of /t/, where the speech sound gets pronounced as a glottal stop (Boberg, 2008). Similarly, this feature is found in the Caribbean (Schneider, 2008). CanE has a surplus of consonants, such as /θ/ and /ð/. JamC, however, has fewer consonant clusters and will often use replacements. The use of /d/ for the voiced interdental fricative (e.g. /ðɪs/ as [dɪs]) and /t/ for the voiceless interdental fricative (e.g. /tiθ/ as [tit]) has long been recognized as a feature of JamC speech production in adults and in children and has remained in more recent observations (Harry, 2006; Washington *et al.*, 2017, 2023). This is because dental fricatives are not an inherent feature of this language. As a result, voiced and voiceless dental fricatives are replaced. For example, *think* may become [tɪŋk] or *this* will become [dɪs]. Devonish and Harry (2004) noted in their study that some phonological differences in JamC can be classified according to Western and Eastern varieties. One speech difference is that Eastern varieties have an absence of the phoneme /h/, whereas the Western variety doesn't since it classifies it differently (Harry, 2006). In the Eastern varieties, the [h] sound still appears in cases of hypercorrection.

JamC has 21 consonant phonemes as indicated in recent studies (Devonish & Harry, 2004; Harry, 2006; Washington *et al.*, 2025). It's a non-rhotic variety, although other methods of speech on the continuum (such as Jamaican English) contain at least r-coloring (Farquharson, 2013). There is ongoing debate about whether JamC contains consonant phonemes that aren't also in English's inventory (see Table 6.2). Word-final consonant clusters (e.g. schwa, or [ə]) are simplified and often dropped from JamC (Gooden, 2023; Patrick, 1999). The voiced stops /b/, /d/ and /g/ are occasionally spoken as their implosives /ɓ/, /ɗ/ and /ɠ/ based on word-initial position in consonantal allophones (Farquharson, 2013). The frequency of these changes is similar to that of voiceless stops /p/ and /k/ and even /t/, where the aspirated [p^h], [k^h] and [t^h] occur in the onset of prominent syllables (Devonish & Harry, 2004). Otherwise, the unaspirated [p], [k] and [t] are produced elsewhere (Devonish & Harry, 2004).

Table 6.2 The phonemic consonants of Jamaican Creole

	Bilabial	Labio-dental	Alveolar	Post-alveolar	Palatal	Velar	Glottal	Labial-velar
Nasal	m		n			ŋ		
Plosive	p b		t d			k g		
Affricate				ʧ ʤ				
Fricative		f v	s z	ʃ			(h)	
Approximant			ɹ		j			w
Lateral approximant			l					

Source: Harry, 2006: 126.

Grammar, Syntax and Tenses

Syntax can be both systematic and sporadic when speaking any language.

(Bailey, 1966)

Deuber (2009) as cited in Gooden's article (2023) lists past marking, agreement marking on verbs, copula forms, main verb negation, noun morphology, pronoun morphology and direct *wh-* questions as morphosyntactic variables that cover the most important Creole features. The following observations are explored below. Pre-verbal variables and marking distinguishes time (Durrleman-Tame, 2008). The tense system in JamC is limited (Bailey, 1966), and there is no subject-verb agreement. Conversely, CanE marks the past and present tense but uses the present or progressive forms of the verb with adverbs like *tomorrow* to indicate the future. JamC uses pre-verbal particles such as 'done' to indicate the past (e.g. *Mi done talk* vs *I'm finished speaking)* or 'a' for the present continuous tense (e.g. *Mi a eat dinner* vs *I am eating dinner*) (Durrleman-Tame, 2008; Gooden, 2023). Further, 'a' will go before an uninflected verb (e.g. *She a run* vs *She is running)*, or in some cases, a null copula is used (e.g. *Mi tired* vs *I am tired*) (Gooden, 2023). Copula use is complex and variable in JamC. Scholars such as John R. Rickford have begun to study the parallels between JamC and other English varieties, particularly African American Vernacular English (AAVE). In a 1996 study, Rickford replicated low zero copula percentages for a following noun phrase or locative verb, and a high zero copula percentage for following adjectives. However, the differences were also made clear when the subject and tense did not operate the same in JamC as AAVE, nor did JamC prioritize Person (despite it being crucial to AAVE's copula use) (Rickford, 1996).

Next, differences between CanE and JamC appear in negation, pronouns and nouns. Negation in CanE is indicated through auxiliary verbs and the word 'not'. Meanwhile, in JamC, markers are used once again. *No*, *nuh*, *neva* and *duon* are employed (e.g. *Mi nuh know* vs *I don't know*) (Karem *et al.*, 2021). Personal pronouns and nouns do not have a case system, nor is there a distinction of sex in third-person pronouns (Bailey, 1966). This is often due to *dem* being used to express the plural form, added as a marker after the noun (e.g. *Di gyal dem pretty, enuh* vs *The girls are pretty, you know?*). In contrast, English nouns need either a singular form with an article (e.g. *Over there is the chair*) or a plural form without an article (e.g. *Over there are chairs*) (Bailey, 1966).

Wh- questions and focus constructions are examined by Joseph T. Farquharson. In the first of his survey's examples, the question word may be preceded by the focus marker /a/ (1). Based on whether objects or adjuncts are the focused element, speakers will move the marker (2) or for predicates, move it and then repeat it (3). Declarative sentences use rising intonation to transform them into yes-no questions (4), (5).

(1) *A wen yu a go to de shop?*
'When are you going to the grocery store?'
(2) *A di man Piita biit op kaaz im iizi a beks.*
'Peter beat up the man because he is easily irritated'.
(3) *A biit Piita biit op di man kaaz im iizi a beks.*
'Peter beat up the man because he's easily irritated'.
(4) *Amy gaan a wok.*
'Amy has gone to work'.
(5) *Amy gaan a wok?*
'Has Amy gone to work?'

Taryn Malcolm conducted a study to investigate the morphosyntactic structures of bilingual JamC and Jamaican English speakers who live in Jamaica and the United States. The evidence indicated that there was bidirectional influence in the verb tense marking, subject-verb agreements and copula use of the participants (Malcolm, 2021). L2 grammatical and semantic differences were clear examples of L1's influence, such as when a zero-marked verb was used, e.g. saying *Him wash him hands* instead of *He washed his hands* (Malcolm, 2021: 57). This is consistent with the belief that mesolectal speakers use a mixture of grammar from both languages. Vivian Cook's theory of multicompetence (2003) is applicable here, where bilingual speakers' languages begin to influence one another as soon as L2 acquisition begins. Regarding other sociolinguistic factors, Peter Patrick (1995) as cited in Mair (2002) recognizes that for Jamaicans, speaking English in certain contexts results in others viewing the speaker as snobbish or uptight. Social value among Jamaicans is awarded when speakers have linguistic range, where they can comfortably use the basilect and at least one other English variety (Mair, 2002). In this way, multilingual Black Canadians (whether Jamaican or otherwise) are set up to undergo cross-linguistic interactions which will alter their speech patterns.

Cross-linguistic influence

It's important to consider how regional and social variation affects Canada's linguistic structure. In Ontario, JamC's linguistic practices are increasingly being recognized as a means of Black Canadian speech and being adopted by other Black speakers (Baxter & Peters, 2011; Hinrichs, 2014). As a result, JamC is being used by second-generation Torontonians as a means of solidifying racial groups as opposed to an ethnic/cultural distinction. One prominent area where this is happening is among young adolescents who live within the Greater Toronto Area (GTA). Derek Denis, a Linguistics Professor at the University of Toronto Mississauga, oversaw research about dialect and linguistic varieties within the GTA. His team concluded that teens in Brampton, Ontario, a region of the GTA, had their own way of speaking, one that he referred to as Multicultural Toronto English (MTE). The speech was most apparent in immigrant youth communities who borrowed words from their heritage languages. Speakers in Toronto use these borrowings alongside local slang to create new phrases. Denis *et al.* (2023) suggested that the language of GTA adolescents (including their dialects and borrowed terms) may act as a means of linguistic resistance.

While this may be the case, it's again important to note that Toronto's Black and immigrant community is not a monolith. This linguistic difference is also a reflection of the individuals who are establishing their identities while living in a diaspora. As previously mentioned, Toronto's culture is largely influenced by its JamC-speaking population. Non-speakers of the language have adopted terms such as *wagwaan* and *ahlie*, indicating how pervasive JamC vocabulary has become. Additional words that are popular in Toronto slang with an origin in JamC include *bare*, *dutty* and *vex*. This is growing evidence of how Canadian Black English draws on Caribbean linguistics, as Toronto's Jamaican population regularly interacts with residents from other diasporas. Somali and Arabic are two linguistic communities whose word borrowings have also been added to the cities' vocabulary. In this way, language exchange is fluid and is regularly adopted by Torontonians. By using a different means of communication from their parents, Torontonians are carving out a space in the city for their hybridized identities. Both in CanE and JamC, speakers exercise their cultural agency by changing linguistic patterns. This act is working to distinguish Jamaican diaspora populations from one another while changing the landscape of contemporary Canadian English.

Laura Baxter and Jacqueline Peters (2011) were curious about this evolution, resulting in a conference paper titled 'Black English in

Toronto: A New Dialect?'. Black speakers from non-Jamaican backgrounds were found to have adopted Toronto's Jamaican-influenced speech. Jamaicans, Somalis and other West Indian participants were interviewed by the duo. Baxter and Peters (2011) found that while the deletion of word-final consonant clusters occurs in English varieties worldwide, there is still local variation between ethnic populations in the GTA. In Black neighborhoods such as Jane and Finch, those who regularly encountered other Black residents had affected speech. Within this ethnic enclave, instances of t/d deletion occurred 51% of the time (Baxter & Peters, 2011). Opposingly, non-enclave speakers had a t/d deletion rate only 15% of the time (Baxter & Peters, 2011). Although there were differences in frequency, the authors noted that both groups had a similar pattern in their overall results and chose to group them together for the purpose of further analysis.

Baxter and Peters (2011) compared the t/d deletion of second-generation Black Torontonians to second-generation Irish, Italian and Chinese populations as studied by Hoffman and Walker in their 2010 study, 'Ethnolects and the City: Ethnic Orientation and Linguistic Variation in Toronto English'. Black Torontonians had a higher rate of deletion in preceding fricatives and stops. However, the lowest rate of t/d deletion for the other ethnicities was in the preceding nasals. Black Torontonians do not share the same linguistic assimilation as the other ethnicities presented in the study. Instead, the results resembled a 1999 study by Peter Patrick which referred to mesolectal JamC. For Jamaicans who speak Patwa, fricatives and stops favored t/d deletion, whereas nasals and laterals disfavored it. This reinforces the observation that in the current linguistic context in Canada, the Black diaspora population in Toronto uses features of JamC as both a heritage language and a means of cultural agency. For researchers and practitioners to accurately treat their clients, it is essential they have a solid understanding of the language's grammar and its speakers' attitudes.

Clinical Implications for Researchers

By understanding JamC's grammatical features, researchers can validate the assessment tools that they use in clinical practice. Washington and colleagues (León *et al.*, 2021; Washington *et al.*, 2017, 2023) conducted studies with the ICS and created the ICS-JC to confirm whether these tools were a functional measure of speech for Jamaican children with a suspected speech sound disorder. By validating that the resource could be used for bilingual children and their parents, the tool's use was extended beyond its intended purpose, and its applicability broadened (Washington *et al.*, 2023). Reviewing studies like these and compiling data ensures that the resources available are reliable. By updating assessment tools and regularly reviewing findings, JamC speakers with speech impediments can receive adequate care. Further, researchers can develop specific strategies to target the linguistic needs of Canada's Jamaican population, such as programs focused on interdental fricatives. By doing so, they improve therapeutic outcomes and modernize intervention procedures. Researchers also play a significant role in establishing normative data for bilingual speakers. Caesar and Kohler (2007) surveyed SLPs in the United States and found that many relied on formal standardized practices to assess bilingual children, despite there being evidence that this was inadequate. JamC bilingual children with speech disorders are underrepresented in studies and may then be subjected to bias. By establishing normative data for the Creole speakers, future policies can be designed that keep this group in mind (Washington *et al.*, 2023).

In addition to modernizing tools, linguistically relevant research can be shared with other fields (e.g. social science, neurobiology, etc.) since secondary information may be revealed during these studies. A few examples include information about the neural pathways of bilinguals or the functional communication abilities of JamC individuals with acquired communication disorders. Additionally, social determinants benefit from an empirically supported basis, so evidence can be used to make broader statements about patterns in language or in a specific community. Research exists already that recognizes how national environments adapt an immigrant's speech patterns (Dereck-Martins Akachukwu, 2018). There is evidence here to support the belief that JamC speakers share similar linguistic traits with those in their home country. In due time, researchers can even expand their work to compare what specific patterns affect the diaspora internationally. The field of World English is constantly looking to identify linguistic patterns that arise between diaspora populations.

Academics interested in language revitalization projects can collaborate with The University of West Indies or the Centre for Reparation Research to strengthen efforts that preserve Kromanti or JamC. Kromanti is a minority language spoken by the elderly Maroons of Moore Town (Jackson, 2022). The World Directory of Minorities and Indigenous Peoples (WDMIP) recognizes the Maroons of Jamaica as Indigenous Peoples (Shepherd, 2022). Although still being used, the movement of JamC varieties away from the basilect and towards the acrolect could lead to decreolization (Holm, 2000). By positioning JamC against its substrate languages, researchers can better document minority languages and work to limit cultural loss. Whether Kromanti or JamC, speakers must use the language regularly to keep it alive and pass aspects along to diaspora populations. Otherwise, descendants lose the cultural knowledge that each language carries. Medicinal knowledge, local ecological or geographical knowledge, and language behaviors have the capacity to be disrupted. When one considers how Canadian English is prioritized in schools and workplaces, as well as how closely some JamC's varieties resemble the acrolect, it's evident that in some way a change is occurring. Mufwene (2020) notes that since grammar changes are not monolithic, people must work to incorporate mesolectal varieties into their day-to-day lives to preserve it. This action would not just be for cultural agency but as a means of language planning. If speakers are to continue using their language, decisions must be made that incorporate the mesolectal variety into schools and public administration (Mufwene, 2020), and in the case of this chapter, into language assessment tools. For these reasons, the theory of decreolization and the creole continuum are currently being debated in the field (Jourdan, 2021).

Clinical Implications for Practitioners

By recognizing the linguistic features of JamC, SLPs can better consider which speech attributes are unique to the child's background and which tools best draw on these skill sets (León *et al.*, 2023). Speakers can be reached through early intervention programs with cross-lexical tasks, thereby lowering the chance of misdiagnosis. To give proper diagnoses to JamC speakers, there needs to be a basic level of understanding of the language (Washington *et al.*, 2023). Additionally, the speaker's attitude about JamC is relevant as well since speakers are encouraged to speak the acrolect in the workplace both in Jamaica and abroad (Mufwene, 2020). SLPs are steadily creating resources to describe JamC's linguistic nuances, such as the Intelligibility in Context Scale – Jamaican Creole (ICS-JC; McLeod *et al.*, 2012b). This allows physicians to become familiar with how their patients adjust their communication styles to chat with friends or family members. In doing so, they can better understand whom they are trying to help. Further, the effect of speech therapists extends not just through families but into schools, where students can be assessed to determine whether they are facing literacy, communication or speech challenges (Halldorson *et al.*, 2020).

When practitioners create lexical tasks/dialect surveys that first consider a speaker's autonomy, patients can feel at ease when voicing their concerns. Practitioners can improve clinician-patient relationships by effectively discussing their expectations for the appointment. This communication allows the patient or parents of the patient to gain a stronger understanding of the testing process. This will limit the client's need to expend additional energy if they are code-switching when seeking care. Often, code-switching is key to navigating Western spaces for diaspora populations (Washington *et al.*, 2023). Clinicians build stronger relationships by building trust with children and adults alike, which can encourage a willingness for treatment plans (McLeod *et al.*, 2017). Family-based therapy approaches allow professionals to better explore treatment goals, especially when they are 'in the language of the family and expressed in terms of their view of the problem' (Andrews &

Andrews, 1986: 362). This interactive collaboration allows for trust to be maintained. Practitioners also strengthen their procedures by designing cross-cultural assessments that encourage collaboration with other experts (e.g. language specialists, interpreters, etc.).

Speech therapists continue their clinical learning and professional development by engaging with Creoles and their varieties. Easton and Verdon (2021) examined whether linguistic bias still contributes to the diagnoses of nonstandard dialect speakers of Australian English. Some Australian SLPs made the call to document any variation from the standardized language as an error, despite a few recognizing certain linguistic features as those from Aboriginal Australian English or other local varieties (Easton & Verdon, 2021). If this is the case for a country considered to be a part of the Global North, it's crucial to question how SLPs may misconstrue varieties that are born out of the Global South. One benefit of Easton and Verdon's (2021) study was that it pointed out the benefits of continued learning. Those with more clinical experience and those who had received professional development were less likely to document that a nonstandard dialect speaker was undergoing speech difficulty.

With this awareness, SLPs can better determine which speech production patterns in JamC speakers are reflective of differences versus disorders. SLPs gain knowledge about new languages and can feel confident about their decisions by expanding their learning with validated assessment tools and additional resources. As immigration rates grow in Canada, replication studies are necessary to identify where non-standard varieties sit on the post-Creole continuum. Equally, technological advancements are continuously being made, so culturally competent SLPs are key to combating bias (Easton & Verdon, 2021; McLeod *et al.*, 2023). The increasing demand for artificial intelligence-powered tools makes it crucial that practitioners do what they can to limit linguistic bias from settling further into their field. Already, tele-diagnosis and telemonitoring are more frequent, speech and language data are being used by computer scientists for natural language processing, and there are budding conversations about the use of AI to update augmentative and alternative communication (AAC) methods.

Conclusion

The purpose of this chapter was to explore language patterns in JamC and CanE speakers as a means of determining the language's influence in Canada. By examining this topic, researchers and practitioners can reflect on how Jamaican Canadian populations develop their speech patterns. The study of JamC in diaspora populations is steadily rising. Its contributions to England's Multicultural London English (MLE) or Costa Rica's Limonese Creole offer researchers a look at how sociocultural influences contribute to the way these populations communicate.

For more information about MLE, Cheshire *et al.* (2011) go in depth about the recreolized variety used in England in 'Contact, the Feature Pool and the Speech Community: The Emergence of Multicultural London English'. Meanwhile, Robert Bell's (2019) 'Limón Patwa: A Perceptual Study to Measure Language Attitudes Toward Speakers of Patwa in Costa Rica' highlights how negative attitudes towards the speakers (and other political factors) contribute to a loss of the language.

Jamaican Creole speakers do not have much established research regarding which shared patterns occur internationally, so this is one direction that future researchers can work towards. In reviewing both Canada and Jamaica's prominent linguistic features, SLPs can consider how diaspora populations draw on both racial and linguistic means to establish their identities in their respective nations. Linguists can use this review to expand discussions about the post-Creole continuum as they continue to question which pole Toronto's diaspora populations veer closer to. One limitation of this review is the amount of existing literature that is primarily focused on JamC's effect in Toronto's CanE populations. Thankfully, researchers continue to add to the amount of existing JamC studies by validating their assessment tools. This ensures that there are culturally responsive practices moving forward. Practitioners therefore have an accessible knowledge base with which they can continue their learning. In addition to creating accurate assessments that recognize JamC as a heritage language, increasing literature is of great importance to validating its speakers' cultural identities.

References

Andrews, J. and Andrews, M. (1986) A family-based systemic model for speech-language services. *Seminars in Speech and Language* 7 (4), 359–365. https://doi.org/10.1055/s-0028-1085234

Bailey, B.L. (1966) *Jamaican Creole Syntax*. Cambridge University Press.

Baxter, L. and Peters, J. (2011) 'Black English in Toronto: A new dialect?'. *Proccedings of Methods in Dialectology XIV*, Canada, Academia Edu. https://www.academia.edu/2966441/Black_English_in_Toronto_A_New_Dialect?source=swp_share

Beckford-Wassink, A. (1999) A sociophonetic analysis of Jamaican vowels. Doctoral dissertation, The University of Michigan. University of Michigan's Library.

Beckford-Wassink, A. (2001) Theme and variation in Jamaican vowels. *Language Variation and Change* 13 (2), 135–159. https://doi/.org/10.1017/S0954394501132023

Bell, R. (2019) Limón Patwa: A perceptual study to measure language attitudes toward speakers of Patwa in Costa Rica. PhD dissertation, University of Kentucky. University of Kentucky's Institutional Repository. https://doi.org/10.13023/etd.2019.352

Bickerton, D. (1973) The nature of a creole continuum. *Language* 49 (3), 640–669. *JSTOR*. https://doi.org/10.2307/412355

Bickerton, D. (1975) *Dynamics of a Creole System*. Cambridge University Press.

Bigham, D.S. (2010) Correlation of the low-back vowel merger and trap-retraction. University of Pennsylvania Working Papers in Linguistics. *Proceedings of New Ways of Analyzing Variation*, USA 15 (2). https://stanford.edu/class/linguist159/restricted/readings/Bigham2010

Boberg, C. (2008) Regional phonetic differentiation in Standard Canadian English. *Journal of English Linguistics* 36 (2), 129–154. https://doi.org/10.1177/0075424208316648

Caesar, L.G. and Kohler, P.D. (2007) The state of school-based bilingual assessment: Actual practice versus recommended guidelines. *Language, Speech, and Hearing Services in Schools* 38 (3), 190–200. https://doi.org/10.1044/0161-1461(2007/020)

Cassidy, F.G. and Page, R.B.L. (2002) *Dictionary of Jamaican English*. University of the West Indies Press.

Cheshire, J., Kerswill, P., Fox, S. and Torgersen, E. (2011) Contact, the feature pool and the speech community: The emergence of Multicultural London English. *Journal of Sociolinguistics* 15 (2), 151–196. https://doi.org/10.1111/j.1467-9841.2011.00478.x

Clachar, A. (2005) Creole English speakers' treatment of tense-aspect morphology in English interlanguage written discourse. *Language Learning* 55 (2), 275–334. https://doi.org/10.1111/j.0023-8333.2005.00305.x

Cook, V. (2003) Chapter 1. Introduction: The changing L1 in the L2 user's mind. In V. Cook (ed.) *Effects of the Second Language on the First* (pp. 1–18). Multilingual Matters.

Coy, A. and Watson, S. (2020) Acoustic similarity of inner and outer circle varieties of child-produced English vowels. *Journal of Speech Language and Hearing Research* 63 (3), 722–737. https://doi.org/10.1044/2019_JSLHR-19-00179

Decamp, D. (1977) The development of pidgin and creole studies. In A. Valdman (ed.) *Pidgin and Creole Linguistics*. Indiana University Press.

Denis, D., Elango, V., Nor Kamal N.S., Prashar, S. and Velasco, M. (2023) Exploring the vowel space of Multicultural Toronto English. *Journal of English Linguistics, Sage Journals* 51 (1), 30–65. https://doi.org/10.1177/00754242221145164

Dereck-Martins Akachukwu, O. (2018) Language adaptability in immigrant situations. *Igwebuike: An African Journal of Arts and Humanities* 4 (3), 42–59. https://ezenwaohaetorc.org/journals/index.php/IJAH/article/view/675/639

Deuber, D. (2009) 'The English we speaking': Morphological and syntactic variation in educated Jamaican speech. *Journal of Pidgin and Creole Languages* 24 (1), 1–52. https://doi.org/10.1075/jpcl.24.1.02deu

Devonish, H. and Harry, O. (2004) Jamaican Creole and Jamaican English: Phonology. In B. Kortmann and E. Schneider (eds) *A Handbook of Varieties of English: A Multimedia Reference Tool. Volume 1: Phonology. Volume 2: Morphology and Syntax* (pp. 450–480). De Gruyter Mouton.

Durrleman-Tame, S. (2008) *The Syntax of Jamaican Creole*. John Benjamins Publishing Company.

Easton, C. and Verdon, S. (2021) The influence of linguistic bias upon speech-language pathologists' attitudes toward clinical scenarios involving nonstandard dialects of English. *American Journal of Speech-Language Pathology* 30 (5), 1973–1989. https://doi.org/10.1044/2021_AJSLP-20-00382

Farquharson, J.T. (2013) Survey chapter: Jamaican. In S.M. Michaelis, P. Maurer, M. Haspelmath and M. Huber (eds) *The Survey of Pidgin and Creole Languages, Volume 1: English-based and Dutch-based Languages* (pp. 81–91). Oxford University Press.

Gooden, A. (2023) The perception of mixed utterances by Jamaican bilinguals. Doctoral dissertation, York University. York University's Library.

Halldorson, S., Dowling, S., Kelly, D., Lemieux, G., Miller, A., Ukrainetz, T. and Speech-Language and Audiology Canada (2020) SAC position paper on speech-language pathology service delivery models in schools. In *Speech-Language and Audiology Canada*. See https://www.sac-oac.ca/wp-content/uploads/2023/02/SAC-OAC_S-LP_In_Schools_Delivery_Models_EN_V1.pdf

Hall-Lew, L. (2009) Ethnicity and sound change in San Francisco English. In I. Kwon, H. Pritchett and J.Spence (eds) *Proceedings of Berkeley Linguistics Society* (pp. 111–122). Sheridan Books. https://linguistics.berkeley.edu/bls/previous_proceedings/bls35.pdf

Harry, O.G. (2006) Jamaican Creole. *International Phonetic Association Journal of the International Phonetic Association* 36 (1), 125–131. https://doi.org/10.1017/S002510030600243X

Hinrichs, L. (2014) Diasporic mixing of World Englishes: The case of Jamaican Creole in Toronto. In E. Green and C.F. Meyer (eds) *The Variability of Current World Englishes* (pp. 169–198). De Gruyter Mouton. https://doi.org/10.1515/9783110352108.169

Hoffman, M.F. (2010) The role of social factors in the Canadian Vowel Shift: Evidence from Toronto. *American Speech* 85 (2), 121–140. https://doi.org/10.1215/00031283-2010-007

Hoffman, M.F. and Walker, J.A. (2010) Ethnolects and the city: Ethnic orientation and linguistic variation in Toronto English. *Language Variation and Change* 22 (1), 37–67. https://doi.org/10.1017/S0954394509990238

Holm, J.A. (1988) *Pidgins and Creoles: Volume 1, Theory and Structure (Vol. 1)*. Cambridge University Press.

Holm, J. (2000) *An Introduction to Pidgins and Creoles*. Cambridge University Press.

Irvine, A. (2004) A good command of the English language: Phonological variation in the Jamaican acrolect. *Journal of Pidgin and Creole Languages* 19 (1), 41–76. https://doi.org/10.1075/jpcl.19.1.03irv

Jackson, R. (2022) The pain in my voice: The reformation of Jamaican Creole in the twenty-first century. MA thesis, The University of Guelph.

Jourdan, C. (2021) Pidgins and creoles: Debates and issues. *Annual Review of Anthropology* 50 (1), 363–378. https://doi.org/10.33422/ntssconf.v1i1.108

Karem, R.W., Washington, K.N. and Crowe, K. (2021) Cross-linguistic interactions in the spontaneous productions of preschoolers who speak Jamaican-Creole and English. *Speech, Language and Hearing* 25 (3), 325–337. https://doi.org/10.1080/2050571X.2021.1936914

León, M., Washington, K.N., Fritz, K.A., Leon, M., Basinger, M. and Crowe, K. (2021) Intelligibility in context scale: Sensitivity and specificity in the Jamaican context. *Clinical Linguistics & Phonetics* 35 (2), 154–171. https://doi.org/10.1080/02699206.2020.1766574

León, M., Washington, K.N., McKenna, V.S., Crowe, K., Fritz, K. and Boyce, S. (2023) Characterizing speech sound productions in bilingual speakers of Jamaican Creole and English: Application of durational acoustic methods. *Journal of Speech, Language, and Hearing Research* 66 (1), 61–83. https://doi.org/10.1044/2022_JSLHR-22-00304

Mair, C. (2002) Creolisms in an emerging standard: Written English in Jamaica. *World-Wide Englishes* 23 (1), 31–58. https://doi.org/10.1075/eww.23.1.03mai

Malcolm, T.R. (2021) Cross-linguistic morphosyntactic influence in bilingual speakers of Jamaican Creole and Jamaican English. PhD thesis, City University of New York.

McLeod, S., Harrison, L.J. and McCormack, J. (2012a) The intelligibility in context scale: Validity and reliability of a subjective rating measure. *Journal of Speech, Language, and Hearing Research* 55 (2), 648–656. https://doi.org/10.1044/1092-4388(2011/10-0130)

McLeod, S., Harrison, L.J. and McCormack, J. (2012b) *Mezha fi omoch ada piipl kyan andastan di pikni: Jamiekan* [Intelligibility in Context Scale: Jamaican Creole]. (K.N. Washington and H. Devonish, Trans.). See http://www.csu.edu.au/research/multilingual-speech/ics (accessed 29 August 2024).

McLeod, S., Verdon, S. and International Expert Panel on Multilingual Children's Speech. (2017) Tutorial: Speech assessment for multilingual children who do not speak the same language(s) as the speech-language pathologist. *American Journal of Speech-Language Pathology* 26 (3), 691–708. https://doi.org/10.1044/2017_AJSLP-15-0161

McLeod, S., Verdon, S., Margetson, K., Tran, V.H., Wang, C., Phạm, B., To, L. and Huynh, K. (2023) Multilingual speech acquisition by Vietnamese-English speaking

Vietnamese-Australian children and adult family members. *Journal of Speech, Language, and Hearing Research* 66 (7), 2184–2229. https://doi.org/10.1044/2023_JSLHR-21-00669

MFAFT – Jamaica (n.d.) *Jamaica and Costa Rica Commit to Strengthening Cooperation.* Ministry of Foreign Affairs and Foreign Trade – Jamaica. See https://mfaft.gov.jm/site/jamaica-and-costa-rica-commit-to-strengthening-cooperation-2/#:~:text=Costa%20Rica%20is%20home%20to,the%20coastal%20province%20of%20Lim%C3%B3n (accessed 11 March 2025).

Mufwene, S.S. (2020) Decolonial linguistics as paradigm shift. A commentary. In A. Deumert, A. Storch and N. Shepard (eds) *Colonial and Decolonial Linguistics – Knowledges and Epistemes* (pp. 287–298). Oxford University Press.

Patrick, P.L. (1999) *Urban Jamaican Creole: Variation in the Mesolect.* John Benjamins Publishing Company.

Rickford, J.R. (1996) Copula variability in Jamaican creole and African American vernacular English. In G.R. Guy, C. Feagin, D. Schiffrin and J. Baugh (eds) *Towards a Social Science of Language: Papers in Honor of William Labov* (pp. 357–372). John Benjamins Publishing Company.

Roeder, R.V. and Jarmasz, L.G. (2010) The Canadian shift in Toronto. *Canadian Journal of Linguistics* 55 (3), 387–404. https://www.ling.upenn.edu/nwav/abstracts/nwav36_roeder_jarmasz.pdf

Sadlier-Brown, E. and Tamminga, M. (2008) *The Canadian Shift: Coast to Coast**. Proceedings of *The 2008 Association canadienne de linguistique,* Canada. See https://www.meredithtamminga.com/pdf/2008_Sadlier-BrownTamminga.pdf

Schneider, E. (2008) Synopsis: Phonological variation in the Americas and the Caribbean. In B. Kortmann and E. Schneider (eds) 2 *The Americas and the Caribbean* (pp. 383–400). De Gruyter Mouton.

Shepherd, V. (2022) The Maroons of Jamaica and their rights as Indigenous Peoples. *The Jamaica Gleaner,* 16 January 2022. See https://jamaica-gleaner.com/article/focus/20220116/verene-shepherd-maroons-jamaica-and-their-rights-indigenous-peoples (accessed 17 July 2024).

Statistics Canada (2022) Ethnic or cultural origin by generation status: Canada, provinces and territories, census metropolitan areas and census agglomerations with parts. https://doi.org/10.25318/9810033801-eng

Tucker, S.K.D. and Murphy, V.A. (2023) Beyond "Sea, Sun, and Fun": Exploring the viability of Jamaican Creole Heritage language education in Toronto. *Canadian Modern Language Review* 79 (1), 59–76. https://doi.org/10.3138/cmlr-2021-0073

Washington K.N. (2025) Creole languages and American Englishes: Multilingualism and pediatric speech-language pathology. *Seminars in Speech and Language* 46 (2), 75–86. https://doi.org/10.1055/s-0044-1801362

Washington, K.N., McDonald, M.D., McLeod, S., Crowe, K. and Devonish, H. (2017) Validation of the intelligibility in context scale for Jamaican Creole-speaking preschoolers. *American Journal of Speech-Language Pathology* 26 (3), 750–761.

Washington, K.N., Karem, R.W., Kokotek, L.E. and León, M. (2023) Supporting culturally responsive assessment practices with preschoolers: Guidance from methods in the Jamaican context. *Journal of Speech, Language, and Hearing Research* 66 (12), 4716–4738. https://doi.org/10.1044/2023_JSLHR-23-0010

Washington, K.N., Crowe, K., Basinger, M. and Farquharson, J. (2025) Jamaican Creole speech development. In S. McLeod (ed.) *The Oxford Handbook of Speech Development in Languages of the World.* Oxford University Press.

Winford, D. (1988) The Creole continuum and the notion of the community as locus of language. *International Journal of the Sociology of Language* 1988 (71), 91–106. https://doi.org/10.1515/ijsl.1988.71.91

7 Jamaican Language Influence in Multiethnic Toronto English

Clive Forrester

Introduction

Jamaican Creole (JC), or 'Patwa' as its speakers call it, is an English-lexified Creole with a rich history and complex sociolinguistic structure. Emerging on 17th-century plantations from the interactions between British colonists and enslaved Africans speaking diverse languages, JC developed a unique linguistic profile. However, it is crucial to recognize that this linguistic development was not a simple byproduct of contact. Rather, the deliberate and brutal practice of forcibly congregating individuals from disparate African linguistic backgrounds served as a tool of control, intended to impede communication and solidarity among the enslaved. Despite this oppressive context, the creation of JC stands as a testament to the resilience and agency of those who were subjected to this system. While its vocabulary is primarily English-derived, its grammatical framework reveals significant influence from West African languages.

JC exists on a post-creole continuum, encompassing varieties that range from the basilectal form, heavily influenced by West African grammar, to the acrolectal form, closely resembling Standard Jamaican English, and a range of intermediate varieties between those two poles referred to as mesolectal varieties (Mair, 2002; Patrick, 2012). DeCamp (1971b: 355) eloquently describes this continuum:

> In Jamaica, there is no sharp cleavage between Creole and standard. Rather, this is a continuous spectrum of speech varieties ranging from 'bush talk' or 'broken language' of Quashie to the educated standard of Phillip Sherlock and Norman Manley. Many Jamaicans persist in the myth that there are only two varieties; the patois (Creole) and the standard... Each Jamaican commands a span of this continuum, the breadth of the span depending on the breadth of the social contacts.

DeCamp (1971b) introduced the concept of the creole continuum as a method for describing this language situation, and linguists such as Rickford's (1987) study of Guyanese Creole and Patrick's (1999) on JC have since expanded upon it extensively. The JC continuum is a linguistic phenomenon that reflects the social stratification and complex history of Jamaica. It is characterized by a spectrum of speech varieties, ranging from the basilect (most distant from standard English) to the acrolect (standard Jamaican English). These two poles are connected by a series of minimally differentiated grammars, forming a seamless web of linguistic variation. The basilect is considered to have undergone abrupt creolization, while the acrolect is a result of normal transmission from British input dialects. The mesolect is the most important variety in Jamaica, spoken by most Jamaicans in most situations. It is characterized by the systematic presence and integration of English forms and rules in a partial and variable manner. The mesolect is considered to be a part of JC, sharing many constraints and organizing principles with the basilect.

A distinguishing feature of JC is its unique tense, mood and aspect marking system. Unlike English, which employs inflections and auxiliary verbs, JC utilizes preverbal particles to express these grammatical categories. For example, past tense in JC is often indicated by markers like *did* or *neva* before the verb stem (Brown, 1968). The past tense marker *did* is primarily reserved for action verbs e.g. *run*, *play*, *cook*, etc. It is important to note, however, that marking the simple past tense (preterite) is optional in JC since the default interpretation for unmarked action verbs is the past tense. Thus, the sentences in (1) and (2) below could have identical interpretations, specifically, the simple past tense:

(1) Mi run go home.
(2) Mi did run go home.

This syntactic feature is in sharp contrast with English, which obligatorily indicates past tense on the verb. The per-verbal marker *neva*, on the other hand, is a combination of the negator *no* + past tense. It is typically used with stative verbs (verbs describing a mental state). For instance:

(3) Mi no know.
(4) Mi neva know.

The sentence in (3) is describing a current state of not knowing, congruent with the time of speaking – it receives a present tense interpretation. The adjustment in (4) suggests that the state of not knowing existed in the past and is true up to, and including, the time of speech. This same distinction is paralleled by the use of *don't* and *didn't* with stative verbs in English.

Linguist Frederic Cassidy spearheaded the standardization of JC orthography in the 1960s. His phonemic writing system aimed to capture the unique sounds of JC, differentiating it from English spelling conventions. In 2009, the Jamaican Language Unit (JLU) further refined this system with the publication of *Writing Jamaican the Jamaican Way*, a manual providing comprehensive guidance on JC spelling and grammar rules. Despite its linguistic significance and cultural importance, JC has struggled to gain official recognition and acceptance. The historical legacy of colonialism has led to the perception of JC as less prestigious than Standard Jamaican English, resulting in resistance to efforts to introduce JC instruction in schools and encourage its use in formal settings (Jamaican Language Unit, 2005: 5).

Immigration history

Jamaicans constitute a significant portion of the immigrant population in Canada. The 2021 Canadian census revealed that approximately 249,070 Canadians are of Jamaican origin (Statistics Canada, 2023). The immigration of Jamaicans to Canada dates back to the 19th century when Jamaican Maroons were brought to Halifax to suppress a rebellion. These Maroons were descendants of Africans brought to Jamaica to work as slaves on plantations, and their arrival marked an early chapter in the history of the Jamaican diaspora in Canada. It is important to note that approximately 76% of present-day Jamaicans are of African origin (University of the West Indies, 2024).

Large-scale immigration of Jamaicans to Canada commenced in the 1960s and continues to this day. The 2016 Canadian Census indicated a substantial increase in the Jamaican-Canadian population, growing by over 40% between 2006 and 2011. Many Jamaican-Canadians maintain strong cultural ties to Jamaica, including the use of JC across generations (The Jamaican Community in Canada, 2007). This sustained migration has resulted in a significant imprint of Jamaican culture and language on Black communities in Canada. While the linguistic influence of JC on English-speaking Black Canadians warrants further investigation, researchers have identified the emergence of a distinct variety of English, often referred to as Canadian Black English or Multiethnic Toronto English (MTE) (Hinrichs, 2014a).

Geographical locations

The Jamaican presence in the Greater Toronto Metropolitan Area (GTMA) is a notable feature of the city's multicultural landscape, with a significant population and distinct cultural identity (Hinrichs, 2014b: 170). In 2010, 150,840 out of 4,682,897 inhabitants in the GTMA claimed Jamaican nationality, representing 3.2% of the population, though the number of people of Jamaican heritage is expected to be higher (Hinrichs, 2014b).

Jamaicans in Toronto tend to have high cultural visibility, especially within mixed immigrant contexts. While people of Jamaican descent reside across the Toronto area, certain wards have especially high numbers of West Indian residents. These areas, though diverse, are known as 'Jamaican' due to the cultural dominance of Jamaican traditions. For example, Eglinton West is recognized as 'Little Jamaica' by Toronto residents. Since the 1970s, Jamaica has consistently been the country providing the highest annual numbers of immigrants out of all West Indian countries (Hinrichs, 2014b: 170) leading to a very vibrant and visible 'boon to the city'. as one *Toronto Star* journalist puts it (James, 2012). Research indicates that residing in high-density Jamaican neighborhoods in Toronto correlates with a greater use of certain linguistic features, such as higher rates of *t/d*-deletion (Baxter & Peters, 2011). Furthermore, the concept of 'dread talk' within the Rastafarian faith, which is itself conceptualized as diasporic, plays a role in the community's representation of diasporic experience, with cultural brokers mediating between the diasporic community and the Canadian public sphere (Hinrichs, 2015: 65).

MTE is also prominent in Toronto. This distinct dialect, spoken by Black Canadians in the city, shares various linguistic features with African American English (AAE) used in the United States. With over 65% of the Black Canadian population residing in Ontario, and the Greater Toronto Area boasting the highest concentration within the province (according to the 2016 Canadian census), the widespread use of MTE in the Greater Toronto Area (GTA) reflects the significant influence of Jamaican culture and language on Black communities in Canada (Hinrichs, 2014b). The geographical concentration of Jamaican immigrants in Canada, especially in the GTA, has facilitated both the preservation and evolution of JC. It has become an integral part of the linguistic landscape of Toronto and its surrounding areas, contributing to the rich tapestry of language and culture in the region. While smaller pockets of Jamaican communities exist in Vancouver and Ottawa, these have garnered less scholarly attention to date.

Language attitudes

In Canada, JC often faces negative perceptions, being viewed as a substandard or inferior variant of the English language. Similarly, Multiethnic Toronto English frequently encounters stigmatization and marginalization. These negative attitudes toward JC and MTE can lead to significant discrimination against their speakers in various settings, including the workplace and educational institutions. The historical legacy of colonialism and the perceived lower prestige of these language varieties contribute to the persistence of this problematic linguistic discrimination.

However, there is a growing recognition and appreciation of the cultural and linguistic richness of the Jamaican language and its varieties within the Jamaican-Canadian community. Many Jamaican-Canadians actively maintain and celebrate their linguistic heritage, viewing it as an integral part of their cultural identity. Furthermore, the spread of Jamaican popular culture, including music and dance, has helped to increase the visibility and acceptance of JC and MTE in Canada (Patrick, 1995, 1999, 2012).

While attitudes toward JC are evolving in Canada, it is crucial to acknowledge that JC has also faced negative perceptions within Jamaica itself. The collapse of the plantation economy led to urbanization and the migration of many JC speakers to Kingston, where societal pressures often favored Standard Jamaican English. It is noteworthy that only in the 21st century has the Jamaican government begun to explore language planning and the recognition of JC as a national language.

Interestingly, attitudes toward JC appear to be more positive in Toronto, where many community members view it as an important part of their identity (Farquharson, 2014). This highlights the dynamic and context-dependent nature of language attitudes. It is essential for practitioners working with JC and MTE speakers to avoid stigmatizing these varieties. In cases where comprehension challenges arise due to unfamiliarity with these language varieties, seeking assistance from colleagues or interpreters is crucial.

Despite the growing recognition of JC and MTE, the linguistic influence of JC on MTE requires further investigation. While researchers have identified the emergence of a distinct variety of English in Toronto that shares features with both JC and African American Vernacular English, the specific dynamics of this linguistic interplay remain an area ripe for exploration (Poplack & Tagliamonte, 1991; Rickford *et al.*, 2015).

Formal and Sociolinguistic Features of Jamaican Creole-Influenced Multiethnic Toronto English

In Toronto, the variety of MTE, known colloquially as 'Toronto Slang', exhibits a fascinating dynamic: it is heavily influenced by just two immigrant languages, Jamaican Patwa and Somali. This concentrated influence provides a unique opportunity to examine language contact and change in an urban setting.

Phonology and lexis

Several phonological features distinguish Jamaican-influenced MTE, contributing to its unique sonic signature. One prominent feature is the pronunciation of the diphthong vowel /aʊ/, as in *house*. In Jamaican-influenced MTE, this vowel is often realized as a monophthong, [oː], a pattern also observed in the Midland and Southern dialects of American English. Interestingly, León *et al.* (2023) found that JC-English bilingual children produce VOT, vowel duration and whole-word duration similarly across both JC and English, suggesting potential cross-linguistic influence. Another salient feature is *th*-stopping, where the voiceless and voiced <*th*> sounds, /θ/ and /ð/, are realized as [t] and [d], respectively (e.g. *thin* pronounced as 'tin', and *that* pronounced as 'dat'). This feature, prevalent in JC, has become emblematic of MTE, serving as a marker of both solidarity and cultural identity. *Th*-stopping illustrates how linguistic features of JC persist in diaspora communities and integrate into local speech patterns, contributing to the dynamism of language change. Notably, these phonological traits, while rooted in JC, are often used by speakers of diverse ethnic backgrounds in Toronto, signaling the broader appeal and adoption of Jamaican-influenced linguistic practices. This process is also prevalent in AAE, highlighting the interconnectedness of language variation across different communities.

Hinrichs (2014) provides a detailed analysis of the variation in the FACE vowel. In JC, this vowel typically surfaces as a falling diphthong /ɪɛ/ contrasting with the raising diphthong /ɛɪ/ found in Canadian English. Speakers in Toronto's Jamaican diaspora often produce a compromise realization, effectively blending these two patterns. This variation, however, is not merely phonetic; it carries significant sociolinguistic weight, indexing both Jamaican heritage and local belonging. It underscores the complex negotiation of identity within the Jamaican diaspora in Toronto, showcasing how language embodies the interplay between heritage and adaptation. The FACE vowel variation also serves as a marker of linguistic hybridity. Research indicates that second-generation speakers, who are often bicultural, strategically employ these vowel realizations depending on the context (Hinrichs, 2014a: 235). For instance, some speakers utilize Jamaican-influenced vowel patterns in informal or in-group settings, while adopting more Canadian-like patterns in formal contexts. This strategic variation demonstrates how phonological features can function as flexible tools for navigating multiple identities and social spaces.

Morphology and syntax

Beyond phonology, Jamaican-influenced MTE exhibits several distinctive morphosyntactic features that contribute to its unique character. The influence of JC on the MTE lexicon is undeniable, with numerous words and expressions being adopted into the vernacular. Terms such as *gyal* 'girl' and *mans* 'man' (or a generalized pronoun) exemplify this influence. These terms, initially markers of Jamaican heritage, have undergone semantic shifts and are now widely recognized as integral components of Toronto's urban slang, highlighting the dynamic interplay between language and identity.

The case of *mans* is particularly intriguing, illustrating a fascinating instance of grammatical innovation. In MTE, *mans* has evolved from a plural noun to a first-person singular pronoun in certain contexts, a clear example of ongoing grammaticalization. This development mirrors similar processes observed in Multicultural London English (MLE), where *man* serves as a pronoun. However, the morphological and functional trajectory of *mans* in Toronto reveals distinct local adaptations, underscoring the role of community-specific factors in language change. The use of *mans* in speech often signals in-group identity and solidarity, while also functioning as a stylistic marker of urban youth culture (Denis, 2016).

Interestingly, Jamaican-influenced MTE also incorporates lexical items from other languages spoken within Toronto's diverse communities. One such example is the word *bucktee*. Derived from the Somali word *bakhti*, meaning 'corpse' or 'dead thing', which initially served as a pejorative term to refer to an underclass, often houseless, drug user. However, in Toronto, it has undergone semantic expansion, becoming a general personal pejorative (Denis, 2021). This case illustrates how language contact can lead to lexical borrowing and semantic change, reflecting the complex linguistic interactions within a multicultural urban environment.

Sociolinguistic features

The social meaning of words like *bucktee* is indeed complex. Despite being a loanword from Somali, a language with a relatively small number of speakers in the city, it has become associated with MTE, colloquially known as 'Toronto Slang'. This variety is predominantly used by racialized youth, especially those with Jamaican and Somali backgrounds. This association is partly due to its use by high-profile figures such as Drake and other Somali-Canadian hip-hop artists, who have effectively amplified its presence in the local vernacular. For young people in Toronto, particularly males, the use of Somali loanwords, like *bucktee*, carries a certain social currency. It is perceived as cool, masculine and ultimately desirable, reflecting the intricate ways in which language intersects with identity and social dynamics (Denis, 2021).

The integration of JC features into MTE is inextricably linked to the negotiation of identity within Toronto's Jamaican diaspora. Language serves as a form of symbolic capital, enabling speakers to navigate the complexities of racial and cultural identity in a multicultural urban environment. For many second-generation Jamaicans, the use of Jamaican Creole-influenced linguistic features allows them to assert their heritage while simultaneously signaling belonging within the broader Toronto community. It's a way of maintaining a connection to their roots while actively participating in the construction of a shared urban identity.

This dynamic is particularly salient in the performative use of language in music, media and social interactions. JC features are frequently employed in Toronto's vibrant hip-hop scene, where they serve as markers of authenticity and cultural pride. Interestingly, these features are also adopted by non-Jamaican speakers, illustrating their broader appeal and the role of JC as a cornerstone of MTE. This cross-cultural adoption speaks to the power of language to transcend ethnic boundaries and create a sense of shared identity.

Jamaican Creole's influence on MTE exemplifies the intricate interplay between language, identity and culture in Toronto's multicultural context. Phonological features like the FACE vowel and *th*-stopping, grammatical innovations such as *mans* and the integration of Jamaican-origin lexical items all highlight the linguistic creativity and adaptability of Toronto's diverse communities. Sociolinguistically, MTE serves as a site for negotiating identity and belonging, illustrating the power of language as both a cultural artifact and a tool for social connection. The study of Jamaican-influenced MTE not only sheds light on the linguistic dynamics of diaspora communities but also offers broader insights into the ways in which language evolves in multicultural urban settings. It provides a compelling case study of how language contact, social interaction and identity construction shape the linguistic landscape of a city.

Jamaicans in 'Canada Data Set'

Farquharson's (2014) study of Jamaicans who immigrated to Canada during the 1970s provides invaluable insights into the experiences of individuals navigating the linguistic landscape of Toronto, particularly the presence and influence of JC. One key theme that emerges from the transcripts is the intricate nature of language attitudes surrounding JC and the ways in which these attitudes intersect with broader issues of identity, belonging and marginalization.

One of Farquharson's interviewees articulates the societal pressures that can lead to the perception of JC as 'Other', forcing individuals to grapple with their own identity constructions:

Speaker A: *...I was born in England, aahm there you were not defined as British, you were defined as Jamaican, and you were defined as black and you were defined as Other. So, that means that if somebody was white and British back then they would have be defined as Canadian. If I was British and Black they... I would have be defined as Other. I may be confused about other what but I definitely would be Other.*

Interviewer: *Yes.*

Speaker A: *And then that externality of aahm of the society then forces the individual to define for themself who do they think they are. So, in that regard aahm the the struggle for identity aah then aah resulted in a real desire to be able to have a strong expression of both Jamaican culture and*

> *Patwa and aah a real latching on to aahm the Rastafarian culture. And a lot of that interestingly enough aahm aahm was exhibited or maybe infused first not necessarily by interaction with people but through the music.*
>
> *(Transcript code: jamaican0001, recorded August 29, 2014; Toronto)*

The provided excerpt powerfully illustrates the ways in which language and perceived identity become intertwined with racialization, shaping the experiences of individuals of Jamaican descent within diasporic contexts. The speaker's personal journey, born in England to Jamaican parents, highlights how external forces can influence an individual's relationship with their language and culture, even fostering a desire for strong expressions of Jamaican identity as a means of asserting belonging and resisting marginalization. This experience of 'othering', a common phenomenon for individuals of diasporic backgrounds, created a sense of displacement, preventing the speaker from fully identifying as British. The speaker's analogy to a white British person being labeled Canadian underscores the arbitrary nature of these imposed identities, revealing a speaker grappling with the complexities of identity formation within a racially stratified society. The complex interplay between language, identity and social context is thus underscored, demonstrating how imposed categorizations can disrupt an individual's sense of self and belonging.

This lack of a clear, ascribed identity appears to have propelled the speaker towards a self-defined identity rooted in their Jamaican heritage. The transcript suggests that this search for belonging manifested in a 'latching on' to Rastafarian culture and the embrace of Jamaican Patois. Interestingly, the speaker notes that this connection to Jamaican culture was initially mediated not through direct interpersonal interaction, but rather through music. This suggests the powerful role of cultural products in identity formation, particularly for individuals navigating complex social landscapes. The music served as a conduit, connecting the speaker to a cultural heritage that provided a sense of grounding in the face of societal othering.

The Farquharson (2014) interviews also shed light on the importance of intergenerational transmission of JC, even in diaspora settings. Another interviewee reveals that she learned JC from her father and through visits to Jamaica, indicating that both formal and informal learning environments contribute to language acquisition and maintenance:

A: *Does he get upset with you at all?*
B: *Sometimes.*
A: *Sometimes. What language does he use when he's upset?*

B: *He [/] he speaks English, but [/] and sometimes I hear him speak, erm, Jamaican.*
A: *Okay. Alright, good. ow, do you speak Jamaican at all?*
B: *Yeah.*
A: *You do?*
B: *Yeah.*
A: *You Sure?*
B: *Yeah.*
A: *Where did you learn it from? [03:30]*
B: *I learned it from my dad and when we went to Jamaica.*
A: *Okay, you've been to Jamaica?*
B: *Yeah.*
A: *Erm, how often?*
B: *Er... # Probably, like, two or three times XXX.*

(Transcript code: jamaican0003, recorded September 9, 2014; Toronto)

This brief exchange aligns with research demonstrating the vital role of family and community in language socialization. Speaker B's acquisition of JC, learned from their father and reinforced through visits to Jamaica, underscores the crucial role of family and heritage tourism in language maintenance. While Speaker B's primary language appears to be English, the mention of their father occasionally using JC, and Speaker B's own self-attested fluency, suggests an ongoing connection to the language, even if it's not the dominant language in their daily life.

The interviewer's repeated questioning about Speaker B's JC proficiency ('You sure?') could indicate a perceived tension between the speaker's claim and the interviewer's assumptions about language use in the diaspora. It's possible the interviewer expected less fluency or usage. However, Speaker B's consistent affirmation demonstrates a clear sense of their linguistic identity. The fact that Speaker B learned JC from their father emphasizes the family's role in transmitting cultural and linguistic heritage across generations, strengthening their connection to their Jamaican roots even while living elsewhere. The trips to Jamaica further solidify this connection, creating opportunities for language immersion and cultural reinforcement.

The excerpts from the interviews, while brief, offer a glimpse into the process of language acquisition and the factors that influence language choice. The interviewer's probing questions and the interviewee's responses reveal the nuances of language use within the family and the broader community. Further analysis of this and other interviews could provide richer insights into the dynamics of language variation and change within the Jamaican diaspora in Toronto. By centering the voices of Jamaican immigrants, Farquharson's study offers a nuanced and compelling perspective on the sociolinguistic realities of this community.

It highlights the complexities of language attitudes, the importance of intergenerational transmission and the role of language in negotiating identity and belonging in a multicultural context.

Implications for Language Researchers

The linguistic complexities of the GTA present significant implications for researchers investigating MTE and its interaction with Standard Toronto English (STE). These implications arise from the multifaceted influences of youth vernacular culture, code-switching practices and the intricate sociolinguistic identities embedded within these varieties.

This linguistic complexity, while fascinating, undoubtedly presents challenges for researchers. It is crucial to be acutely aware of the inherent variation within MTE. Usage is not uniform across all speakers; the extent to which individuals utilize MTE features can vary depending on factors such as age, ethnicity, gender and social network. This intra-speaker variation necessitates a nuanced approach to data collection and analysis, taking into account the individual and social factors that influence language use.

In addition to variation across speakers, intra-speaker variation is also prevalent. A single speaker may employ more or fewer MTE features depending on the context. The formality of the situation, the topic of conversation and the interlocutor can all influence the use of MTE. Researchers must be attuned to these subtle nuances of language use in order to fully capture the sociolinguistic complexity of MTE and its relationship to the city's diverse linguistic landscape. This requires a keen awareness of the social and interactional dynamics that shape language variation.

Furthermore, the influence of JC on MTE underscores the need for researchers to consider the role of language contact and diaspora in shaping urban vernaculars. The incorporation of Jamaican linguistic features into MTE reflects the transnational flows of people, cultures and linguistic practices that characterize Toronto's multiculturalism. Understanding these broader sociolinguistic forces is essential for a comprehensive analysis of MTE and its place within the linguistic ecosystem of Toronto. Investigating MTE requires a multi-faceted approach, drawing on quantitative and qualitative methods to capture both the patterns and nuances of language variation. Ethnographic observation, sociolinguistic interviews and detailed linguistic analysis are all crucial tools for unraveling the complexities of MTE and its role in the construction of identity and community in Toronto. By embracing this multifaceted approach, researchers can contribute to a deeper understanding of the dynamic interplay between language, culture and identity in a multicultural urban setting.

Implications for Clinical Practitioners in the GTA

The linguistic landscape of the GTA presents unique opportunities and challenges for clinical researchers interested in language acquisition, variation and contact. The presence of JC and its influence on MTE requires researchers to adopt nuanced approaches that account for the dynamic interplay between these language varieties.

A key implication for researchers stems from the inherent variability within MTE. The use of MTE features is not uniform across speakers and can be influenced by factors such as age, ethnicity, gender and social network. Researchers need to be aware of this variability and develop research designs that adequately capture the diverse ways in which MTE is used. This necessitates a move away from traditional, monolithic views of language and toward an appreciation of the heterogeneity within linguistic communities.

In addition to inter-speaker variation, researchers must also consider intra-speaker variation, where individuals may adjust their use of MTE features depending on the context. The formality of the situation, the topic of conversation and the interlocutor can all influence the extent to which a speaker uses MTE. By being attuned to these nuances, researchers can gain a deeper understanding of the social and linguistic factors that govern MTE use. This requires a sensitivity to the social and pragmatic factors that shape language variation, recognizing that language is not simply a static system but a dynamic tool for social interaction.

Given the variability within MTE, researchers need to employ methodologies that can effectively capture and analyze this complexity. Ethnographic approaches, which involve prolonged engagement with the community and careful observation of language use in natural settings, can provide rich insights into the social meanings and functions of MTE. This immersive approach allows researchers to move beyond superficial observations and delve into the intricate ways in which language is embedded in social practices and cultural norms. Quantitative methods, such as sociolinguistic interviews and surveys, can also be valuable for gathering data on language attitudes, usage patterns and the distribution of linguistic features across different social groups. These quantitative approaches can complement ethnographic work, providing a broader picture of language variation and its social correlates.

Investigating the influence of Jamaican Creole

The influence of JC on MTE underscores the need for researchers to investigate the role of language contact and diaspora in shaping urban vernaculars. The presence of JC features in MTE reflects the transnational flows of people, cultures and linguistic practices. This phenomenon presents a unique opportunity to examine how languages adapt and evolve in multicultural contexts, challenging traditional notions of language boundaries and offering insights into the processes of creolization and language change.

Researchers can also focus on understanding the mechanisms through which JC is transmitted and maintained within the GTA. Studies can examine the role of family, community and peer networks in language socialization, as well as the impact of language attitudes and ideologies on language use and transmission. This line of inquiry can shed light on the dynamics of language maintenance and shift within diaspora communities, highlighting the interplay between individual agency and societal pressures.

Examining the specific ways in which JC features are integrated into MTE can shed light on the processes of language change and the emergence of new linguistic varieties. Studies can investigate the phonological, lexical and grammatical features of JC that are most salient in MTE and explore the motivations behind their adoption. This detailed linguistic analysis can reveal the intricate ways in which languages interact and influence each other, providing evidence for the creative and adaptive nature of language use.

Considering clinical implications and culturally responsive practices

The presence of MTE poses challenges for speech-language pathologists in terms of differential diagnosis. Features of MTE, such as *th*-stopping and unique vowel patterns, may be misconstrued as speech sound disorders if clinicians are not familiar with these variations. This highlights the critical need for culturally and linguistically informed clinical practice. Research is needed to develop assessment tools and protocols that can accurately distinguish between typical language variation and speech or language impairment in speakers of MTE.

If a child is diagnosed with a speech or language disorder, it is crucial that intervention approaches are culturally and linguistically appropriate. This involves considering the child's language background, cultural experiences and communication styles. Collaborating with families and community members can ensure that intervention is tailored to the child's individual needs and preferences. This collaborative approach recognizes the importance of cultural sensitivity and the value of local knowledge in developing effective intervention strategies.

Community-based participatory research (CBPR) emphasizes the importance of collaboration in ensuring ecological validity and cultural sensitivity in research and clinical practice (Washington *et al.*, 2023). By involving community members in all stages of the research process, from design to dissemination, researchers can gain valuable insights into the lived experiences and perspectives of the population being studied. This approach can also enhance the relevance and impact of research findings for the community. Furthermore, researchers should consider adapting existing assessment tools or developing new tools that are specifically designed for speakers of MTE. This process should involve consulting with community members and language experts to ensure that the tools accurately reflect the linguistic features and communication norms of the target population.

Finally, it is crucial to focus on evaluating functional communication, which encompasses the ability to use speech and language effectively in everyday social interactions. Researchers can develop measures that assess a child's ability to communicate their needs, participate in conversations and navigate different social situations. This focus on functional communication can provide a more holistic understanding of a child's communication abilities and challenges, moving beyond standardized assessments to consider the child's communicative competence within their natural environment. The study of JC and its influence on Multiethnic Toronto English offers a rich and complex field of inquiry for clinical researchers. By embracing the dynamism and diversity of these language varieties and adopting culturally responsive practices, researchers can contribute valuable insights into language acquisition, variation, contact and the development of appropriate clinical assessment and intervention approaches. This research has the potential to not only advance our understanding of language but also to improve the lives of individuals from diverse linguistic backgrounds.

Conclusion: The Enduring Influence of Jamaican Creole in Multiethnic Toronto English

This chapter has explored the intricate relationship between JC and MTE, highlighting the profound influence of JC on the linguistic landscape of Toronto. From its historical roots in the transatlantic slave trade to its contemporary presence in the vibrant streets of the GTA, JC has left an indelible mark on the speech of Toronto's diverse communities. This linguistic legacy speaks to the enduring impact of migration, cultural contact and the resilience of language in the face of social and historical challenges.

The influence of JC on MTE extends beyond mere lexical borrowings; it encompasses a range of phonological, morphological and syntactic features that have become integral components of this dynamic urban vernacular. Features such as *th*-stopping, the distinctive realization of the FACE vowel, and the innovative use of *mans* as a pronoun exemplify the creative adaptation and integration of JC elements within MTE. These linguistic innovations not only reflect the enduring legacy of Jamaican culture in Toronto but also highlight the dynamism and fluidity of language in contact situations. They provide compelling evidence for the ways in which languages interact, adapt and evolve in multicultural contexts, challenging traditional notions of linguistic boundaries and enriching the linguistic tapestry of the city.

The social and cultural significance of JC in Toronto cannot be understated. For many speakers, particularly those of Jamaican descent, JC serves as a powerful symbol of identity, heritage and community belonging. It represents a linguistic bridge that connects them to their ancestral roots while simultaneously allowing them to navigate the complexities of a multicultural urban environment. JC acts as a marker of cultural identity, a vehicle for expressing solidarity and a means of negotiating belonging within a diverse social landscape. However, we must acknowledge the challenges and complexities associated with JC in Toronto. Negative attitudes and societal prejudices, often rooted in the historical legacy of colonialism and linguistic discrimination, continue to marginalize JC and its speakers. The struggle for recognition and acceptance of JC as a legitimate language variety remains an ongoing battle, highlighting the need for greater understanding and appreciation of linguistic diversity and the dismantling of linguistic hierarchies.

The interview transcripts discussed in this chapter offer compelling insights into the experiences of individuals navigating the linguistic landscape of Toronto. They provide tangible examples of the ways in which JC is used, perceived, and valued within families and communities. The transcripts reveal the complex interplay between language attitudes, acquisition and identity, demonstrating how JC can serve as a source of both pride and prejudice. The stories shared by the interviewees underscore the importance of acknowledging and respecting the diverse linguistic repertoires of Toronto's residents and challenge us to move beyond simplistic notions of language and identity.

The presence of MTE, with its unique features often influenced by JC, poses both opportunities and challenges for clinical researchers and practitioners. These features have significant implications for speech-language pathologists in terms of assessment and intervention. It is crucial for clinicians to develop culturally and linguistically responsive practices that account for the variability and complexity of MTE. Misinterpreting features of MTE as speech sound disorders can have detrimental consequences for speakers, highlighting the need for greater awareness and training among professionals. Accurate assessment and effective intervention require a deep understanding of the linguistic features of MTE, its sociolinguistic context and the individual needs of each speaker.

The research highlighted in this chapter underscores the need for continued investigation into the multifaceted dimensions of JC and its impact on MTE. Further exploration of the linguistic features, social meanings and clinical implications of JC in Toronto will contribute to a deeper understanding of this dynamic language variety and its role in shaping the city's linguistic and cultural landscape. By embracing the richness and complexity of JC's influence, researchers and practitioners can foster greater appreciation for linguistic diversity and promote more equitable and inclusive language practices. This research has the potential to not only advance our understanding of language but also to contribute to a more just and inclusive society.

Acknowledgments

I would like to thank Dr Joseph Farquharson for graciously allowing me to use transcripts from his sociolinguistics interviews of Jamaicans living in Canada, which were funded by a fellowship at the University of Bielefeld, Germany.

References

Baxter, L. and Peters, J. (2011) *Black English in Toronto: A New Dialect?* Ontario.

Brown, E.K. (1968) *Beryl Loftman Bailey, Jamaican Creole Syntax: A Transformational Approach*. Cambridge University Press, 1965 (pp. xv + 164). *Journal of Linguistics* 4 (2), 296–298. https://doi.org/10.1017/s002222670000195x

DeCamp, D. (1971a) Introduction: The study of pidgin and Creole languages. In *Pidginization and Creolization of Languages* (pp. 13–39). Cambridge University Press.

DeCamp, D. (1971b) Toward a generative analysis of a post-Creole continuum. In D. Hymes (ed.) *Pidginization and Creolization of Languages* (p. 349). Cambridge University Press.

Denis, D. (2016) A note on mans in Toronto. *Toronto Working Papers in Linguistics* 37. https://doi.org/10.33137/twpl.v37i0.26973

Denis, D. (2021) Raptors vs. bucktees: The Somali influence on Toronto Slang*. *Journal of Multilingual and Multicultural Development* 42 (6), 565–578. https://doi.org/10.1080/01434632.2021.1895181

Farquharson, J. (2014) *Transcript of Sociolinguistics Interviews: Jamaicans in Canada* (J. Farquharson, Interviewer) [Personal communication]. University of Bielefeld.

Forrester, C. (2024) Language policy in the Caribbean. In *The Wiley Blackwell Encyclopedia of World Englishes* (1st edn). John Wiley & Sons, Ltd.

Hinrichs, L. (2014a) Diaspora and sociolinguistic space: The Jamaican community in Toronto. *Presses Universitaires de La Méditerranée EBooks* 1, 235–268. https://doi.org/10.4000/books.pulm.9040

Hinrichs, L. (2014b) Diasporic mixing of World Englishes: The case of Jamaican Creole in Toronto. In E. Green and C. Myer (eds) *The Variability of Current World Englishes (Topics in English Linguistics 87.1)* (pp. 169–194). de Gruyter.

Hinrichs, L. (2015) Tropes of exile in everyday Caribbean-Diasporic speech: The reindexicalization of Dread Talk in the Jamaican diaspora. In J. Hartmann and H. Zapf (eds) *Censorship and Exile*. Vandenhoeck & Ruprecht.

Jamaican Language Unit (2005) *The Language Attitude Survey of Jamaica Data Analysis*. See https://www.mona.uwi.edu/dllp/sites/default/files/dllp/The%20Language%20Attitude%20Survey%20of%20Jamaica%20-%20Data%20Analysis.pdf

James, R. (2012) Most Torontonians of Jamaican descent a boon to the city. *Toronto Star*, 3 November. See https://www.thestar.com/news/insight/2012/11/03/most_torontonians_of_jamaican_descent_a_boon_to_the_city.html

León, M., Washington, K.N., McKenna, V.S., Crowe, K., Fritz, K. and Boyce, S. (2023) Characterizing speech sound productions in bilingual speakers of Jamaican Creole and English: Application of durational acoustic methods. *Journal of Speech, Language, and Hearing Research* 66 (1), 61–83. https://doi.org/10.1044/2022_jslhr-22-00304

Mair, C. (2002) Creolisms in an emerging standard: Written English in Jamaica. *English World-Wide* 23 (1), 31–58. https://doi.org/10.1075/eww.23.1.03mai

Patrick, P.L. (1995) Recent Jamaican words in sociolinguistic context. *American Speech* 70 (3), 227. https://doi.org/10.2307/455899

Patrick, P.L. (1999) Urban Jamaican Creole: Variation in the mesolect. In *Varieties of English around the World*. https://doi.org/10.1075/veaw.g17

Patrick, P.L. (2012) Jamaican Creole. In *The Mouton World Atlas of Variation in English*. https://doi.org/10.1515/9783110280128.222

Poplack, S. and Tagliamonte, S. (1991) African American English in the diaspora: Evidence from old-line Nova Scotians. *Language Variation and Change* 3 (3), 301–339. https://doi.org/10.1017/s0954394500000594

Rickford, J.R. (1987) *Dimensions of a Creole Continuum: History, Texts and Linguistics Analysis of Guyanese Creole*. Stanford University Press.

Rickford, J.R., Duncan, G.J., Gennetian, L.A., Gou, R.Y., Greene, R., Katz, L.F., Kessler, R.C., Kling, J.R., Sanbonmatsu, L., Sanchez-Ordoñez, A.E., Sciandra, M., Thomas, E. and Ludwig, J. (2015) Neighborhood effects on use of African American Vernacular English. *Proceedings of the National Academy of Sciences* 112 (38), 11817–11822. https://doi.org/10.1073/pnas.1500176112

Statistics Canada (2019) *The Jamaican Community in Canada*. Statcan.gc.ca. See https://www150.statcan.gc.ca/n1/pub/89-621-x/89-621-x2007012-eng.htm

Statistics Canada (2023) *Jamaica and Canada: Connected by People, Travel and Trade*. Www.statcan.gc.ca, 2 February. See https://www.statcan.gc.ca/o1/en/plus/2880-jamaica-and-canada-connected-people-travel-and-trade

University of the West Indies (2024) *Jamaica | The University of the West Indies*. See www.uwi.edu. https://www.uwi.edu/jamaica.php

Washington, K.N., Karem, R.W., Kokotek, L.E. and León, M. (2023) Supporting culturally responsive assessment practices with preschoolers: Guidance from methods in the Jamaican context. *Journal of Speech Language and Hearing Research* 66 (12), 1–23. https://doi.org/10.1044/2023_jslhr-23-00106

8 From Us to Us: Mapping Blaxican Spanish toward Community Solidarity

Aris Moreno Clemons

Introduction

To situate this chapter, I invite the reader to imagine a scene. I am a Black American, born to an immigrant mother from the Caribbean and an African American father whose family migrated to California from Louisiana. Though I have often been misidentified in terms of my ethnicity, for most, it is quite clear that I am Black. I am 19 years old and despite speaking relatively no Spanish, I have decided that I am moving to Spain from California. If I learn the language within three months, I will transfer schools and complete the majority of the necessary credits to get my bachelor's degree. While in Spain, I have quickly become conversational and I've made a group of friends who would be classified as heritage Spanish speakers (i.e. an individual who is raised in a home where a language other than the dominant societal language is spoken, and who has some degree of proficiency in that heritage language). As a result, I have integrated myself into a community that feels much the same as my communities at home. On Tuesdays, we have what we have affectionately called 'Taco Tequila Tuesdays' and we switch seamlessly between California English and several varieties of Spanish. We all live in the same building, and we share apartments with international students from all over the world – Brazil, Mexico, Bulgaria, Italy and more as time goes on. While these roommates are welcome to join our festivities, most do not make it a habit as we sing and dance and cook. One night, I am speaking to my friend, a Mexican American woman born and raised in San Diego. We are speaking in Spanish about how her mother taught her to make Mexican rice. '*Añade un* bouillon cube whole', she says. I respond, '*chale*' while crumbling the cube up into the onions that are sautéing in the pan. As the interaction is happening, a Brazilian roommate is grabbing some water from the kitchen. He turns to me, and with a tone of surprise, he says, 'Hey, you're Mexican too?' At that moment, my friend and I look at each other, our own conceptions of Blackness and Mexicanness as mutually exclusive categories etched in our minds, and we fall into a fit of laughter. I tell him that I am just from California, and

I guess that means kind of. We grow up in such close contact that often we adapt to each other's cultures, and with this comes the sharing of language practices. In my case, and the case of Inglewood rapper D-Smoke, who I will discuss later in this chapter, the sharing of space and culture has resulted in novel linguistic practices that have yet to be fully mapped within the field of linguistics.

Over the past two decades, linguistic researchers have begun to take seriously the ways in which language not only functions as a tool for communication but also as a mechanism that shapes experiences, interactions, identities and allegiances (Bucholtz & Hall, 2005; Eckert, 2018). Importantly, these studies have also explored the pivotal role that language plays in understanding how power dynamics are enacted and reinforced within society. Building on the widely accepted understanding that race is a social construct that shapes and is shaped by power dynamics within postcolonial societies (Omi & Winant, 2014), it is crucial to examine how the construction of racial categories and the power structures that uphold them are deeply intertwined with both the production and perception of the language practices of racialized populations. In the emerging field of raciolinguistics, scholars emphasize that language is not merely a neutral medium of communication but a 'central role in the construction, maintenance, and transformation of racial and ethnic identities' (Alim *et al.*, 2016: 7). This view challenges us to recognize language as a site of ideological struggle, where competing understandings of race and identity are both formed and contested. However, this analysis also acknowledges the existence of alternative viewpoints, recognizing that language's role in identity formation can be viewed through various lenses, including those that prioritize individual agency and resistance to dominant narratives.

In the United States, Spanish sits firmly in the realm of racialized language (Mena & García, 2021). However, linguistic research on English and Spanish in California has disproportionately focused on non-Black Hispanic populations, framing Spanish as a language that belongs almost exclusively to these communities. This essentializing view situates Spanish as a marker of Hispanic identity, implicitly excluding Black populations, even though many Black individuals, including Afro-Latinxs, also speak Spanish. Thus, power dynamics within the perception and use of language reveal how linguistic categories (or even features) are mediated through racial perceptions. In contrast to the perceived notions of who Spanish belongs to in the US context, English varieties such as African American English (AAE) are often conceived as being shared by both long-established African American communities and more recent migrants from other parts of the world (Paris, 2009). This dynamic reflects a racialized conception of language, where Spanish is racialized as 'belonging' to Hispanic populations, while AAE is seen as encompassing a broader spectrum of identities. Fought's (2003) seminal work on

Chicano English (ChE), a variety of English associated with Mexican and Mexican American communities in California and other western regions, highlights numerous phonological, syntactic and sociolinguistic features that characterize this variety. However, it's important to note that ChE has developed alongside AAE in California, shaped by shared spaces and interactions. Despite this, discussions about Spanish-language contact and bilingualism frequently ignore the experiences of Black communities, focusing instead on non-Black Hispanic populations. This marginalization mirrors broader societal dynamics that limit Spanish to Hispanic speakers, reinforcing monolingual and monoethnic expectations, and often disregarding Black speakers of Spanish. Moreover, the erasure reflects a broader academic tendency to categorize linguistic behaviors along rigid racial and ethnic lines, reinforcing monoracial expectations for multiracial and multiethnic speakers. As Romo (2011: 219) notes, multiracial and multiethnic individuals 'are expected to choose and assert a monoracial identity', erasing the linguistic realities of Black Latinidad and other complex racialized identities. Through a raciolinguistic lens, these dynamics reveal how racial hierarchies shape language ideologies that marginalize Blackness in discussions of both Spanish and English, while reinforcing racialized boundaries that obscure the linguistic diversity within Black communities, particularly when it comes to Spanish.

Importantly, my analysis in this chapter is shaped by what many scholars are terming linguistic justice (Baker Bell, 2020a, 2020b; Charity-Hudley & Flores, 2024). In short, linguistic justice is any action that redresses and seeks to undo linguistic racism and injustice. Linguistic injustice refers to the ways in which language is used to marginalize, oppress or devalue certain groups of people based on their speech patterns, dialects or accents. Historically, this has involved the privileging of certain 'standard' languages or dialects – often those spoken by people in positions of power – while stigmatizing or suppressing others. For example, people speaking African American Vernacular English (AAVE), Indigenous languages or immigrant languages have faced discrimination in education, the workplace and many other social settings (Baugh, 2016). This discrimination can limit opportunities and reinforce social inequalities. To understand this concept fully, it's essential to define linguistic racism, particularly Anti-Black Linguistic Racism, as articulated by April Baker Bell (2020a). She defines Anti-Black Linguistic Racism as the 'linguistic violence, persecution, dehumanization, and marginalization' that Black language speakers face in everyday interactions and educational spaces (Baker-Bell, 2020b: 19). The prevalence of linguistic racism is evident in numerous aspects of society. Historically, the denial of literacy to enslaved African populations in the Americas is a foundational example, one that has lasting impacts today, as we see similar exclusions in the refusal to recognize or support literacy in people's mother tongues and a recent call to make English the official language of the United States (The White House, 2025). Consider also the ways that technology, like Siri or Google Assistant, often fails to understand varieties of English spoken by racialized communities (Sundar, 2023), privileging a narrow, dominant linguistic standard. Another striking example is the racial discrimination that occurs in housing markets, where individuals with racialized accents are three times more likely to have their housing inquiries rejected (Wright, 2023). These examples are only a few of the many ways linguistic racism permeates daily life, and they underscore the urgent need for equity and justice. If we are committed to advancing justice, we must critically engage with how we understand, evaluate and conceptualize minoritized languages, ensuring that these linguistic forms are seen as legitimate and valued in all spheres of society. Importantly, this also has clinical implications for how we diagnose and treat patients from minority language backgrounds.

To further explore the intersection of language, identity and racialized communities, scholars and language practitioners alike must consider how specific ethnoracial terms are used in the context of linguistic practices. Understanding these terms, which carry both political and cultural weight, allows for deeper analysis of how language functions within these communities. For the purposes of this chapter, I will use varying ethnoracial terms such as Black and African American interchangeably. Additionally, I will use Mexican and Chicano to refer to Mexican Americans and Hispanic and Latinx to refer to wider populations with Latin American heritage. Each of these terms is political and fraught; thus, I use them to understand that race is mutable and contextual. In particular, the term Blaxican extends beyond its use in describing individuals of mixed Black and Mexican heritage; instead, it captures a broader cultural fusion of Black and Mexican social practices. This concept reflects how shared spaces are not only geographic meeting points but also cultural ones, where traditions, languages and ways of being intertwine. In these neighborhoods, Black and Mexican communities often come together in collective expressions of identity, creating hybrid forms of music, language and art that resist simplistic, monoracial labels. In this sense, Blaxican is not just a term for mixed-race individuals, but a lens through which we can understand the cultural landscape of Los Angeles, a city shaped by cross-racial solidarities and the creative blending of diverse traditions.

The chapter has the following structure – first, I will review how Black and Mexican relationships have shaped the sociohistorical context by which a Blaxican variety emerges. Then, I will provide a brief overview of how Blaxican or Black Chicano Spanish emerges as a contact variety, followed by a case study of one song written and performed by the Inglewood, California, native, Daniel Anthony Farris (aka D-Smoke). Importantly, the chapter argues for moves away from practices that pathologize language practices that don't conform to canonical understandings of Spanish or English grammar as they have been defined in the literature. In other words, the chapter asks researchers and practitioners to lead their investigations with questions about the social and psychological conditions that produce varying linguistic production.

Context and Culture

Black Mexican relationships in the greater Los Angeles region

According to the most recent data (US Census Bureau, 2022), Los Angeles County holds a population of roughly 10 million, with Hispanics comprising nearly 49%, and Black residents about 8%. Of the Hispanic population, those of Mexican descent form a clear majority, making up around 75%. The multiracial population, though still a smaller percentage at 3%, continues to rise, signaling increasing racial mixing across the region. Yet, despite these shifts, neighborhoods like South Central, Inglewood and Boyle Heights remain shared by Black and Latinx communities, spaces where the lines of racial identity blur and become more complex. In these areas, people navigate the convergence of shared histories within their distinct racial and ethnic experiences. Various scholars have examined the ongoing interactions between Black and Mexican populations in Southern California, highlighting historical alliances in civil rights movements, union activism and demographic shifts (Johnson, 2002; Ortiz, 2018; Rivera, 2010). In October 2022, a scandal erupted when Los Angeles council members were recorded using derogatory terms about a Black boy and Indigenous Oaxacan immigrants, revealing anti-Black and anti-Indigenous sentiments in parts of the Latinx community (Hernández, 2022). The incident highlighted tensions between Black and Latinx communities, which had been managed through a ‘fragile alliance’ based on a shared history in labor and civil rights (Garrison *et al.*, 2022).

At the same time, political and social coalition building between Black and Latinx communities in California is deeply rooted, with histories of shared struggle and solidarity against white supremacy and oppressive labor systems (Ortiz, 2018). In the context of Los Angeles, the Black and Latinx community has been shaped by political activism, the shared use of public spaces like parks and schools, and, as I am arguing, a distinctive Blaxican sonic landscape (Clemons *et al.*, 2025). D-Smoke, a former teacher and musician, uses his platform to highlight these issues through music that fosters Blaxican solidarity, particularly in Inglewood and greater Los Angeles. D-Smoke’s music and the resultant engagement with his music point to the emergence of a unique Black Spanish, which emerges as a symbol of these enduring coalitions.

Grammar of Language: Approaching Blaxican Spanish as a Contact Variety

A contact variety of language emerges when speakers of different linguistic backgrounds come into sustained interaction, leading to the creation of a new, hybrid linguistic system. Weinreich (1953) describes these varieties as products of language contact, wherein elements of multiple languages combine, forming a unique linguistic structure that reflects the social and cultural exchange between communities. These contact varieties are not merely linguistic fusions but are deeply tied to the power dynamics, historical circumstances and social identities of their speakers. In such contexts, the blending of languages often mirrors broader processes of cultural negotiation and adaptation, with speakers selecting and modifying linguistic features in ways that reflect their social positions and community affiliations. The resulting contact variety is thus not only a linguistic artifact but also a cultural one, embodying the lived experiences of its speakers and their engagement with complex histories of migration, colonization and resistance.

The racial and ethnic diversity in the greater Los Angeles region is not only reflected in its population but also in the linguistic practices of its communities. Drawing on sociolinguistic research, the concept of *linguistic repertoires* can be useful to help us understand linguistic practices in this region. Linguistic repertoires (Poplack, 1980) refer to the full range of language varieties, dialects, registers and styles that individuals use, drawing on these different resources depending on the context or social interaction. Benor's (2010) concept of *ethnolinguistic repertoire* extends the idea of linguistic repertoire by integrating cultural, social and ethnic dimensions into language use. It encompasses not only the various linguistic forms a speaker can employ – such as dialects, registers and styles – but also the sociolinguistic contexts and identities associated with those forms. This approach highlights how individuals draw on their diverse linguistic resources to navigate different social environments, reflecting their cultural backgrounds and community affiliations. Ultimately, ethnolinguistic repertoire emphasizes the dynamic interplay between language and identity in multilingual settings. In the case of Black and Latinx speakers in the greater Los Angeles region, the available repertoires are and have been shaped by the city's unique history of racial mixing and shared neighborhoods.

In spaces where Black and Latinx communities live side by side, the concept of *translanguaging* also becomes particularly relevant. Translanguaging (García & Li, 2015) refers to the dynamic process by which bilingual or multilingual individuals fluidly engage their linguistic repertoires to make meaning, assert identity and communicate in ways that challenge traditional notions of separate, bounded languages. In neighborhoods like South Central and Boyle Heights, where African American English (AAE), Chicano English (ChE) and Chicano Spanish (ChS) coexist, translanguaging reflects the social realities of racial and linguistic exchange. Nonetheless, the established racial scripts in the region often obscure who speaks what dialect and how.

Blaxican or Black Chicano Spanish

Blaxican Spanish will undoubtedly contain linguistic features from Chicano English (ChE), Black Southern California English (BSCE) and Chicano/Mexican Spanish (ChS). Following Bayley and Santa Ana's (2004) definition, ChE can be defined as an ethnolect spoken by people who either have English as their first language, English and Spanish as their simultaneously acquired first languages or those who began to acquire English in school or around the age of five. The ethnolect does not include speakers who are of Mexican descent that have acquired Anglo varieties of English as their first language – generally those who come from middle- or upper-class settings and do not have strong connections with their Spanish-speaking relatives or community members. Additionally, this dialect is not some sort of mixed language or interlanguage of those who are in the process of acquiring English.

ChE exhibits a variety of distinctive linguistic features that reflect both its cultural heritage and regional influences. Intonation patterns often include uptalk in neutral declaratives, giving the impression of questioning where certainty is expected (Metcalf, 1974). While Chicano vowels are generally not directly influenced by Spanish, they can reflect overgeneralizations of perceived differences. ChE also shares innovative trends with California English. For example, speakers often raise the vowel sound [ɛ] before nasals, so *ten* may sound more like *tin* (Holliday, 2024). There's also a fronting of the [aʊ] diphthong, leading to *out* being pronounced more like [æʊt]. Furthermore, many ChE speakers may lose the distinction between /o/ and /a/, providing for a *caught* and *cot* merger that has been found in many ethnolects.

Since the 1960s, the majority of research on AAE has been conducted in the East and Midwest, providing much of the information we have on how it differs from mainstream English as a rule-governed dialect (Labov, 1968; Spears, 2008; Wolfram, 1969). The English spoken by Black people in California was also a topic of interest, adding to the literature on differences between AAE and mainstream American English (Legum, 1971; Rickford, 2014, 2015). Nonetheless, in the early 2000s, regional differences in Black English dialects became a topic of interest and mostly noted phonological and lexical differences, while maintaining notions of structural or grammatical similarity cross-regionally (Charity, 2007; Gooden & Eberhardt, 2007). BSCE, while exhibiting many of the features explored in the longstanding research on African American English, displays some unique features which can appear in Blaxican Spanish. While simplification rates for past-tense clusters are similar across Black Englishes, Los Angeles shows significantly lower rates for non-past-tense clusters (Rickford, 2014). Additionally, Black speakers in California seem to use the invariant habitual be more frequently than Black speakers in other regions. Alongside these structural differences, differences in lexical items abound in California (the term *hella* is quintessentially linked with AAE in California).

Lastly, ChS exhibits several distinguishing features that reflect its unique sociolinguistic context. Phonologically, it often shows simplification in consonant clusters, similar to patterns observed in English, and vowels may be tenser than in standard varieties of Spanish, influenced by English phonetics. Additionally, the aspiration or dropping of the /s/ sound at the end of syllables is common in certain areas. Morphologically, Chicano Spanish frequently incorporates code-switching, alternating between Spanish and English within sentences, a practice known as *Spanglish*. It also often uses diminutive forms to convey affection or familiarity and may regularize irregular verbs, influenced by English structures (Gutiérrez, 1994). Syntactically, Chicano Spanish commonly employs double negation (e.g. *no tengo nada* for 'I don't have nothing'), similar to AAE; and subject pronoun dropping, similar to other varieties of Spanish. Sentence structures may reflect English syntax, particularly in contexts of code-switching. Lexically, the dialect includes many English loanwords, especially for concepts and items that lack direct Spanish equivalents, such as *computadora* for 'computer' or *lonche* for 'lunch' (Gutiérrez, 1994). Certain words may also have meanings that differ from standard Spanish due to local cultural influences. Pragmatically, Chicano Spanish may exhibit different norms of politeness or directness, shaped by its bilingual context. Overall, these features illustrate how Chicano Spanish serves as a dynamic linguistic expression of identity, culture and community among speakers in the United States (Fought, 2010).

The features outlined above provide a foundation for understanding the complexities of Blaxican Spanish. While I have only reviewed a small sample, the unique features associated with each ethnolect emphasize the broadness of linguistic material available for analysis within Blaxican Spanish. In the sections that follow, I highlight the dynamic interplay of influences from both Black and Mexican linguistic traditions that make D-Smoke's language an exemplar for Blaxican Spanish in the region. In the case of Blaxican Spanish or Black Chicano Spanish, three key features can help us to situate its speakers: (1) linguistic dexterity; (2) translanguaging; and (3) increased free variation in phonetic production across language systems.

A key feature of Blaxican linguistic production is indeed a social and linguistic dexterity. In other words, where linguists may look for stability in mapping or defining a particular variety, I argue here that much of the linguistic production of Black Spanish speakers may look like what we would call free variation or shifts not triggered by any intralinguistic conditions. These shifts more often happen in ways that allow a speaker to draw on cultural nuance in the production of their identity and thus in their linguistic production. As a result of the longstanding [oppression] faced by Afro-descendant communities in the Americas, linguistic dexterity has long been a characteristic of Black languaging.

An additional key feature of Blaxican Spanish is translanguaging. Unlike code-switching, this concept does not suggest that speakers move between two bounded language systems but rather draw from a unitary system that has different functions for individual features of the system. For example, a Blaxican speaker may have the words *abuela* and *Mimi* for their maternal and paternal grandmothers. The words are not a one-to-one translation in each system but have different functions to indicate whole experiences with one or the other. The speaker would indeed not switch to using Mimi for their *abuela* when speaking in English or *abuela* for Mimi when speaking in Spanish but, instead, count each term as an individual lexical item.

The acoustic features of 'El Rey' highlight the fluid and dynamic nature of the Blaxican ethnolect, a variety shaped by the sociohistorical position of being in-between. D-Smoke's vocal production navigates the phonetic spaces between English and Spanish, while at times distinctly occupying phonetic territories belonging to neither fully, and yet both at once. These acoustic nuances reflect the sociopolitical identity work inherent in Blaxican linguistic practices, embodying the ethno- and raciolinguistic negotiations that define what it means to claim a Blaxican identity through voice and sound. The phonetic variability here underscores how Blaxican speakers resist and reframe traditional linguistic boundaries, engaging in complex, identity-driven linguistic performance.

Language Sample: D-Smoke's 'El Rey' as a Case Study

Methodology

The following discussion proceeds from a larger analysis of the 2022 song and video, 'El Rey', by D-Smoke. Though the song represents a performance, written and practiced prior to its production, due to the musical genre in which it is performed, we can expect the style used in this song to be more consistent with casual speech than formal speech. As a result, this song is used as a case study in describing a potential emergent variety, Blaxican Spanish. Importantly, the variety being described is something developed over time due to the increased contact between peer groups who use a variety of linguistic tools to perform their identity. Though these features may show up in childhood speech samples, they would most likely appear during the developmental stages where peer language influence has the most impact (Tagliamonte & Molfenter, 2007).

Song description (data)

On 16 September 2022, the song 'El Rey' premiered as a visual album on D-Smoke's official YouTube page (https://www.youtube.com/watch

?v=eKAl3unUOco). Produced by DemJointz, 'El Rey' is a three-minute musical and visual celebration of racial pride, faithfulness and solidarity for Mexican Independence Day (September 15). The song not only features a sample from the classic Ranchera, 'El Rey', but also includes a cameo from an unnamed Mexican man, who we call Tio Chava throughout the analysis. Between the sample, D-Smoke's own use of Spanish, and Tio Chava's explanation of what Mexican Independence Day means to him and his community, the song stands as an audiovisual representation of Inglewood as Blaxican both visually and linguistically.

Procedure and analysis

In the original study, we first conducted a critical discourse analysis applied through a raciolinguistic lens, considering the sociohistorical context of Los Angeles. The approach focused on both the enregistered linguistic choices and visual representations within the song, highlighting the ways D-Smoke disrupts established notions of language, race and identity. Using the theoretical frameworks of 'sounds of crossing' (Chávez, 2017) and 'phonographies' (Weheliye, 2005), the analysis examined the song's discursive and sonic elements to uncover how language shifts in the context of a Blaxican imagined community. Our analysis was then supported by a sociophonetic analysis. For this analysis, we focused on two key variables that highlight perceptual differences between Spanish and English: the production of rhotics and voice onset time (VOT) for voiceless stops /p, t, k/. VOT, which refers to the time between the release of a stop and the onset of the following vowel, is an important feature in distinguishing between languages. Spanish typically features shorter VOT for /p, t, k/, while English shows longer VOT, often referred to as 'long lag'. This variable serves as a useful tool for understanding how the speech in 'El Rey' aligns with the norms of each language.

Raciolinguistic analysis

D-Smoke's track 'El Rey' is emblematic of his broader artistic incursion into Blaxican linguistic and cultural innovation, serving as a critical space for exploring the intersectionality of race, language and social formations. In this song, he enacts a raciolinguistic process that destabilizes the rigid boundaries typically drawn between Blackness and Mexicanness, making clear the fluidity of these identities (Rosa & Flores, 2017; Urciuoli, 1995). Through cultural and linguistic switching, D-Smoke navigates these constructs in ways that both align and juxtapose historically distinct cultural repertoires. Take, for instance, the opening verse of the song.

> *Black is beautiful, brown is born of the earth*
>
> Found a love for the people that's down to stomp on the turf (what?)

Count 'em, all the reasons we in the dirt

'Til we on top, *build pyramids, still could live in a yurt*

...

Here, D-Smoke immediately establishes a parallel between Black and Brown experiences. By invoking the phrase 'Black is beautiful', he taps into a longstanding African American cultural affirmation that emerged from movements to counteract anti-Black racism. He follows this powerful declaration with a phrase that grounds Brownness as similarly essential, asserting, 'Brown is born of the earth'. This linguistic choice connects Black and Brown communities not only through the experience of oppression but also through a shared historical and cultural affirmation of worth.

This alignment is further deepened through the juxtaposition of pyramids – ancient symbols of power and ingenuity in Black diasporic imagination, particularly in relation to Egypt – with yurts, a symbol of indigenous, often nomadic, dwelling practices. These cultural symbols, historically associated with different regions and peoples, are brought into conversation with one another, illustrating how D-Smoke denaturalizes racial and cultural boundaries. The juxtaposition, in this context, emphasizes the shared struggles of Black and Indigenous peoples while also celebrating their resilience and adaptability. In denaturalizing these boundaries, D-Smoke disrupts racial essentialism, instead positing a raciolinguistic fluidity that allows for a more expansive understanding of what it means to be both Black and Mexican in contemporary society. This process not only challenges monolithic representations of Blackness and Brownness but also reaffirms the social and cultural realities of a Blaxican identity that thrives in the intersection of these worlds. Through 'El Rey', D-Smoke offers an example of how raciolinguistic processes can transcend the limitations of traditional identity categories, embracing instead a dynamic and ever-shifting understanding of race and language. Importantly, D-Smoke shows how categorization may complicate the ways practitioners engage Black Spanish speakers in therapeutic contexts.

Sociophonetic analysis

The Blaxican Spanish ethnolect, as observed through D-Smoke's sonic expressions, reflects the intricate sociopolitical interplay between language, race and identity. Through his careful manipulation of phonetic elements, D-Smoke disrupts the linguistic binaries that often attempt to separate English from Spanish, and Blackness from Mexicanness. An acoustic analysis of voice onset time (VOT) data reveals the nuanced ways in which D-Smoke's productions fall between typical English and Spanish phonetic patterns. Comparing his Spanish VOT to that of Tío

Table 8.1 Mean VOT of /p, t, k/ by speaker and named language

	English	Spanish	English	Spanish	English	Spanish
	/p/	/p/	/t/	/t/	/k/	/k/
D'Smoke	46.20ms (5)	64.5ms (2)	80.20ms (5)	20.50ms (2)	54.50ms (6)	33.60ms (5)
Tío Chava	–	18.50ms (2)	–	–	–	25.50ms (2)

Chava, who speaks in a more traditional monolingual Mexican Spanish style, D-Smoke's average Spanish VOT of 37.55ms reflects greater variability than Tío Chava's 22ms average. Meanwhile, D-Smoke's English productions exhibit a higher average VOT of 59.94ms, demonstrating a subtle phonetic shift towards English.

The data in Table 8.1 further break down the VOT measurements across different plosive consonants (/p, t, k/) for both D-Smoke and Tío Chava, highlighting D-Smoke's fluid movement between linguistic boundaries. Additionally, examining the production of intervocalic rhotics (the Spanish /r/), Tío Chava's taps average 18ms, while D-Smoke's slightly shorter taps (17ms) suggest minimal deviation in their Spanish realizations. However, D-Smoke's more variable rhotic productions throughout the song, particularly his longer word-final /r/ realizations, illustrate his cross-linguistic dexterity. For example, in the word 'catorce', D-Smoke's 32ms tap impressionistically resembles an English retroflex, [ɹ], and his final /r/ before pause extends to 59ms, a feature characteristic of Spanish phrase-final lengthening. These intricate phonetic details provide evidence of a Blaxican Spanish that both adheres to and resists monolingual norms, capturing the in-betweenness of this ethnolect. The sonic landscape of 'El Rey' serves as a form of sociopolitical identity work. D-Smoke's linguistic practices challenge the rigid boundaries of named languages and racialized identities, using sound to embody and assert the Blaxican experience. His fluid alternation between English and Spanish, and the phonetic variation within each, resists monolithic understandings of language and culture. Through the sonic performance of his Blaxican identity, D-Smoke engages in the racial and linguistic negotiations that continue to shape his community, demonstrating how Spanish and English, Blackness and Mexicanness, are not just in contact – they are inextricably intertwined.

Translanguaging analysis

D-Smoke's use of translanguaging in 'El Rey' reveals a complex interplay between English and Spanish, navigating the linguistic and cultural identities tied to the Blaxican experience. In the 377-word song, approximately 37% are in Spanish, notably during moments where José Alfredo Jiménez's voice and Tío Chava's Spanish monologue are used. D-Smoke's use of Spanish is minimal but purposeful, often manifesting in lexical switches, such as the reference to culturally significant food items like 'carne asada' and 'arroz y frijoles'. These examples align with Delgado's (2020) and López's (2020) notions of 'common currency' words in code-switching, where culturally charged words remain untranslated due to their deep symbolic value. This careful linguistic choice also mirrors the juxtaposition within the Blaxican identity, where Black and Mexican heritages intersect and are expressed through a shared cultural lexicon.

For instance, D-Smoke's alignment of 'ribs' with 'carne asada' and 'potato salad' with 'arroz y frijoles' reflects a blending and, simultaneously, a distinction of these cultural food items, indexing both Black and Mexican identities in the diaspora. His use of 'jerk', a Jamaican dish, further illustrates the diasporic connections that expand beyond the immediate Blaxican experience, embracing broader Afro-diasporic connections. Phonologically, D-Smoke demonstrates flexibility in his handling of Spanish rhotics, moving between English-like realizations and more traditional Spanish trills and taps. For instance, his pronunciation of 'carne' incorporates a retroflex /ɹ/, while 'arroz' features a fully trilled /r/, highlighting the fluidity of his bilingualism. This linguistic dexterity is a marker of Blaxican identity, a negotiation of place and ethnicity that resists singular racial and linguistic categorizations. D-Smoke makes a compelling argument for the mutability of both linguistic and racial perception when, at the end of the song, he asserts that this is 'from us to us'. In doing so, he centers Black/Mexican sonorities and redirects the ear toward sounds that 'claim space physically and culturally in ways that rebuke politically motivated nationalist and segregationist epistemologies' (Chávez, 2017: 20). Through translanguaging, D-Smoke's work sonically resists monolingual and monoracial frameworks. His shifts between English and Spanish emphasize that these languages are both integral to Black identity, particularly within his Los Angeles community, where racial and linguistic boundaries are porous and continuously redefined.

Implications for Researchers

For researchers, the analysis of phonetic variation and raciolinguistic processes highlighted in the case of 'El Rey' has significant implications for shifting the focus from purely linguistic features to broader sociocultural frameworks. Researchers should first examine the cultural and racial histories that shape language use, particularly in their local environments, understanding that linguistic production is deeply rooted in sociohistorical contexts. The alignment of Black and Brown identities in the Blaxican soundscape, for instance, reflects a fusion of cultural and racial histories that must be considered when analyzing language. This approach departs from the traditional focus on discrete linguistic elements and encourages interdisciplinary perspectives, such as those found in sound studies and ethnic studies, to explore how language operates as a social and cultural practice. By considering the sociohistorical implications and adopting frameworks that account for the interaction between race and sound, rather than named language and identity categories, researchers can offer more holistic and nuanced analyses of language production. Importantly, the analysis suggests the need for researchers to consider societal perceptions of language practices rather than focusing purely on observed linguistic production, a focus that has historically dominated the field of linguistics and speech language pathology.

Implications for Practitioners

Clinical practitioners, particularly in speech-language pathology, must consider the dynamic interplay between race, language and multilingualism when working with both monolingual and bilingual speakers. The analysis of phonetic variables such as voice onset time (VOT) and rhotic production in bilingual speakers, as seen in the case of 'El Rey', challenges the static understanding of race and language. Monolingual speakers, particularly in racially diverse communities, may exhibit multilingual influences that blur traditional linguistic boundaries. For bilingual speakers, the shifting VOT patterns and phonetic features suggest that their language production is not confined to strict monolingual norms but is shaped by cultural and social alignments, such as those seen in Blaxican Spanish. By moving beyond rigid categorizations of language tied to race, practitioners can adopt more flexible diagnostic and therapeutic approaches that accommodate the fluid linguistic identities of their clients. This perspective is critical for recognizing the full linguistic repertoire of individuals, avoiding over-pathologization and promoting culturally responsive care.

Of note is that much of the research on linguistic features within varying ethnolects has been conducted in the subfield of dialectology, which gained prominence in the field of linguistics in the late 1960s and early 1970s. Since this time, dialectology has expanded to include notions of race and identity not previously allowed by the methodological approaches preferred in the study of language. To understand Blaxican Spanish as an emerging ethnolinguistic variety, scholars and practitioners alike must be aware of the potential for an integration and use of varying linguistic features that may or may not be typically associated with named linguistic varieties and the speakers who have been traditionally attributed with the usage of said features.

Conclusion

D-Smoke's linguistic performance – spanning phonological, lexical and discursive dimensions – embodies Black Spanish, Black Spanish speakers and transnational identities. The translanguaging and phonetic variability highlighted in this paper are well-documented in the literature on language contact and bilingualism. However, the social, political and historical movements from which these features emerge, and to which they are ascribed social value, are deeply rooted in a distinctly Black repertoire, intertwined with visual semiotic resources and aural identities and practices. Importantly, D-Smoke's work challenges the ideological divide between what it means to be Black and what it means to be Mexican in Inglewood, California. The case study presented in this chapter represents the opportunity for researchers to shift the ways in which they have traditionally conceptualized the language production of minoritized populations. By focusing on Blaxican Spanish, I ask how considering sociohistorical implications can highlight language practices developed in community rather than insisting on available linguistic features within a dialect. In the case of D-Smoke, who naturally acquired his Spanish among neighborhood peers, translanguaging, phonetic variability and linguistic dexterity provide an example of an emerging multiethnolect.

References

Alim, H.S., Rickford, J. and Ball, A. (2016) *Raciolinguistics: How Language Shapes) Our Ideas about Race*. Oxford University Press. https://doi.org/10.1093/acprof:oso/9780190625696.001.0001

Baker-Bell, A. (2020a) *Linguistic Justice: Black Language, Literacy, Identity, and Pedagogy* (1st edn). Routledge. https://doi-org.utk.idm.oclc.org/10.4324/9781315147383

Baker-Bell, A. (2020b) Dismantling anti-black linguistic racism in English language arts classrooms: Toward an anti-racist black language pedagogy. *Theory Into Practice* 59 (1), 8–21.

Baugh, J. (2016) Linguistic profiling and discrimination. In O. García, N. Flores and M. Spotti (eds) *The Oxford Handbook of Language and Society* (pp. 349–368). Oxford University Press.

Bayley, R. and Santa Ana, O. (2004) Chicano English grammar. In E.W. Schneider, K. Burridge, B. Kortmann, R. Mesthrie and C. Upton (eds) *A Handbook of Varieties of English: Morphology and Syntax* (2nd edn, pp. 167–183). De Gruyter.

Benor, S.B. (2010) Ethnolinguistic repertoire: Shifting the analytic focus in language and ethnicity. *Journal of Sociolinguistics* 14 (2), 159–183. https://doi.org/10.1111/j.1467-9841.2010.00440.x

Bucholtz, M. and Hall, K. (2005) Identity and interaction: A sociocultural linguistic approach. *Discourse Studies* 7 (4–5), 585–614.

Charity, A.H. (2007) Regional differences in low SES African-American children's speech in the school setting. *Language Variation and Change* 19 (3), 281–293.

Charity Hudley, A.H. and Flores, N. (2022) Social justice in applied linguistics: Not a conclusion, but a way forward. *Annual Review of Applied Linguistics*. 42, 144–154. https://doi.org/10.1017/S0267190522000083

Chávez, A.E. (2017) *Sounds of Crossing: Music, Migration, and the Aural Poetics of Huapango Arribeño*. Duke University Press.

Clemons, A.M., Callesano, S. and Torres Castro, C. (2025) D-Smoke's, El Rey: An interdisciplinary approach toward a Blaxican soundscape. In M. Amengual and A. Dalola (eds) *Interdisciplinary Approaches to Romance Linguistics: In Honor of Barbara E. Bullock and Almeida Jacqueline Toribio* (pp. 211–239). John Benjamins.

Delgado, R. (2020) Gender and phonetics in the Spanish/English code-switched determiner phrase. Thesis, University of Illinois at Chicago. https://doi.org/10.25417/uic.13476114.v1

Eckert, P. (2018) *Meaning and Linguistic Variation: The Third Wave in Sociolinguistics*. Cambridge University Press.
Fought, C. (2003) *Chicano English in Context*. Springer.
Fought, C. (2010) Language as a representation of Mexican American identity. *English Today* 26 (3), 44–48.
García, O. and Li, W. (2015) Translanguaging, bilingualism, and bilingual education. In xxx (eds) *The Handbook of Bilingual and Multilingual Education* (pp. 223–240).
Garrison, J., Vives, R., Gerber, M. and Zahniser, D. (2022) Can L.A.'s fragile Black-Latino alliance survive racist recording? *Los Angeles Times*. https://www.latimes.com/california/story/2022-10-16/in-la-politics-latino-and-black-alliances-are-strong-and-complicated
Gooden, S. and Eberhardt, M. (2007) Local identity and ethnicity in Pittsburgh AAVE.U. *Penn Working Papers in Linguistics* 13 (2), 81–94.
Gutiérrez, M.J. (1994) Simplification, transfer, and convergence in Chicano Spanish. *Bilingual Review/La Revista Bilingüe* 19 (2), 111–121.
Hernández, T.K. (2022) *Racial Innocence: Unmasking Latino Anti-Black Bias and the Struggle for Equality*. Beacon Press.
Holliday, N. (2024) Sociophonetic properties of Southern California English among Black and Latinx teens. *Journal of English Linguistics* 52 (3), 183–212.
Johnson, K.R. (2002) The struggle for civil rights: The need for, and impediments to, political coalitions among and within minority groups. *Louisiana Law Review* 63, 759.
Labov, W. (1968) A study of the non-standard English of Negro and Puerto Rican speakers in New York City. Volume I: *Phonological and Grammatical Analysis*.
Legum, S.E. (1971) *The Speech of Young Black Children in Los Angeles*. Southwest Regional Educational Lab., Inglewood, CA. Office of Education (DHEW), Washington, DC.
López, L. (2020) *Bilingual Grammar: Toward an Integrated Model* (1st edn). Cambridge University Press. https://doi.org/10.1017/9781108756181
Mena, M. and García, O. (2021) 'Converse racialization' and 'un/marking' language: The making of a bilingual university in a neoliberal world. *Language in Society* 50 (3), 343–364.
Metcalf, A. (1974) The study of California Chicano English. *Linguistics* 12 (128), 53–58. https://doi-org.utk.idm.oclc.org/10.1515/ling.1974.12.128.53
Omi, M. and Winant, H. (2014) *Racial Formation in the United States*. Routledge.
Ortiz, P. (2018) *An African American and Latinx History of the United States*. Beacon Press.
Paris, D. (2009) "They're in my culture, they speak the same way": African American Language in multiethnic high schools. *Harvard Educational Review* 79 (3), 428–448.
Poplack, S. (1980) Sometimes I'll start a sentence in Spanish y termino en español: Toward a typology of code-switching. *Linguistics* 18 (7–8), 581–618.
Rickford, J.R. (2014) An early study of the speech of young Black children in California: Why it matters. *American Speech* 89 (2), 121–142.
Rickford, J.R. (2015) African American Vernacular English in California. In S. Lanehart (ed.) *The Oxford Handbook of African American Language* (pp. 299–315). Oxford University Press.
Rivera, R.Z. (2010) Ghettocentricity, Blackness, and Pan-Latinidad. In M.J. Román and J. Flores (eds) *The Afro-Latin@ Reader: History and Culture in the United States* (pp. 373–386). Duke University Press.
Romo, R. (2011) Between Black and Brown: Blaxican (Black-Mexican) multiracial identity in California. *Journal of Black Studies* 42 (3), 402–426. https://doi.org/10.1177/0021934710376172
Rosa, J. and Flores, N. (2017) Unsettling race and language: Toward a raciolinguistic perspective. *Language in Society* 46 (5), 621–647. https://doi.org/10.1017/S0047404517000562

Spears, A.K. (2008) Directness in the use of African American English. In S. Lanehart (ed.) *Sociocultural and Historical Contexts of African American English* (pp. 239–260). John Benjamins.

Sundar, P. (2023) Listening with an accent—or How to Loeribari. In P. Rangan, A. Saxena, R. Tharoor Srinivasan and P. Sundar (eds) *Toward a New Object, Method, and Practice* (1st edn, pp. 281–297). University of California Press.

Tagliamonte, S.A. and Molfenter, S. (2007) How'd you get that accent?: Acquiring a second dialect of the same language. *Language in Society* 36 (5), 649–675.

The White House (2025) Designating English as the official language of the United States. The White House, 13 March. See https://www.whitehouse.gov/presidential-actions/2025/03/designating-english-as-the-official-language-of-the-united-states/

Urciuoli, B. (1995) Language and borders. *Annual Review of Anthropology* 24 (1), 525–546. https://doi.org/10.1146/annurev.an.24.100195.002521

US Census Bureau (2022) *American Community Survey 1-year Estimates.* See Census Reporter Profile page for Los Angeles County, CA http://censusreporter.org/profiles/05000US06037-los-angeles-county-ca/

Weheliye, A. (2005) *Phonographies: Grooves in Sonic Afro-Modernity.* Duke University Press.

Weinreich, U. (1953) *Languages in Contact. Findings and Problems.* Linguistic Circle of New York.

Wolfram, W.A. (1969) *A Sociolinguistic Description of Detroit Negro Speech.* Urban Language Series, No. 5.

Wright, K.E. (2023) Housing policy and linguistic profiling: An audit study of three American dialects. *Language* 99 (2), e58–e85.

9 Language Acquisition in Spanish–English Bilingual Children in Texas

Stefanie N. Becerril and Raul F. Prezas

Introduction

Context and culture

Ethnography of the bilingual community in Texas

Texas has one of the largest bilingual populations in the United States, driven largely by its proximity to Mexico and the significant Latine presence in the state. The ethnography of the Spanish-English bilingual community in Texas reveals a complex intersection of language, culture and social networks that shape the experiences of bilingual individuals, particularly children. This community's linguistic diversity reflects broader patterns of migration, cultural identity and social interaction.

Demographics of Spanish-English bilingual children in Texas

Spanish-English bilingual children represent a significant portion of the Texas population. As of 2020, Texas had the second-highest number of Spanish speakers in the United States, and roughly 30% of the state's population speaks a language other than English at home, with Spanish being by far the most common (Pew Research Center, 2020). The state's Latine population, which makes up nearly 40% of the overall population, plays a crucial role in the prevalence of bilingualism, particularly among children (Pew Research Center, 2020).

The Texas Education Agency (TEA) reports that about 18% of public-school students are classified as English Language Learners (ELLs), with the vast majority speaking Spanish as their first language (Texas Education Agency, 2020). Many of these children grow up in homes where Spanish is spoken primarily, but they also acquire English through schooling and social interactions. These students are not only learning two languages but are often navigating between two cultural identities – balancing their heritage language and the dominant English-speaking environment.

Bilingualism among children in Texas is more common in urban areas and regions along the US-Mexico border, such as El Paso, Laredo and Brownsville, where Spanish-speaking communities are more concentrated. In cities like Houston and San Antonio, large immigrant and Latine communities sustain a robust bilingual culture, providing children with exposure to both languages in various social contexts.

Overview of Mexican-American and Latine cultural influences on language use

Mexican-American and Latine cultures have a profound impact on language use in Texas, shaping the way bilingual individuals navigate both Spanish and English. For many Mexican-American families, Spanish serves as a crucial link to cultural identity, family traditions and community connections. It is often the language used in the home, in religious settings and in social gatherings, while English is used in formal settings like school and work. This dual use of languages reflects a broader cultural practice where bilingual individuals shift between languages depending on the context.

Cultural celebrations, such as Día de los Muertos, Las Posadas and Cinco de Mayo, often occur in Spanish, embedding the language deeply in cultural practices. These events not only reinforce language use among younger generations but also serve as important cultural transmission points, preserving traditions within the community. Mexican-American families often emphasize the importance of Spanish to maintain connections with relatives in Mexico or other Spanish-speaking countries, which fosters intergenerational bilingualism (Fishman, 2001).

At the same time, English is increasingly prominent among younger generations, particularly those who grow up attending US schools. This dynamic creates what scholars often refer to as code-switching, where bilingual individuals switch between languages in conversation depending on the context or subject matter (Poplack, 1980). Code-switching is a common linguistic practice in Texas's bilingual communities, highlighting how language use is both a reflection of cultural identity and a practical response to bilingual environments. Texas Spanish-English bilingual children live in a linguistically diverse environment, with speakers from backgrounds of several Spanish-speaking countries. Use of both languages is very common among family members and not only assists family members but also supports the development of biliteracy skills (Lara *et al.*, 2025).

The role of family, community and social networks in language development

The development of bilingualism in Texas is deeply influenced by family, community and social networks, which provide children with the foundation for language acquisition and use. Family is often the primary domain where Spanish is spoken and transmitted to children. Many Mexican-American and Latine families view Spanish not only as a communication tool but also as a key aspect of cultural heritage and identity (Orellana, 2009). In these households, parents, grandparents and extended family members play a vital role in ensuring that younger generations maintain their Spanish fluency, even as they become proficient in English through school and external environments.

Social networks within the community, such as churches, local businesses including local community language schools, and community centers, also reinforce bilingualism. These spaces often serve as bilingual hubs where Spanish is regularly spoken, creating a linguistic environment where children and adults alike can practice both languages. Churches, for example, frequently offer services in Spanish, and community events are often conducted in both languages, allowing bilingual individuals to navigate between cultural and linguistic worlds seamlessly (Pew Research Center, 2020).

Communities in Texas often rely on intergenerational social networks, where children learn from older relatives who may be more fluent in Spanish, while younger family members often help with English-language tasks, such as translating for non-English-speaking relatives. This reciprocal language exchange is a crucial component of language development in bilingual households (Orellana, 2009).

Political Landscape and Educational Policy in Texas: Bilingual Education

Texas, with its rich cultural diversity and proximity to Mexico, has a long history with bilingual education. The state's political landscape – shaped by its conservative leanings, demographic shifts and complex relationship with immigration – has had a significant influence on educational policies. This is particularly evident in bilingual education, where policies such as House Bill 3 (HB 3) and historical sociopolitical factors have shaped the availability and quality of bilingual programs in Texas schools.

Overview of Texas' bilingual education policies

Bilingual education in Texas has a unique place in the state's educational policy, largely because of its large Latine and Mexican-American population. The Texas Bilingual Education Act of 1973 mandated bilingual education programs for public schools with significant populations of students with limited English proficiency (LEP). This legislation aimed to ensure that non-English-speaking students, particularly Spanish speakers, had access to an equitable education by receiving instruction in both their native language and English (San Miguel, 2004).

A key development in recent years has been the passage of House Bill 3 (HB 3) in 2019, a major school finance reform that included provisions aimed at improving bilingual education. HB 3 increased state funding for bilingual programs, offering additional resources for districts based on the number of students in bilingual or dual-language programs. The bill also incentivized dual-language immersion programs, which aim to foster fluency in both English and another language, recognizing the benefits of bilingualism in an increasingly globalized economy (Texas Education Agency, 2019).

These programs are particularly relevant in Texas, where Spanish is the primary language for a significant portion of the population. Dual-language programs, unlike traditional transitional bilingual education, emphasize long-term bilingualism and biliteracy rather than simply transitioning students to English as soon as possible (Thomas & Collier, 2017). Dual-language immersion programs and transitional bilingual education models are common in districts with large Latine populations. These programs acknowledge the cognitive and cultural benefits of bilingualism and aim to maintain a child's Spanish skills while facilitating English acquisition. By supporting these initiatives, HB 3 acknowledges the value of bilingualism not only for language minority students but for all students (Thomas & Collier, 2017).

The impact of sociopolitical factors on bilingual education

Despite the advancements made through legislation like HB 3, bilingual education in Texas faces significant challenges due to sociopolitical factors. One of the most influential factors has been the rise of English-only movements in the United States, which have periodically led to the restriction of bilingual education programs. In Texas, there have been efforts by some policymakers to prioritize English as the primary language of instruction, reflecting broader national trends (Crawford, 2000). While Texas has resisted enacting strict English-only legislation like California's Proposition 227 (1998), the political climate often pushes for English language acquisition as the primary focus in education, which can marginalize bilingual programs.

Funding disparities further complicate the landscape for bilingual education. Texas's school finance system, heavily reliant on local property taxes, creates inequities between wealthy and low-income districts. Schools in low-income areas, which often serve large numbers of English Language Learners (ELLs), tend to have fewer resources for implementing comprehensive bilingual education programs (Johnson, 2020). These disparities mean that while legislation like HB 3 provides additional funding for bilingual programs, the benefits are unevenly distributed, leaving students in poorer districts at a disadvantage.

The political debate around immigration also impacts bilingual education in Texas. Anti-immigrant rhetoric and policies can influence public perception of bilingualism and ELL students. As the state's immigrant population grows, particularly from Latin American countries, some conservative lawmakers have framed bilingual education as a threat to the dominance of English, despite evidence that bilingual education benefits both ELL students and English-speaking students in dual-language programs (Gándara & Escamilla, 2017).

Historical lens: Immigration patterns and their influence on bilingual communities

Texas's long history of immigration has played a crucial role in shaping its bilingual education policies. Throughout the 20th century, large waves of Mexican immigration, particularly after the Mexican Revolution and during periods of US labor demand, established strong bilingual communities in Texas, especially in cities like Houston, San Antonio and along the US-Mexico border (Montejano, 1987). These communities have continuously advocated for bilingual education as a means of preserving cultural heritage while promoting academic success.

In response to these demographic shifts, Texas became one of the first states to implement large-scale bilingual education programs in public schools. The Texas Bilingual Education Act of 1973 was a direct result of activism by Latine communities, who fought for the right to receive instruction in their native language. This historical context underscores the relationship between immigration patterns and the development of bilingual education, as growing immigrant populations have often driven the demand for language support in schools (San Miguel, 2004).

Geographical Distribution of Bilingualism in Texas

Bilingualism in Texas is a complex and dynamic phenomenon, influenced by geographic, social and cultural factors. The state's vast size and its proximity to Mexico contribute to significant regional differences in how Spanish and English are spoken and maintained. Urban centers like Houston, Dallas and San Antonio, along with the rural Rio Grande Valley, serve as key areas where bilingualism flourishes. Additionally, geographic location influences dialectal variations, such as Tex-Mex and Spanglish, which reflect the blending of languages in border and urban communities.

Urban vs rural linguistic diversity

Bilingualism is more prevalent in urban areas than in rural regions of Texas, though both contexts exhibit unique characteristics. Cities such as Houston, Dallas, San Antonio and Austin are home to large, diverse Latine populations, contributing to a strong bilingual presence. Houston, the most populous city in Texas, is a major hub for Spanish-speaking communities, with 38% of its population speaking a language other than

English at home, primarily Spanish (Pew Research Center, 2020). Bilingualism in these urban areas is often facilitated by access to resources such as bilingual education programs, Spanish-language media and social networks that maintain both English and Spanish.

These cities often provide dual-language programs in public schools that promote bilingualism from a young age, making it easier for children to grow up proficient in both languages (Thomas & Collier, 2017). Additionally, the diversity of the Latine population in urban areas introduces a variety of Spanish dialects and accents from across Latin America, contributing to a rich linguistic environment.

By contrast, rural areas in Texas, particularly in the Rio Grande Valley, exhibit a different pattern of bilingualism. The Rio Grande Valley, which borders Mexico, is one of the most densely Spanish-speaking regions in the state. In towns like McAllen, Brownsville and Laredo, more than 80% of the population speaks Spanish at home (US Census Bureau, 2020). Here, bilingualism is more deeply rooted in everyday life, often with Spanish serving as the primary language for many residents. The region's proximity to the US-Mexico border facilitates continuous cross-border cultural exchange, which sustains strong bilingual communities.

However, rural areas further away from the border, particularly in West Texas and the Texas Panhandle, tend to have lower rates of bilingualism. In these regions, Latine populations are smaller, and English dominates in public life. While Spanish may still be spoken in homes or within smaller communities, the lack of institutional support, such as bilingual education programs, and the isolation from larger Spanish-speaking populations mean that bilingualism is less prevalent compared to urban areas or the border region.

Influence of geographic location on dialectal variations

Geographic location in Texas not only influences the prevalence of bilingualism but also shapes dialectal variations. In regions like the Rio Grande Valley and urban centers, the interaction between Spanish and English has given rise to unique linguistic forms, such as Tex-Mex and Spanglish.

Tex-Mex, a blend of Spanish and English with influences from both Mexican and American cultures, is a distinctive dialect spoken primarily in the border regions of Texas. It reflects the historical and ongoing cultural exchange between Texas and Mexico. Tex-Mex incorporates English words and phrases into Spanish, often adapting English grammar to fit Spanish structures. For example, speakers may use English verbs conjugated in Spanish, such as '*parquear*' (to park), which reflects the hybrid nature of the language (Billings, 2015). Tex-Mex is not just a linguistic adaptation but also a reflection of the bicultural identities of many people in South Texas, who straddle both Mexican and Texan cultures.

Spanglish, a broader term that refers to the mixing of Spanish and English, is common in urban areas like Houston and Dallas, where bilingual individuals often switch between the two languages depending on the context. Spanglish can involve code-switching within a single conversation or even within a sentence, where speakers fluidly move between Spanish and English. This linguistic practice is a way for bilingual individuals to navigate their dual cultural identities and reflect their lived experiences in multicultural environments (Zentella, 1997). For example, a speaker might say, '*Voy al* mall *para comprar* clothes', seamlessly blending Spanish and English.

Urban areas, with their larger and more diverse Latine populations, tend to exhibit more variation in Spanglish usage, as speakers from different parts of Latin America bring their own dialectal influences. Meanwhile, in the border regions, Tex-Mex is more prominent and reflects the deep historical ties between Texas and Mexico.

The influence of geographic location on these dialects demonstrates how bilingualism in Texas is not a monolithic experience but rather a diverse and regionally specific phenomenon. In cities, the constant flow of immigrants from Latin America introduces new linguistic variations, while in rural and border areas, long-established bilingual communities have developed their own distinctive language patterns.

Grammar of the Language

Phonology

Unique phonological features of Spanish-English bilingual children

Spanish-English bilingual children in Texas often display distinctive phonological features that reflect their bilingual experiences. One notable feature is the pronunciation of vowels. Spanish has five pure vowels (/a/, /e/, /i/, /o/, /u/), while English has a more extensive inventory of vowel sounds, including diphthongs (Goldstein & Prezas, 2026). Bilingual children may simplify their vowel production by reducing English vowel contrasts when speaking Spanish. For instance, they might pronounce the English word *cat* as *cot* [kɑt], merging the vowel sounds due to their reliance on the Spanish vowel system (Sanchez & Valdes, 2018).

Consonant clusters are another area where bilingual children exhibit unique phonological patterns. In English, consonant clusters at the beginning of words (e.g. *street*, *blast*) are more common, whereas /s/ clusters in Spanish do not exist within the syllable; rather, they occur across syllable boundaries as consonant sequences (Prezas, 2025). Bilingual children may insert vowel sounds, such as the schwa, in front of the cluster, resulting in pronunciations such as [eskul] or [estar] when attempting to articulate English words. This phenomenon, known as epenthesis, can also occur between cluster consonants and when bilingual children attempt to pronounce complex words in Spanish, reflecting the influence of English phonological patterns on their speech. It is important to note that the occurrence of a schwa before the cluster is common and should be viewed as a dialectal difference as part of honoring the perspective of the speaker (Prezas, 2025).

Other dialectal differences that may occur between Spanish speakers include differences between /ʃ/ and /tʒ/ (*share* [ʃɛɚ] versus *chair* [tʒɛɚ]); /b/ and /v/ (*base* [bes] versus *vase* [ves]); and /dʒ/ and /j/ ([dzodzo] versus [jojo]). The noted differences may occur in Spanish (shared phonemes or loanwords) and/or English (Kester, 2014; Prezas, 2025). Moreover, idiosyncratic differences are possible among bilingual Texas speakers. For example, some speakers may produce the trilled /r/ cross-linguistically in English words (e.g. *car* produced as /kar/, Prezas, 2025).

Another phonological feature often observed in bilingual children is the realization of certain consonants. For example, the interdental fricatives /ð/ and /θ/ that exist in English (as in this or think) do not exist in Spanish. Consequently, bilingual children may substitute them with /d/ or /t/, pronouncing this as dis [dɪs] or think as tink [tɪŋk] or even tink [t̪ɪŋk] (note the dentalized [t̪], which is common among many bilingual speakers) (Gildersleeve-Neumann & Goldstein, 2022). This substitution highlights how the phonetic inventory of the first language influences the articulation of sounds in the second language (Sanchez & Valdes, 2018).

Dialectal differences between Mexican Spanish and other Latine varieties in Texas

Texas is home to a rich tapestry of Spanish dialects, with Mexican Spanish being the most prevalent due to the state's proximity to Mexico. However, the dialectal landscape is further enriched by the presence of other Latine varieties, which exhibit distinct phonological features. Mexican Spanish, particularly as spoken in northern Mexico and regions of Texas, tends to have specific phonological characteristics, such as the pronunciation of the <s> sound, which is generally retained in syllable-final positions. In contrast, some Caribbean Spanish varieties, such as Cuban or Puerto Rican Spanish, exhibit a phenomenon known as 's-aspiration', where the /s/ is often aspirated or dropped altogether (Prezas, 2025; Goldstein & Prezas, 2026).

Moreover, Mexican Spanish speakers tend to articulate their vowel system compared to other dialects. For example, the vowel /e/ in the word *mesa* 'table' is often pronounced with more duration in Mexican Spanish, while speakers of other dialects, such as those influenced by Caribbean Spanish, may produce vowel sounds with less duration and may not produce weak syllables (Goldstein & Prezas, 2026). This variation highlights how regional influences shape the phonological landscape of Spanish in Texas.

In bilingual communities, the interaction of these dialectal differences with English can lead to unique phonological blends. For instance, bilingual speakers might code-switch between dialects depending on the social context, which can create distinctive speech patterns. For example, in predominantly Mexican-American communities, speakers might combine aspects of Mexican Spanish phonology with English pronunciations, resulting in a hybrid dialect often referred to as Tex-Mex or Chicano English.

To summarize, the phonological features of Spanish-English bilingual children in Texas reflect a complex interplay of linguistic influences from both languages. The simplification of vowel pronunciations, adjustments to consonant clusters and substitutions of phonemes are all part of the bilingual experience. Additionally, the dialectal differences between Mexican Spanish and other Latine varieties further enrich the phonological landscape of bilingual communities, showcasing the diversity and dynamism of language in Texas.

Morphology

Developmental progression of morphological structures

The developmental progression of morphological structures in bilingual children typically follows a similar trajectory to that of monolingual children, but the interaction between Spanish and English can lead to distinct patterns of development. In both languages, the mastery of verb conjugation and tense agreement is part of effective communication.

In English, children usually begin to use simple past tense forms (e.g. *walked*) and the progressive aspect (e.g. *is walking*) between the ages of two and three. As they develop, they learn to apply more complex morphological rules, such as the use of irregular verbs (e.g. *went* instead of **goed*). However, bilingual children may exhibit variability in this progression due to the influence of their home language. For example, in Spanish, verb conjugation is more complex, with a wider array of endings that vary by subject pronouns, mood and aspect. This can lead bilingual children to initially overgeneralize rules from one language to the other. For instance, a child might say 'he go' in English, applying the simpler present tense structure of Spanish, which does not mark the third-person singular differently (Cohen, 2017). Researchers have found that bilingual Spanish-English-speaking children may need more time to develop both their languages compared to monolingual children. However, there is evidence that bilingual children's speech sound skills approximate those of their monolingual peers within a relatively short period of time (approximately 9–12 months; Gildersleeve-Neumann & Goldstein, 2022). Each child's language acquisition, including strengths and weaknesses, will vary (Prezas & Jo, 2017), and development may be minimal at first, especially in the language used less often in their environment.

This is evident in verb conjugation, where bilingual children may struggle with tense agreement due to the differences in tense marking between Spanish and English. In Spanish, tense is often marked through verb endings (e.g. *habló* for 'he spoke'), whereas English relies more heavily on auxiliary verbs and changes in the verb form (e.g. 'has spoken'). This difference can lead to confusion and variability in the use of tense in English as bilingual children attempt to transfer their knowledge from Spanish (Genesee *et al.*, 2004).

Common morphological errors seen in bilingual children

Bilingual children often display specific morphological errors that can impact their language development and communication. One common difference is the omission of tense markers in English, particularly among children who are still developing their English skills. For example, a bilingual child might say, 'I go to the store yesterday', omitting the past tense auxiliary *went* (Cohen, 2017). This phenomenon is often attributed to the influence of Spanish, which relies on different morphological structures for indicating tense.

Another difference involves the overgeneralization of morphological rules. For instance, bilingual children might apply regular past tense endings to irregular verbs, producing forms like **eated* instead of *ate* or **goed* instead of *went*. This overgeneralization occurs as children attempt to apply learned rules across different contexts, reflecting their developing understanding of morphology (Bialystok & Craik, 2010).

Syntax

Typical syntactic structures in bilingual speech

In bilingual speech, particularly among Spanish-English bilingual children, the basic syntactic structure often mirrors that of both languages. Both Spanish and English primarily follow a subject-verb-object (SVO) order, which allows for a relatively smooth integration of the two languages in bilingual communication. For example, a bilingual child might construct sentences like *Yo quiero pizza* 'I want pizza' in Spanish and 'I want pizza' in English, maintaining the same SVO order (Schwartz & Korman, 2011).

However, variations can arise in bilingual speech due to the influence of each language's syntactic rules. For instance, in Spanish, adjectives typically follow nouns (e.g. *casa blanca* for 'white house'), while in English, adjectives precede nouns (e.g. 'white house'). Bilingual children may demonstrate flexibility in these structures, sometimes adopting English adjective-noun order in their Spanish sentences. For example, a child might say *la blanca casa* 'the white house' instead of *la casa blanca*, reflecting the influence of English syntax.

Moreover, Spanish allows for more flexible word order due to its rich inflectional system, whereas English relies heavily on word order to convey grammatical relationships. This flexibility can lead to innovative sentence structures in bilingual children, as they may experiment with different arrangements influenced by their experiences with both languages. For instance, a bilingual child might say, 'Pizza I want' in English when trying to replicate a more flexible Spanish structure, demonstrating a blend of syntactic rules.

Code-switching patterns and their relevance in assessing bilingual children's syntactic abilities

Code-switching, the practice of alternating between two or more languages or language varieties within a conversation or discourse, is a prevalent phenomenon among bilingual speakers. It reflects the dynamic nature of bilingual communication and serves as a valuable resource for understanding bilingual syntax. Code-switching can occur at various levels, including intra-sentential (within a single sentence) and inter-sentential (between sentences).

In bilingual children, code-switching often highlights their syntactic competence as they navigate the rules of both languages. For example, a bilingual child might say, *I want a casa* 'I want a house', where the English and Spanish elements are combined. This switch often adheres to the syntactic norms of both languages, suggesting that the child is aware of the grammatical structures of each language (Myers-Scotton, 1993).

Assessing code-switching patterns can provide insight into bilingual children's syntactic abilities. Children who frequently switch codes might demonstrate a strong understanding of the grammatical rules governing both languages. It is essential for SLPs and educators to recognize that code-switching is a natural part of bilingual language development and should not be viewed solely as a deficit. Instead, it can serve as a window into children's linguistic abilities, showcasing their capacity to maneuver between languages and apply different syntactic rules (Becerril, 2019).

In evaluating bilingual children's syntactic skills, SLPs should consider the contexts in which code-switching occurs and the motivations behind it. This understanding will help differentiate between typical bilingual language development and potential developmental language disorder (DLD), leading to more accurate assessments and effective interventions.

Semantics

Semantic development in bilingual children: Challenges in vocabulary acquisition across both languages

Bilingual children often face specific challenges in vocabulary acquisition as they learn to navigate two linguistic systems. One major challenge is the 'vocabulary gap', where bilingual children may have a 'smaller' vocabulary in English compared to their monolingual peers, but collectively when considering their vocabulary in Spanish their overall vocabulary is appropriate. This 'gap' can be attributed to several factors, including limited exposure to English, the distribution of language use in different contexts and the cognitive load of managing two language systems (Wong Fillmore, 1991). Research has shown that while bilingual children may acquire a broad vocabulary over time, the depth and richness of their vocabulary in each language may differ from that of monolingual children, particularly in contexts where one language is used less (Gathercole & Thomas, 2009).

Moreover, bilingual children may encounter difficulties with word retrieval and lexical access, which can lead to code-switching. For instance, a child may use a Spanish noun with an English verb, saying *I want un libro* 'I want a book', as a strategy to compensate for gaps in their English vocabulary (Schwartz & Korman, 2011). This phenomenon reflects the children's dynamic negotiation of meaning across languages but can also indicate challenges in semantic processing.

Cross-linguistic influence on word meaning, idiomatic expressions and polysemy

Cross-linguistic influence significantly affects how bilingual children understand and use vocabulary. The semantic properties of words in one language can shape the interpretation and use of corresponding words in another language. For instance, a child may apply the rules or meanings of a word from Spanish when using its English equivalent, leading to potential misunderstandings. This influence is particularly evident in the use of idiomatic expressions, which often do not translate directly between languages. For example, the Spanish idiom *echar agua al mar* (literally, 'to throw water into the sea') conveys the idea of doing something pointless. If a bilingual child attempts to translate this idiom directly into English, it may not carry the same meaning, potentially leading to a breakdown in communication (Grosjean, 1989).

Additionally, bilingual children may develop unique semantic blends that reflect their bilingual experiences. For example, a child might understand the English expression *kick the bucket* 'to die' through the lens of their Spanish knowledge, leading to a more literal interpretation. This phenomenon can affect how they use idiomatic expressions, as they may create hybrid phrases or misunderstand established idioms in one language based on their understanding of the other language (Myers-Scotton, 1993).

Bilingual children also face the complexity of acquiring polysemous words – words with multiple meanings – across both languages. For example, the Spanish word *pasa* can mean 'it happens' or 'pass' depending on context, just like the English word 'bank' can refer to a financial institution or the side of a river. If a bilingual child encounters multiple meanings of a word in one language but is not exposed to the full range of meanings in the other language, they may struggle to use the word correctly in conversation. This complexity can create challenges for bilingual children. This is because bilingual children may struggle to differentiate between the meanings of polysemous words in each language, affecting their overall comprehension and expressive language abilities (Bialystok, 2001). This challenge can complicate vocabulary acquisition and lead to miscommunication, as the child may not be aware of the various contextual meanings of a word across both languages (Gathercole & Thomas, 2009).

In conclusion, the semantic features of bilingual communities in Texas highlight the complexities of vocabulary acquisition and meaning negotiation in children learning both Spanish and English. The challenges associated with semantic development, including vocabulary gaps, polysemy and the influence of idiomatic expressions, underscore the need for targeted support in bilingual education settings. By recognizing these intricacies, educators and SLPs can better assist bilingual children in developing their semantic skills and navigating the rich tapestry of language.

Pragmatics

Pragmatic language use in bilingual contexts

In bilingual communities, pragmatic language use often includes the strategic application of code-switching. As previously discussed, for bilingual children, code-switching serves various communicative purposes, such as clarifying meaning, expressing identity and navigating social dynamics. Children may switch codes to enhance understanding, particularly when discussing topics that are culturally specific to one language. For example, a child might switch to Spanish when discussing a cultural celebration, using *quinceañera* rather than 'fifteenth birthday party' to convey the cultural significance more effectively (Myers-Scotton, 1993).

Conversational repair strategies are also crucial in bilingual communication, as children learn to navigate misunderstandings and clarify their messages. Bilingual children may employ different repair strategies based on the language of their interlocutor or the context of the conversation. For instance, if a child encounters confusion while speaking English, they might switch to Spanish to clarify their point or provide additional context, demonstrating their awareness of their listener's comprehension (Grosjean, 1989). This ability to employ appropriate repair strategies reflects the children's pragmatic competence and their understanding of the conversational dynamics in bilingual settings.

Research indicates that bilingual children often demonstrate a high degree of flexibility and adaptability in their conversational practices. They learn to gauge the linguistic proficiency of their interlocutors and adjust their language use accordingly. For example, a bilingual child might simplify their language or provide explanations when speaking with a non-Spanish speaker, showcasing their pragmatic awareness and social cognition (Tse, 2001).

Cultural influences on pragmatic norms

Cultural influences significantly shape the pragmatic norms that govern communication in bilingual communities. In many Latine cultures, indirectness and politeness are highly valued in communication, which can contrast with the more direct communication style often found in English-speaking contexts. This cultural difference can lead to variations in how bilingual children navigate conversations and express themselves.

For instance, in Spanish-speaking cultures, speakers often use indirect language to maintain politeness and avoid confrontation. Phrases such as *¿Te gustaría...?* 'Would you like...?' are commonly used to soften requests or invitations. In contrast, English speakers may adopt a more straightforward approach, saying 'Do you want...?' This difference can lead bilingual children to exhibit varying degrees of directness based on their cultural context. In settings where they are surrounded by English speakers, they may adopt a more direct style, while in Spanish-speaking contexts, they may revert to more indirect forms (Zentella, 1997).

Politeness strategies also differ across cultures, impacting how bilingual children communicate requests, refusals and disagreements. In Spanish, it is common to use formal address (e.g. *usted*) to show respect, while in English in Texas, the use of *sir* or *ma'am* may fulfill a similar role. Bilingual children must learn to navigate these politeness strategies depending on the language and cultural context, which may involve code-switching to match the social expectations of their interlocutors (Schwartz & Korman, 2011).

Furthermore, cultural norms surrounding turn-taking and interruptions can vary. In some Latine cultures, overlapping speech is more acceptable as a sign of engagement, whereas, in many Anglo-American contexts, it may be perceived as rude. Bilingual children may find themselves adapting their conversational styles to fit the expectations of their interlocutors, demonstrating their pragmatic flexibility and cultural awareness (Tse, 2001).

Clinical Implications for Researchers

With Spanish being the second most common spoken language in the United States, there is an ever-growing body of research on how to conduct culturally sensitive research related to bilingualism. For example, researchers should have a good understanding of second language acquisition so that they are able to value and promote bilingualism, recognize code-switching as a typical bilingual behavior, consider the dynamic and uneven nature of bilingual language development, and maintain cultural humility and bias awareness.

To be culturally relevant, researchers interested in serving the needs of the Spanish-English bilingual community in Texas need to consider the previously discussed implications such as the ethnography of the bilingual community and the political landscape and educational policy in Texas. To accomplish this, researchers are reminded to engage families and communities as linguistic informants, account for sociocultural influences on language use, monitor the impact of educational policy and schooling context, ensure diverse and representative participant samples, and of course use culturally and linguistically appropriate assessment tools that reflect bilingual norms, including code-switching and dialectal variations (e.g. Tex-Mex, Chicano English). There is still a need for context-specific research related to the Spanish-English bilingual community in Texas, such as dialectal varieties in Texas.

Researchers interested in bilingualism, and those interested in the Spanish-English bilingual community in Texas are also urged to consider all three components related to evidence-based practice (EBP): clinical expertise/expert opinion, evidence (external and internal) and client/patient/caregiver perspectives. Especially in the areas of client/patient/caregiver perspectives, research should include qualitative work that can account for their unique set of personal and cultural circumstances, values, priorities and expectations (American Speech-Language-Hearing Association, n.d.).

Clinical Implications for Practitioners

Assessment guidelines for speech-language pathologists

Assessing bilingual children's literacy and language skills presents unique challenges that require a nuanced understanding of bilingual development. Speech-language pathologists (SLPs) play a crucial role in conducting these assessments, and adhering to best practices is essential to ensure accurate evaluations. This section provides guidelines for assessing bilingual children, emphasizing best practices and strategies to avoid misdiagnosis.

Best practices for assessing bilingual children's language skills

(1) Use Culturally and Linguistically Appropriate Assessment Tools: SLPs should prioritize assessment tools that are designed specifically for bilingual populations. These tools should reflect the child's cultural and linguistic background and be validated for use with bilingual children. Utilizing assessments in both languages can provide a more comprehensive picture of a child's abilities (Paradis, 2011). This dual-language approach helps to capture the full extent of a child's linguistic competence, including vocabulary, grammar and discourse skills.

(2) Incorporate Dynamic Assessment Approaches: Dynamic assessment is an evidence-based approach that emphasizes a child's learning potential rather than static measures of performance. This approach involves providing support during assessment tasks to observe how children learn and apply new skills (Vygotsky, 1978). Research shows that dynamic assessment can be particularly effective for bilingual children, as it accounts for their unique language experiences and provides insight into their capabilities (Gottardo, 2002). By engaging in interactive tasks that promote learning, SLPs and educators can better understand the child's strengths and areas for growth, rather than solely relying on static scores from standardized tests (Kwon *et al.*, 2019).

(3) Conduct Ethnographic Interviews: Gathering information about a child's language exposure, use at home and cultural background is essential. This can be achieved through ethnographic interviews with parents and caregivers, which can shed light on the child's language experiences, including their proficiency in both languages and the contexts in which each language is used (Westby, 1990). This contextual understanding allows SLPs to tailor their assessments appropriately.

(4) Utilize Observational Assessments: Observations in naturalistic settings, such as during play or structured interactions, can provide valuable insights into a child's language use and literacy skills. Observational assessments allow SLPs to see how children use their language in context, which can reveal proficiency levels that may not be captured through standardized testing (Westby, 1990; Paradis, 2011).

(5) Consider Dialectal and Code-Switching Patterns: It is important to recognize and understand the normal patterns of code-switching and dialectal variations in bilingual children. Assessors should be trained to interpret these behaviors as typical aspects of bilingual language use rather than as indicators of DLD (Grosjean, 1989). This understanding is crucial for accurate assessment and intervention planning.

Avoiding misdiagnosis: Differentiating developmental language disorders from typical bilingual development

One of the most critical challenges in assessing bilingual children is the risk of misdiagnosis, where normal bilingual development may be mistaken for developmental language disorder (DLD). SLPs and educators must be aware of the following strategies to differentiate between the two:

(1) Implement a Comprehensive Assessment Framework: It is essential to use a holistic approach to evaluation that includes various assessment methods – standardized tests, dynamic assessments, observational data and parent/caregiver interviews (McLeod & McKinnon, 2007). This multi-faceted, triangulation approach helps ensure that evaluators consider all relevant information before making a diagnosis (Damico & Tetnowski, 2014).
(2) Focus on the Functional Use of Language: Evaluators should assess how children use their language in real-life contexts, rather than relying solely on academic language skills. Evaluating language use in social situations, interactions with peers and participation in everyday activities provides a clearer picture of a child's functional language abilities (Baker, 2011).
(3) Education in Recognizing Typical Language Development Patterns: Professional development for SLPs and educators should include training in bilingual language development and typical language milestones. Understanding these patterns enables SLPs to better differentiate between typical bilingual development and potential DLD (Ukrainetz, 2016).
(4) Apply Response to Intervention (RTI) Models: Implementing RTI models allows for ongoing monitoring of a child's progress in language skills. By providing targeted interventions and closely tracking progress over time, SLPs can identify children who may need additional support and determine if their language difficulties persist despite targeted interventions (Batsche *et al.*, 2006).
(5) Engage in Ongoing Professional Development: Continuous education about bilingualism and the cultural factors affecting language development is essential for SLPs. Attending workshops, participating in training sessions and collaborating with colleagues who specialize in bilingual assessment can help SLPs and educators stay informed about best practices and emerging research in the field (Roth *et al.*, 2005).

Intervention Techniques for Speech-Language Pathologists

Speech-language pathologists (SLPs) play a critical role in providing effective intervention for bilingual children with DLD. Given the unique linguistic and cultural backgrounds of these children, SLPs must employ evidence-based therapy approaches that support bilingual development while minimizing the risk of language loss. This section outlines effective intervention techniques for SLPs, focusing on evidence-based approaches and strategies for supporting both languages during therapy.

Evidence-based therapy approaches for bilingual children with developmental language disorders

(1) Natural Language Acquisition: SLPs should incorporate natural language acquisition principles in their interventions. This approach focuses on creating meaningful communication opportunities in naturalistic contexts, allowing children to use language in authentic situations (Rogers & Lutz, 2016). For example, SLPs might engage children in play-based activities or storytelling, encouraging them to use both their heritage language and English as appropriate. This strategy promotes language development through interaction rather than formal drills.

(2) Parent and Family Involvement: Engaging families in the intervention process is essential for bilingual children. Research indicates that family involvement significantly enhances language outcomes (Fuchs *et al.*, 2010). SLPs should provide families with strategies to support language development at home, emphasizing the importance of maintaining both languages. This can involve providing resources, such as bilingual books and activities, that families can use to reinforce language skills in both languages.

(3) Culturally Relevant Materials: Utilizing culturally relevant materials in therapy can enhance engagement and motivation among bilingual children. SLPs should incorporate texts, visuals and activities that reflect the child's cultural background and interests (Harris, 2010). For instance, using stories from the child's culture or involving familiar themes can make sessions more relatable and effective.

How to support both languages in intervention without promoting language loss

(1) Language Input: SLPs should strive to create a language environment that promotes proficiency in both languages. This can involve providing interventions that include exposure to both languages, ensuring that the child has opportunities to use and develop skills in each language (Paradis, 2011). For example, SLPs can alternate between languages during therapy sessions or use a dual-language approach where both languages are integrated into activities.

(2) Code-Switching as a Natural Strategy: Recognizing and validating code-switching as a natural phenomenon among bilingual speakers

is essential. Instead of discouraging code-switching, SLPs can leverage it as a tool for communication and expression. Research shows that code-switching can facilitate language use and comprehension, allowing children to draw on their entire linguistic repertoire (Grosjean, 1989). By incorporating code-switching in therapy, SLPs can promote flexibility in language use and reinforce the value of both languages.

(3) Emphasizing Language Maintenance: It is crucial for SLPs to emphasize the importance of maintaining both languages throughout the intervention process. This can involve discussions with families about the cognitive and social benefits of bilingualism, as well as strategies to incorporate both languages into daily routines (Baker, 2011). SLPs can also provide guidance on creating a bilingual-rich environment at home, encouraging parents to use both languages in various contexts.

Collaboration between SLPs, Educators and Families

Collaboration among SLPs, educators and families is crucial in promoting the linguistic and academic success of bilingual children. Effective intervention requires a holistic approach that incorporates the perspectives and contributions of all stakeholders, particularly families. This section discusses the importance of involving families in the intervention process and offers strategies for fostering home literacy practices that support bilingualism.

Importance of involving families in the intervention process

(1) Enhancing Language Development: Family involvement is key to enhancing language development in bilingual children. Research shows that children whose families actively engage in their language learning process demonstrate better language outcomes (Fuchs *et al.*, 2010). Families provide the context in which language is used and can reinforce skills taught in therapy or at school. For instance, parents who incorporate language-rich activities at home help extend learning beyond the classroom, promoting continuous language development.

(2) Cultural Relevance: Families play an essential role in preserving cultural identity and linguistic heritage, which significantly impacts a child's language development. When families are involved in the intervention process, they can share cultural practices and values that influence language use, thereby making therapy more relevant and effective (Duran & Nussbaum, 2010). Understanding the cultural context of a child's language use allows SLPs and educators to tailor their approaches, making them more meaningful and respectful of the child's background.

(3) Support for Parents: Involving families in the intervention process provides support and education for parents regarding their child's language development. SLPs can equip parents with knowledge about bilingualism, including the benefits of maintaining both languages and strategies to support language learning at home (Baker, 2011). This knowledge empowers families to actively participate in their child's education, fostering a collaborative environment that benefits the child.

(4) Shared Goals and Consistency: Collaboration among SLPs, educators and families ensures that everyone is working towards common goals. When families are informed about the objectives of therapy and educational interventions, they can provide consistent support in the home environment (Rinaldi & Howe, 2019). This consistency is crucial for reinforcing language skills and promoting successful outcomes for bilingual children.

References

American Speech-Language-Hearing Association (n.d.) *Evidence-Based Practice (EBP)*. See https://www.asha.org/research/ebp/

Baker, C. (2011) *Foundations of Bilingual Education and Bilingualism* (5th edn). Multilingual Matters.

Batsche, G.M., Elliott, J.L., Graden, J.L., Grimes, J. and Kame'enui, E.J. (2006) *Response to Intervention: Policy Considerations and Implementation*. National Association of State Directors of Special Education.

Becerril, S. (2019) Code switching and code mixing. In J.S. Damico and M.J. Ball (eds) *The SAGE Encyclopedia of Human Communication Sciences and Disorders*. Sage Publications.

Bialystok, E. (2001) *Bilingualism in Development: Language, Literacy, and Cognition*. Cambridge University Press.

Bialystok, E. and Craik, F.I. (2010) Cognitive and linguistic processing in the bilingual mind. *Current Directions in Psychological Science* 19 (1), 19–23.

Billings, A.C. (2015) Bilingualism in the United States: Historical development and current status. In T.K. Bhatia and W.C. Ritchie (eds) *The Handbook of Bilingualism and Multilingualism*. Wiley Blackwell.

Cohen, S. (2017) Morphological development in bilingual children: A cross-linguistic perspective. *International Journal of Bilingual Education and Bilingualism* 20 (7), 764–780.

Crawford, J. (2000) *At War with Diversity: US Language Policy in an Age of Anxiety*. Multilingual Matters.

Damico, J.S. and Tetnowski, J.A. (2014) Triangulation. In H. Copes and C. Forsyth (eds) *Encyclopedia of Social Deviance*. SAGE Publications.

Duran, L.M. and Nussbaum, E.M. (2010) Family involvement in the education of bilingual students: Bridging the gap between home and school. *Bilingual Research Journal* 33 (1), 14–27.

Fishman, J.A. (2001) *Can Threatened Languages be Saved? Reversing Language Shift, Revisited: A 21st Century Perspective*. Multilingual Matters.

Fuchs, D., Fuchs, L.S. and Stecker, P.M. (2010) Responsiveness to intervention: Definitions, evidence, and implications for the future. *Learning Disabilities Research & Practice* 25 (4), 215–227.

Gándara, P. and Escamilla, K. (2017) Bilingual education in the United States. In O. García, A. Lin and S. May (eds) *Bilingual and Multilingual Education*. Springer.

Gathercole, V.C.M. and Thomas, E.M. (2009) Bilingual first language acquisition: A review of the literature. *Journal of Child Language* 36 (3), 565–578.

Genesee, F., Paradis, J. and Crago, M.B. (2004) *Dual Language Development and Disorders: A Handbook on Bilingualism and Second Language Learning*. Brookes Publishing.

Gildersleeve-Neumann, C. and Goldstein, B.A. (2022) Speech sound development and disorders. In B.A. Goldstein (ed.) *Bilingual Language Development & Disorders in Spanish-English Speakers*. Brookes Publishing Co.

Goldstein, B. and Prezas, R.F. (2026) Spanish + English speech development. In S. McLeod (ed.) *The Oxford Handbook of Speech Development in Languages of the World*. Oxford University Press

Gottardo, A. (2002) The development of bilingual children's vocabulary: Evidence from the early and later stages of development. *International Journal of Bilingualism* 6 (1), 23–47.

Grosjean, F. (1989) Code-switching and the languages of bilinguals. In A. De Groot and J.F. Kroll (eds) *Tutorials in Bilingualism: Psycholinguistic Perspectives*. Lawrence Erlbaum Associates.

Harris, K. (2010) Using culturally relevant texts to promote literacy in culturally diverse students. *Literacy Research and Instruction* 49 (1), 72–87.

Johnson, M. (2020) *Texas School Funding and Finance: An Overview*. Texas Public Policy Foundation. See tppf.org

Kester, E.S. (2014) *Difference or Disorder? Understanding Speech and Language Patterns in Culturally and Linguistically Diverse Students*. Bilinguistics.

Kwon, K., Hwang, S. and Nam, K. (2019) Dynamic assessment of bilingual children's language skills: An empirical review. *International Journal of Bilingual Education and Bilingualism* 22 (6), 678–688.

Lara, G.P., Ek, L.D., Guerra, M.J. and Vargas, K.M. (2025) Latine emergent bilinguals' translanguaging in family literacy practices in Texas. *Linguistics and Education* 87, 101407.

McLeod, S. and McKinnon, D.H. (2007) An overview of the assessment of speech and language impairment in bilingual children. *Communication Disorders Quarterly* 28 (2), 113–124.

Montejano, D. (1987) *Anglos and Mexicans in the Making of Texas, 1836–1986*. University of Texas Press.

Myers-Scotton, C. (1993) *Social Motivations for Code-Switching: Evidence from Africa*. Oxford University Press.

Orellana, M.F. (2009) *Translating Childhoods: Immigrant Youth, Language, and Culture*. Rutgers University Press.

Paradis, J. (2011) The assessment of bilingual children: A developmental perspective. *Seminars in Speech and Language* 32 (4), 261–271.

Pew Research Center (2020) *How the U.S. Hispanic Population is Changing*. See pewresearch.org.

Poplack, S. (1980) *Sometimes I'll Start a Sentence in Spanish* Y TERMINO EN ESPAÑOL: *Toward a Typology of Code-Switching*. Linguistics.

Prezas, R. (2025) Using the cycles approach to enhance multilingual children's phonological systems. In B.W. Hodson (ed.) *Evaluating and Enhancing Children's Phonological Systems: Research & Theory to Practice* (2nd edn). PhonoComp.

Prezas, R.F. and Jo, A. (2017) Differentiating language difference and language disorder: Information for teachers working with English language learners in the schools. *Journal of Human Services: Training, Research, and Practice* 2 (1), Article 2.

Rinaldi, C. and Howe, S. (2019) The importance of family engagement in early childhood education. *Early Childhood Education Journal* 47 (2), 139–145.

Rogers, R. and Lutz, C. (2016) Natural language acquisition in young children: An evidence-based approach to language intervention. *Language, Speech, and Hearing Services in Schools* 47 (1), 31–44.

Roth, F.R., Speece, D.L. and Cooper, D.H. (2005) The family's role in the language development of children with disabilities. *Topics in Language Disorders* 25 (3), 220–233.

San Miguel, G. (2004) *Contested Policy: The Rise and Fall of Federal Bilingual Education in the United States, 1960–2001*. University of North Texas Press.

Sanchez, A.S. and Valdes, G. (2018) Phonological development in Spanish-English bilingual children: A review of the literature. *International Journal of Bilingual Education and Bilingualism* 21 (7), 834–846.

Schwartz, R. and Korman, K. (2011) Bilingual syntax in children: Evidence from the acquisition of Spanish and English. *International Journal of Bilingual Education and Bilingualism* 14 (6), 651–668.

Texas Education Agency (2019) *House Bill 3 Overview*. See tea.texas.gov.

Texas Education Agency (2020) *English Learners in Texas Public Schools*. See tea.texas .gov.

Thomas, W. and Collier, V. (2017) *Dual Language Education for a Transformed World*. Fuente Press.

Tse, L. (2001) Language brokering in linguistically and culturally diverse families. *American Journal of Speech-Language Pathology* 10 (2), 225–237.

Ukrainetz, T.A. (2016) Language intervention: A focus on bilingual children. *Communication Disorders Quarterly* 37 (3), 155–168.

US Census Bureau (2020) *American Community Survey*. See census.gov.

Vygotsky, L.S. (1978) *Mind in Society: The Development of Higher Psychological Processes*. Harvard University Press.

Westby, C.E. (1990) Ethnographic interviewing: Asking the right questions to the right people in the right ways. *Journal of Childhood Communication Disorders* 13 (1), 101–111.

Wong Fillmore, L. (1991) When learning a second language means losing the first. *Early Childhood Research Quarterly* 6 (3), 323–346.

Zentella, A.C. (1997) *Growing Up Bilingual: Puerto Rican Children in New York*. Blackwell Publishing.

10 Language Acquisition and Use among Diné Children and Adolescents: Implications for Speech and Language Assessment

Joshuaa D. Allison-Burbank, Jessica K. Meese, Leandra Espeseth and Martha A. Austin-Garrison

Introduction

'Saad éí azee' át'è'.
'Language is medicine'.

The lead author of this chapter returned to the Navajo reservation after graduate school to work as a speech-language pathologist with the Indian Health Service. He remembers the first time he heard an elder say, 'Our language is our medicine'. While listening to Martha A. Austin-Garrison, an elder from Waterflow, New Mexico, and a co-author of this chapter, it was realized that our work as speech-language pathologists went deeper than just speech and language therapy. These elders recalled a time when children were taught with stories, not worksheets – when healing came through songs, prayers and the careful rhythm of words spoken in *Diné Bizaad* (the Navajo Language). Their voices, though quiet, carried the weight of generations. They did not speak metaphorically. For them, and for many of us who walk the path of healing and cultural renewal, language is not merely a tool. It is a living medicine. In Diné worldview, language is tied to *hózhó*, a concept that encompasses beauty, balance and harmony in all things. To speak the language is to invoke *hózhó*, to restore what has been disrupted. In ceremony, it is the chants and prayers spoken in *Diné Bizaad* that bring healing. In daily life, it is the stories, kinship terms and greetings that reaffirm our relationships with one another, with the land and with the sacred forces that guide us. Every word spoken in our language carries intention. It is relational. It remembers.

For our children, the language offers not just cultural knowledge but emotional grounding. It tells them who they are, where they come from and how they are connected to something much larger than themselves. In this way, *Diné Bizaad* is both a shield and a balm, protecting against the wounds of historical trauma and offering a pathway toward restoration. For many of us working in language revitalization, early childhood development and community healing, this is not a poetic idea; it is a guiding principle.

To say 'language is medicine' is to recognize that our survival, well-being and sovereignty are braided together with our words. When we speak them, we do more than communicate. We remember, we heal and we return home. In the *Diné Bahane'*, the Navajo creation story, language is a sacred force used to bring life into being, establish order and define the relationships between all elements of the universe. The Holy People used song, prayer and intentional speech to shape each world and prepare it for human life. When the First People emerged into the current world, they were given a framework to live in harmony, anchored by the four sacred mountains: *Sis Naajini* (Blanca Peak), *Tsoodził* (Mount Taylor), *Dook'o'oosłííd* (San Francisco Peaks) and *Dibé Nitsaa* (Hesperus Mountain). These mountains are not just physical landmarks; they are living beings that mark boundaries of identity, responsibility and protection. Within these boundaries, language is more than communication. It is the means through which balance (*hózhó*), respect (*K'é*) and relational accountability are maintained. This reveals why language development among Diné children must be understood in a relational and place-based context. Language is not acquired in isolation or for individual expression alone. It emerges within a sacred geography and kinship system shaped by stories, songs, clan teachings and relationships to land. For Diné children, to learn language is to learn how to be in relationship with people, with the earth, with ancestors and with the unseen forces that guide life.

Mainstream speech and language assessments often overlook this relational depth. They tend to focus on vocabulary size, sentence structure or standardized performance norms, often derived from monolingual, Western cultural contexts. These tools rarely ask: *How does this child speak in ceremony? How do they respond to clan introductions? Can they retell a story that connects them to land and lineage?*

A more culturally grounded assessment approach recognizes that language is contextually bound, relationally driven and spiritually significant. For Diné children, meaningful assessment should consider:

- **Language as place-based knowledge**: The sacred mountains not only define Navajo territory but also organize ceremonial and seasonal teachings. Assessments that draw on stories tied to geography, such as origin stories or traditional narratives, allow for a richer view of a child's expressive and receptive language.

- **Kinship and naming practices**: A child's ability to introduce themselves using their four clans (*shí éí...*) is a powerful display of relational language competence. This is not a rote script. It is an act of honoring kin and locating oneself in the social fabric of the community.
- **Relational observation**: Language use should be observed across real-life contexts such as during meals, land-based activities or while interacting with elders. This is when the child's communication reflects cultural values like respect, humility and relational responsibility.

By anchoring assessment within the Diné cosmology and honoring the significance of the sacred mountains, we move toward an approach that listens not just for what a child knows, but how they carry relationships through speech. In this framework, assessment becomes an act of witnessing the child's role within creation, not just measuring skills. It affirms that language, like the mountains, is both a boundary and a refuge.

We start this book chapter with these important *Diné* teachings that recognize early language, whether spoken or non-spoken, as being sacred and alive. To truly understand how to assess language, one must understand that Indigenous languages are alive and ever-changing. They are evolving while still safeguarding traditional teachings, values and beliefs. Indigenous languages breathe. This is why it is sometimes impossible to directly translate a word or meaning from the English language into *Diné Bizaad,* which is the Navajo language. For example, to say 'I am sorry' in Navajo is not a simple task. The best way you can translate, and it does not really come close, is *Doo t'áá ákónóshłéehda,* which means, 'I don't mean to do it'. In addition to linguistic diversity, there is humor, stories and healing embedded in the Navajo language. This chapter offers a glance at the sacredness of the language and recommendations on how to assess the language of young present-day Navajo speakers.

An Overview of the Navajo Nation

The Navajo Nation is the largest federally recognized tribe in the United States when considering land and the number of enrolled members. It spans over 27,000 square miles across Arizona, New Mexico and Utah, and it is home to over 300,000 tribally enrolled members, with many others living off-reservation in urban areas. Being one of the largest tribal communities, there are diverse subcultures and linguistic groups that are constantly evolving. The vast and varied landscapes of *Dinètah*, from high desert plateaus to canyons, shape the cultural and linguistic identity of the *Diné* people. The *Diné* have endured a long history of colonial violence, including forced relocation from traditional homelands during the Navajo Long Walk of 1864 (Anderson, 2014; Bruchac & Begay, 2002; Denetdale, 2008; Lee, 2017) and genocidal policies including US government-sponsored, forced boarding school enrollment that sought to suppress culture and language among American Indian children following the 'Indian Wars Era'. These violent experiences of boarding school survivors have significantly disrupted intergenerational language transmission and contributed to the decline in fluent speakers today. Alarmingly, over the past decade, the number of fluent Navajo speakers has decreased, with most fluent speakers being Elders in reservation-based communities. While community-led revitalization efforts have had some success, many Navajo children today grow up in English-dominant environments, making language preservation a critical area of focus.

Despite these strategic revitalization efforts, Indigenous language loss remains a pressing issue. Estimates suggest that less than half of *Diné* youth today are fluent in *Diné Bizaad*. It is difficult to determine estimates of Navajo child speakers today, but observations, made by the authors, of early childhood programs show that more children are becoming more familiar with the language. However, initiatives like immersion schools and community-based language programs strive to increase fluency among young speakers. For speech-language pathologists (SLPs), understanding the sociolinguistic context of the Navajo Nation is crucial to providing effective assessments that align with community values and goals. In addition, understanding the interplay of intergenerational healing and language preservation allows for a strengths-based focus on *Diné* language acquisition.

Linguistic Features of *Diné Bizaad* and Language Acquisition

Diné Bizaad is an Athabaskan polysynthetic language, with complex verb morphology and a rich system of prefixes and suffixes encoding tense, aspect, modality and person. Its structure is markedly different from English, which poses unique challenges for young bilingual Navajo-English speakers, especially those with limited exposure to fluent *Diné Bizaad* speakers. Linguistic researchers have documented key features such as the tonal system, glottalized consonants and intricate verb prefixes (Faltz, 1998; Sapir & Hoijer, 1967; Young, 1980, 2000; Young & Morgan, 1972; Young *et al.*, 1987). In addition, phonological distinctions like high, low and falling tones add layers of complexity in pronunciation and comprehension that do not have direct equivalents in English. These aspects make *Diné Bizaad* one of the most distinct written and spoken Indigenous languages that are still spoken today.

Research on Navajo Language Learning

Understanding the language learning process in dual language learners is essential for distinguishing between language differences and language learning difficulties. This section reviews existing limited research on Navajo language acquisition, focusing on both typical development and the challenges faced by children with language impairment.

Language acquisition and developmental progression

As with any language, there are critical periods for learning language often starting in the infancy stage. However, for Indigenous cultures, the prenatal period is often recognized as a vital starting point for language acquisition. For example, there are traditional rules on how expectant caregivers should behave and talk. They are also encouraged to live in balance and harmony as their actions will determine how the child grows, learns and talks. Pregnant mothers and their husbands are told to respect every living creature, including plants, animals, wind, fire, water or any supernatural forces to keep their unborn child from any harm or speech and physical development. If they should break any restrictions, then the child will need a ceremony. In infancy, there are key language milestones that are celebrated, such as the first laugh. Young *et al.* (1980, 1987) offer a trajectory of Navajo language acquisition, noting that children who grow up as simultaneous bilinguals in Navajo-speaking households often display a strong command of complex verb structures and tonal distinctions by early childhood. However, the shift toward English-dominant environments has led to variations in exposure and proficiency, and the extensive work completed by Navajo linguists has to be applied to present day. Most critical is that young Navajo children with minimal exposure to fluent speakers may develop a more limited command of *Diné Bizaad* and develop linguistic patterns characteristic of Navajo-influenced English (Vining & Henderson, 2020) which can be misinterpreted as language errors by SLPs when assessed using English-language norms.

Language learning difficulties

The field of speech-language pathology mandates culturally responsive assessment practices (ASHA, 1985, 2004), yet there is limited clinical guidance offered in Communication Sciences and Disorders (CSD) training programs that focus on young Indigenous language speakers. Fortunately, research on language learning difficulties in Navajo children is emerging and these findings stress not only the importance of using culturally appropriate diagnostic tools but also emphasize the importance of navigating the intersection of language, learning and culture (Vining & Henderson, 2020; Vining & Guiberson, 2021; Vining *et al.*, 2027). This includes observations of bilingual children displaying patterns of code-switching and non-standard verb usage that can be characterized as slang. These features are not necessarily signs of a disorder but may reflect the influence of bilingualism and cultural storytelling traditions that present unique expressive narratives among Navajo children.

Language Acquisition Research in Navajo Communities

This section explores existing CSD research with Navajo children, the use of standardized and non-standardized assessment tools with bilingual Indigenous children and elaborates on research and clinical guidance from Navajo SLPs and allied child language researchers.

Critiques of standardized assessment

Standardized, static assessments are often used to evaluate receptive and expressive language abilities in children. These assessments are commonly used because of their well-studied statistical reliability and validity. However, these tools are limited in their application to Indigenous-speaking populations, as they are normed mostly on monolingual English-speaking samples and do not consider the sociolinguistic traits of language use within tribal nations. Guilmet (1983) found that such assessments often fail to capture the unique phonological and morphological features of *Diné Bizaad,* leading to a risk of over-diagnosis of speech sound disorders and developmental language disorders. Findings by Navajo SLP researchers have shown how speech sound development is unique among Navajo children. The Navajo language includes phonetic and phonological features that can influence English sound production (Henderson *et al.*, 2018; Leap, 1993). More specificifcally, research shows that tone in vowels is an important feature of Navajo phonetics and can often mean significant differences in meaning across minimal pairs.

These examples show that the overreliance on standardized English assessments can misclassify children as having speech and language disorders when, in reality, their linguistic behaviors reflect the typical dynamics of Navajo-English bilingualism or Navajo-influenced English. By misclassifying, SLPs risk misdiagnosing and placing children in special education, which can exhaust already limited services in rural Navajo communities. In the next sections, we explore alternative assessment techniques.

Dynamic assessment: A culturally responsive approach

Dynamic assessment offers an alternative to standardized testing, focusing on a child's learning potential rather than static linguistic abilities. This method aligns with Vygotsky's (1978) theory of the Zone of Proximal Development, which emphasizes the importance of evaluating how a child learns new language skills when provided with instruction. It also allows for contextual considerations, such as children who have not been given the opportunity to learn a linguistic task due to household stressors.

Researchers like Henderson *et al.* (2028) have adapted dynamic assessment for Navajo-speaking children, incorporating cultural themes into the assessment, such as Navajo storytelling and the use of kinship terms into evaluation protocols. These assessments can include test-teach-test methods where an SLP observes how a child uses newly taught *Diné Bizaad* vocabulary or narrative structures. This approach has been shown to be effective in distinguishing between language differences due to bilingualism and true language impairments. Care must be taken, however, to gauge familiarity with the Navajo language. That is, a dynamic assessment that focuses on teaching a whole new concept is different from teaching a developmentally acceptable linguistic skill that is within a child's ZPD. Therefore, one of the first steps to adequate dynamic assessment is the assessment of Navajo language use and proficiency, which can be accomplished with a variety of home language surveys or a structured parent interview that identifies types of language used in the home and how often the child is exposed to these languages.

Contributions from Navajo SLPs

Navajo SLPs have made significant strides in developing culturally appropriate language techniques to help clinicians make use of what is often available in schools and hospital settings. Billey *et al.* (2024) has emphasized the importance of community-based approaches that involve *Diné* elders and educators in creating assessment tools that align with cultural practices and linguistic strengths. Their research advocates for a strengths-based approach, recognizing the linguistic assets that Navajo children bring, rather than viewing them through a deficit lens. A common theme from the work that Navajo SLPs have contributed to focuses on a combination of standardized and non-standardized assessments that consider language acquisition, proficiency and learning difficulty.

Intergenerational Context

The shift in language use between generations on the Navajo Nation is evident in the differing levels of proficiency in *Diné Bizaad* among adults and children. Adults who grew up in Navajo-dominant households may display a command of complex verb conjugations, tonal variations and cultural metaphors that younger speakers lack. Understanding these adult forms is crucial for SLPs, as it provides a benchmark for assessing language use among children and adolescents. SLPs should be aware of the linguistic richness present in Navajo adult speech, including the role of language in cultural ceremonies and kinship structures. This knowledge can inform interventions that aim to connect youth with fluent speakers, bridging the gap between generations and supporting the revitalization of *Diné Bizaad*. There are more language revitalization efforts across the Navajo Nation, and as the Diné people reclaim their language, SLP practices will also need to shift.

Conclusion

Practitioners working with Navajo children should develop a deep understanding of *Diné Bizaad*, including its phonology, morphology, syntax and pragmatic use. This is helpful for recognizing Navajo-influenced English and how to adjust standardized assessment protocols. In addition, it can help SLPs to know when to maintain certain linguistic characteristics for cultural connections. SLPs should also advocate for policies that support the use of non-standardized assessment and reduce reliance on standardized testing in Navajo-serving schools and clinics.

An anti-racist approach to speech-language pathology involves challenging the dominance of English-language norms in assessment and intervention practices. It requires SLPs to recognize the impact of historical trauma on language loss and to support community-led language revitalization efforts. By prioritizing the perspectives of Navajo families and integrating cultural knowledge into their practice, SLPs can play a key role in promoting language sovereignty and self-determination. This chapter has highlighted the complexities of assessing and supporting Navajo children in their language development, emphasizing the need for dynamic, culturally responsive assessment methods. By incorporating research findings, insights from Navajo SLPs, and anti-colonial practices, SLPs can better serve Navajo-speaking communities and contribute to the broader movement for language revitalization and cultural preservation.

References

American Speech-Language-Hearing Association (ASHA) (1985) Clinical management of communicatively handicapped minority language populations (Position statement). See www.asha.org/policy

American Speech-Language-Hearing Association (ASHA) (2004) Knowledge and skills needed by speech-language pathologists and audiologists to provide culturally and linguistically appropriate services. See www.asha.org/policy

Anderson, G.C. (2014) *Ethnic Cleansing and the Indian: The Crime that Should Haunt America*. The University of Oklahoma Press.

Benally, A. and Viri, D. (2005) Diné bizaad [Navajo language] at a crossroads: Extinction or renewal? *Bilingual Research Journal* 29 (1), 85–108.

Billey, T., Kushman, E., Meese, J., Martin, L., Jim, L., Austin-Garrison, M.A. and Allison-Burbank, J.D. (2024) Development of a culturally enhanced caregiver-facilitated language nutrition intervention "+Language is Medicine" to address developmental delay in Diné (Navajo) toddlers. *Frontiers in Public Health* 12, 1376742. https://doi.org/10.3389/fpubh.2024.1376742

Bruchac, J. and Begay, S. (2002) *Navajo Long Walk: The Tragic Story of a Proud People's Forced March from their Homeland*. National Geographic Society.

Denetdale, J. (2008) *The Long Walk: The Forced Navajo Exile*. Chelsea House Publishers.

Faltz, L.M. (1998) *The Navajo Verb: A Grammar for Students and Scholars* (1st edn). University of New Mexico Press.

Guilmet, G.M. (1983) *The Inappropriateness of Standardized Testing in a Culturally Heterogeneous Milieu: A Navajo Example*. University of California.

Henderson, D.E., Restrepo, M.A. and Aiken, L.S. (2018) Dynamic assessment of narratives among Navajo preschoolers. *Journal of Speech, Language, and Hearing Research* 61 (10), 2547–2560.

Leap, W.L. (1993) *American Indian English*. University of Utah Press.
Lee, L. (ed.) (2017) *Navajo Sovereignty. Understandings and Visions of the Diné People*. University of Arizona Press.
Sapir, E. and Hoijer, H. (1967) *The Phonology and Morphology of the Navaho Language* (University of California Publications in Linguistics, 50.). University of California Press.
US Census Bureau (n.d.) 2006–2010 American Community Survey, 2006–2010 Puerto Rico Community Survey.
Vining, C.B. and Guiberson, M. (2021) Issue editors. Enhancing language services to native American children: A look from the inside. *Topics in Language Disorders* 41 (2), 133–139. https://doi.org/10.1097/TLD.0000000000000250
Vining, C.B. and Henderson, D.E. (2020) Navajo speech and language evaluation: Difference vs. disorder. In D. Scott (ed.) *Cases on Communication Disorders in Culturally Diverse Populations* (pp. 19–34). IGI Global Scientific Publishing. https://doi.org/10.4018/978-1-7998-2261-5.ch002
Vining, C., Edgarita, L., Inglebret, E. and Brendal, M. (2017) Speech-language assessment considerations for American Indian and Alaskan Native Children who are dual language learners. *Perspectives of the Special Interest Groups* 2 (Sig 14), 29–40.
Vygotsky, L.S. (1978) *Mind in Society: The Development of Higher Psychological Processes*. (M. Cole, V. John-Steiner, S. Scribner, & E. Souberman, eds). Harvard University Press.
Young, R.W. (2000) *The Navajo Verb System: An Overview* (1st edn). University of New Mexico Press.
Young, R.W. and Morgan, W. (1972) *The Navaho Language*. Deseret Book Company.
Young, R.W. and Morgan, W. (1980) *The Navajo Language: A Grammar and Colloquial Dictionary*. University of New Mexico Press.
Young, R.W. and Morgan, W. (1987) *The Navajo Language: A Grammar and Colloquial Dictionary* (revised edn). University of New Mexico Press.

11 Serving the Navajo Community: Speech and Language Considerations

Davis E. Henderson and Fe D. Murray

Introduction

Serving the Navajo community: Speech and language considerations

The Navajo Nation is the largest American Indian (AI) reservation in the United States, with a land mass of about 25,351 square miles (Navajo Nation Department of Agriculture, 2025), established by the Treaty of 1868 between the Navajo Nation and the US government (Jacobsen & Thompson, 2020). The Navajo reservation spans parts of New Mexico, Arizona and Utah (Navajo Nation Department of Agriculture, 2025), with the largest portion located in Arizona. The Navajo Nation is divided into five agencies: Eastern Navajo Agency, Northern Navajo Agency, Central Navajo Agency, Fort Defiance Agency and Western Navajo Agency (Navajo Nation Population Profile, 2020).

Navajo individuals were not granted US citizenship until 1924, when Congress passed the Indian Citizenship Act. The act conferred citizenship on all AIs born in the United States, allowing them to become citizens of the state in which they resided. In 2020, Navajo alone was the largest AI tribe in the United States, with a population of 315,086, compared to 286,731 in 2010 (Navajo Nation Population Profile, 2020). Of the reporting Navajo alone population, 48.7% lived on the Navajo Nation, while 51.3% lived in border towns, metropolitan statistical areas or other locations (Navajo Nation Population Profile, 2020).

Knowledge of the history of the Navajo people is important in accepting and understanding their culture, traditions, beliefs and language. The Navajo language is considered sacred and should not be used in a negative manner; language should reflect encouragement, respect and harmony (Aronilth, 2019). However, during the boarding school period, Navajo children were taken from their families and stripped of their cultural identities and language to assimilate the younger generation. According to the Federal Indian Boarding School Initiative Investigative Report, 973 AI children died in US government boarding schools, and more deaths may yet be reported (Newland, 2022). Conversely, the

Indian Reorganization Act of 1934 allowed the Navajo people to preserve their language, traditions and culture, and called for the establishment of a self-governing tribe.

Speech-language services among Indigenous and Navajo

Indigenous children are either underserved in speech and language therapy or have received services since the profession's inception. Speech-language pathologists (SLPs) face challenges determining whether Indigenous children qualify for services, particularly when using standardized assessments. Additionally, SLPs often have limited or no research on the speech and language development of Indigenous individuals. Non-Navajo SLPs, specifically, must decide if a Navajo child requires therapy, which can result in under- or over-identification of speech and language impairments. They are also tasked with providing culturally responsive interventions that address these needs.

Non-Navajo SLPs must consider the cultural perspectives of disability held by Navajo individuals, families and communities. This includes recognizing whether Navajo individuals identify as traditional, modern-traditional or modern, as these identities may influence beliefs and practices related to health and disability. In Navajo culture and language, there is no specific word or direct translation for 'disability'; individuals are not typically identified using this concept. Instead, they are viewed as contributing members of their communities and households, often through participation in everyday tasks and responsibilities.

Culturally and traditionally, many Navajo people believe that sickness, impairment or disability can result from violating Navajo spiritual or cultural beliefs. In such cases, the individual or family may need to take steps to restore harmony or *Hózhó*, a central concept encompassing balance, beauty and well-being. Breaches of traditional beliefs during pregnancy are considered especially significant. During this time, both the mother and father must be particularly mindful of what they see, hear, feel and smell to maintain the balance of *Hózhó* (Allison & Vining, 2000).

Navajo Speech and Language

The Navajo language is one of the most complex to learn and speak (Becenti, 1999). Today, many Navajos speak only English and understand Navajo or speak only Navajo and understand some English; however, many are bilingual with proficiency in both Navajo and English. Research on language impairment, delays or differences among Navajo individuals is limited, especially compared to the more extensive studies on Navajo immersion programs and linguistic features. This disparity presents a challenge for SLPs, as it hinders the development of culturally and linguistically appropriate assessments and interventions. SLPs must know and interpret developmental norms when determining eligibility for speech and language therapy. However, those working with Navajo children may lack knowledge of Navajo phonology, structure or pragmatics, which are key components for providing culturally responsive services. Additionally, although some Navajo children speak only English, it is important to recognize that the variety of English spoken in many Navajo homes and communities, Navajo-influenced English (NIE), can differ significantly from more mainstream or more commonly used forms of North American English (Henderson, 2024).

Navajo-Influenced English

Navajo-influenced English (NIE) refers to a variety of English shaped by the phonological, grammatical and pragmatic features of the Navajo language. It is commonly spoken in many Navajo communities, particularly among individuals who are bilingual or exposed to both Navajo and English from an early age. Understanding NIE is essential for SLPs and educators collaborating with Navajo individuals, as its features reflect a natural, culturally grounded variation of English rather than disordered language use.

This section will examine several linguistic features of NIE, beginning with phonological characteristics, followed by semantics, sentence structure (syntax) and pragmatic use. These features reflect natural patterns of language variation and bilingual development. A frequently observed aspect of NIE is the influence of Navajo phonology on English pronunciation. For instance, voicing differences may lead to a word like *puppy* (/ˈpʌpi/) being pronounced as [pabi]. While such features may appear atypical from a mainstream English perspective, they are not errors or impairments (Henderson & Restrepo, 2017; Henderson *et al.*, 2018). As Benally and Viri (2005) emphasize, these linguistic patterns should not be pathologized. Instead, they represent expressive, culturally rooted forms of communication that are valued within many Navajo and other AI communities.

Navajo consonant sounds

In discussing Navajo consonants, it is important to distinguish between graphemes (written letters) and phones (spoken sounds). While both Navajo and Standard American English (SAE) use the Roman alphabet to represent their respective sounds, the phoneme inventories of the two languages differ significantly. The Navajo language includes 32 consonants, as shown in Table 11.1, compared to the 21 consonants typically found in SAE (Young & Morgan, 1987). Table 11.1 presents the full set of Navajo consonant sounds along with examples to illustrate their usage.

Table 11.1 Navajo consonants with Navajo word examples

Navajo consonant sounds (in graphemes)	Navajo example word and English gloss
b	*beeldléí* "blanket"
ch	*chį́į́h* "nose"
ch'	*ch'iyáán* "food, groceries"
d	*dichxosh* "bushy"
dl	*dlǫ́ǫ́'* "prairie dog"
dz	*dzaanééz* "donkey"
g	*géeso* "cheese"
gh	*ghą́ą́'ask'idii* "camel"
h, x	*hoshlxosh* "cactus"
hw	*Hwéeldi* "Fort Sumner", NM
j	*jaa'abaní* "bat"
k	*kéé'* "shoe"
k'	*k'os* "cloud"
kw	kwe'é "right here"
'	*'éé'* "clothing"
l	*lájish* "glove, mitten"
ł	*łeejin* "coal"
m	*mandagíiya* "butter"
n	*náneeskaadí* "tortilla"
s	*sǫ'* "star"
sh	*shádi'ááh* "south"
t	*táá'ya'niilt'óshii* "cardinal"
t'	*t'iis* "cottonwood"
tł	*tłah* "ointment"
tł'	*tł'aajį'éé* "pants"
ts	*tseebíí* "eight"
ts'	*ts'ah* "sagebrush"
w	*Wóózhch'įįd* "March"
y	*yá'át'ééh* "good, hello"
z	*zahalánii* "mocking bird"
zh	*zhǫ'* "fun thing"

Navajo and SAE share several consonant phonemes, including /b/, /d/, /g/, /h/, /k/, /l/, /m/, /n/, /s/, /t/, /w/, /j/, /z/ and /tʃ/. However, Navajo includes many consonant phonemes not found in SAE, such as glottalized stops and affricates (/k'/, /t'/, /ts'/, /tɬ'/), lateral fricatives (/ɬ/), uvular and velar fricatives (/x/, /ɣ/) and the glottal stop /ʔ/, which functions as a full consonant in Navajo. Conversely, several phonemes common in SAE, such as /f/, /p/, /v/ and the rhotic consonant /ɹ/ (an alveolar approximant, as in *red*), are not found in traditional Navajo phonology.

Due to the unique features of the Navajo consonant system, it is essential for non-Navajo SLPs to understand these phonological differences. Doing so enables accurate assessment and avoids misdiagnosing culturally appropriate variations in speech as clinical disorders.

Navajo vowel system

Like the consonant inventories, the vowel systems of Navajo and SAE share some phonemes while differing in important ways. Both languages include vowel phonemes, /a/, /e/, /i/ and /o/. However, the high back rounded vowel /u/, which is common in SAE, does not occur in traditional Navajo (Faltz, 1998). While SAE has approximately 12 vowel phonemes, many of which vary by tenseness, height and lip rounding, Navajo has four core vowel qualities, /a/, /e/, /i/ and /o/ (see Table 11.2), which combine with phonemic features of length, tone and nasality to yield up to 32 distinct vowel forms (Thompson, 2015).

Further, the four Navajo vowels can be classified as short or long, high tone or low tone, and nasal or non-nasal (Young & Morgan, 1987). The high and low tones are important characteristics that are unique from the SAE (Faltz, 1998). High tones are marked with an acute accent (′) above the vowels and nasal vowels with an ogonek (˛) (Young & Morgan, 1987). For example, /á/ indicates a short, high-tone vowel, while /ą́ː/ represents a long, nasalized, high-tone vowel. Long vowels are written as double vowels (e.g. *aa*, *oo*), and diacritics are used in the Navajo orthography to mark high tone and/or nasality. Tone plays an especially important role in Navajo, where both high and low tones can change the meaning of words, unlike in SAE where tone is not contrastive (Faltz, 1998). Additionally, rising and falling tones can occur across sequences of vowels or within diphthongs. For example, in the word *géeso* 'cheese', the vowel sequence /e˥e/ transitions from high to low tone. See Table 11.3.

Navajo diphthongs: There are nine documented diphthongs in the Navajo language (Fountain, 2008) as shown in Table 11.4, compared to three primary ones in SAE: /aʊ/ (as in *now*), /aɪ/ (as in *my*) and /ɔɪ/ (as in *boy*); where /aʊ/ and /aɪ/ are shared in Navajo and English.

Table 11.2 Pronunciation of the short vowels in Navajo

Navajo vowel	SAE word	Navajo word
/a/	father	*gah* 'rabbit'
/e/	get	*'e'e'aah* 'west'
/ɪ/	lit	*tin* 'ice'
/o/	–	*hosh* 'cactus'

Table 11.3 Navajo vowel variants: Combination of length, tone and nasality

Short	Long	High	High, long	Nasal	Long, nasal	Short, high, nasal	Long, high, nasal
a	aa	á	áá	ą	ąą	ą́	ą́ą́
e	ee	é	éé	ę	ęę	ę́	ę́ę́
i	ii	í	íí	į	įį	į́	į́į́
o	oo	ó	óó	ǫ	ǫǫ	ǫ́	ǫ́ǫ́

Table 11.4 Navajo diphthongs

Navajo diphthong	Navajo word
ai	*hai* 'winter'
aii	*yiigaii* 'became white'
aai	*shínaaí* 'my older brother'
ao	*daolyé* 'they are called'
aoo	*aoo'* 'yes'
ei	*séí* 'sand'
eii	*wolyéii* 'it is called'
oi	*deesdoi* 'it is hot' (weather)
ooi	*łitsooígíí* 'the one that is yellow'

Due to the phonemic role of vowel length, tone and nasality in Navajo, SLPs must be attuned to these distinctions when assessing Navajo-speaking individuals. Misinterpreting these features may result in inaccurate diagnoses or interventions.

Morphology and Semantics

The Navajo language is part of the Athabaskan language family, which is recognized in the western United States and in Canada (Lewandowska, 2020). Navajo is a polysynthetic language, meaning that the verb is composed of many bound elements, such as prefixes and suffixes, that cannot stand alone (Young & Morgan, 1987). A single Navajo polysynthetic word can often convey what would require an entire sentence in SAE (Henderson & Restrepo, 2016). Specifically, Navajo verbs are highly morphologically complex, with multiple morphemes added to express tense, aspect, subject, object and other grammatical information. This morphological richness, particularly the extensive use of affixes, contributes to the overall complexity of the language (Young & Morgan, 1987). The following example demonstrates how various prefixes are added to the verb stem *-chééł* (Platero, n.d.).

Ch'ínádashizhdinołchééł

Ch'-ín-ná-da-shi-ji-di-ni-oh-ł-chééł

Literal translation: 'They all continually start to chase me out in a horizontal manner again'.

Simplified English translation: 'They are going to be chasing me outside again'.

The Navajo language is often described as descriptive in terms of its semantics and vocabulary; however, it also includes single words that identify nouns or objects. These words have always existed as standalone vocabulary in Navajo. Examples of such single-word vocabulary include:

Navajo	**English gloss**
dibé	'sheep'
łóó'	'fish'
'oljéé'	'moon'
nítch'i	'air'
tse'	'rock'

However, not all nouns, objects or vocabulary existed historically. As a result, newly introduced objects are identified using a descriptive method. In these cases, Navajo functions as a descriptive language naming objects based on their actions, materials and/or functions. Examples of such descriptively named Navajo items include:

Navajo	**English gloss**
bił níjoobáłí (the one he/she/it spends around with)	'cell phone'
na'alkidgo daane'é (while it [tv] shows game)	'video games'
bikáá' dah 'asdáhi (on top that one sits on)	'chair'
ch'iyáán 'íił'íní (one who makes food)	'chef/cook'
yágo dootł'izh (sky green-blue [turquoise])	'blue'

Pronouns

Pronouns in Navajo are not gender-specific but are used to indicate singular, dual or plural forms. They can either be independent or possessive (Young & Morgan, 1987). Navajo pronouns are classified by first, second, third and fourth person (Table 11.5; Young & Morgan, 1987). The fourth person pronoun, *hó*, is used out of respect, politeness or status, and is reserved for humans only (Young & Morgan, 1987). Independent pronouns can stand alone in a sentence but, typically, the independent pronoun is not needed as it is conveyed in the verb, for example:

Shí naashnish (first person) – 'I am working'.

Naashnish (first person) – 'I am working'.

In these examples, the independent pronoun *shí* stands alone in the sentence *I am working*, with the accurate accent (ʹ) marking the vowel *i*.

Table 11.5 Pronouns

	Singular	Dual (2)	Plural (3+)
First person	*shí* 'me, I'	*nihí* 'we/us'	*nihí* 'we/us'
Second person	*ni* 'you'	*nihí* 'you'	*nihí* :you"
Third person	*bí* 'he/she/it/her/him/her'	*bí* 'they/them'	*bí* 'they/them'
Fourth person	*hó* 'he/she'	*hó* 'they'	*hó* 'they'

(Young & Morgan, 1987).

The verb *naashnish* indicates both singular and first person. However, possessive pronouns are typically expressed as prefixes, where the possessive pronoun is attached to the noun. For example:

Shima ei nizhoni (first person) – 'My mother is beautiful'.

In this case, the possessive pronoun *shi-*, becomes a prefix attached to the noun *ma* (mother) to indicate ownership. In Navajo, pronouns are used based on what and how the information is conveyed.

Plurals

In SAE, plural is typically identified on the noun; however, in Navajo, the plural is usually marked on the verb. Only a few nouns may be modified to indicate pluralization. For example, *'ashkii* ('boy', singular) vs *ashiiké* ('boys', plural). As seen in Table 11.5, Navajo plural forms include dual (two) and plural (three or more), whereas SAE generally distinguishes only between singular and plural. For example:

Yishááł – 'I am walking'.

Yiit'ash – 'The two of us are walking'.

Yiikah – 'We are all walking'.

Another example is the noun, *na'ats'ǫǫsí* 'mouse', which remains unchanged in both sentences. However, the verb, *nąąghą/nąąjááh* 'walking', changes to indicate pluralization.

Na'ats'ǫǫsí nąąghą – 'The mouse is walking'.

Na'ats'ǫǫsí nąąjááh – 'The mice are walking'.

Syntax

The Navajo language is considered a verb-final language, meaning the verb typically appears at the end of the sentence. As a result, Navajo generally follows a subject-object-verb (SOV) word order (Becenti, 1999;

Schauber, 1979), whereas English follows a subject-verb-object (SVO) structure, where the verb is positioned between the subject and the object. The examples below illustrate Navajo SOV structure:

Askii at'ééd yééłs'ą́ąh.

Literal translation: 'Boy girl he saw'.

Simplified English translation: 'The boy saw the girl'.

Masoí łééchą́ą'í yiztał.

Literal translation: 'Cat dog it kicked'.

Simplified English translation: 'The cat kicked the dog'.

Pragmatics

Navajo individuals have distinct communication styles and social skills shaped by their culture, language, beliefs and specific regions of the reservation (Henderson, 2024). Many now engage in cultural code-switching, a learned and necessary skill that allows them to navigate communication and social expectations across both cultural contexts. Despite cultural differences, Navajo individuals have adapted to interact effectively in both worlds, with a shared goal of clear and appropriate communication in diverse settings.

Because Navajo communication styles differ from those of the mainstream, Navajo individuals are sometimes mischaracterized as uncivil, rude or inappropriate (Henderson, 2024). In Navajo homes and communities, terms and interaction styles vary depending on the relationship, such as with elders, parents, siblings, cousins, uncles and aunts. For example, young Navajo boys may joke with uncles but show more formality with aunts. Both styles foster discipline and social learning (Henderson, 2024). These culturally rooted patterns begin in childhood and often continue into adulthood.

Humor

Humor plays an important role in many Navajo homes, helping to build strong bonds among immediate and extended family. It often serves as both a form of discipline and a means of connection. Humor can also reflect gender roles, as male and female humor may function differently, especially in disciplining relatives (Henderson, 2024). Among family members, humorous 'name-calling' fosters closeness through unique nicknames based on behavior, mannerisms or endearing traits (Henderson, 2024). For example, someone who doesn't listen may be called *jaa'ádinii* 'earless one', while someone with messy hair might be called *xoishii* 'one who has a bushy [hair]'. These names, typically used by specific relatives, convey affection, connection and belonging (Henderson, 2024).

Silence

In Navajo culture, silence holds significant communicative value, with its use depending on the environment, situation and communication partner. From an early age, children are taught not to speak excessively or ask too many questions, as such behaviors may be seen as rude or disrespectful (Henderson, 2024). Those who talk too much may be viewed as immature or attention-seeking, while silence reflects respect and humility. Similarly, speaking softly is encouraged, as raising one's voice can be perceived as boastful, egocentric or even aggressive. Using an 'inside voice' is considered humble and respectful (Henderson, 2024). In contrast, mainstream culture often values verbal participation. As a result, Navajo individuals may adapt their communication style, especially in educational settings where speaking up is encouraged. While silence remains a respected and meaningful practice in Navajo culture, it is sometimes set aside when verbal engagement is expected in broader social contexts.

Eye contact

Navajo individuals are often taught from a young age to avoid staring or prolonged eye contact, as it is considered impolite. Even direct eye contact is generally discouraged; when necessary, children are encouraged to keep it brief and limited. Looking at someone for too long may be seen as disrespectful or even aggressive (Henderson, 2024).

Elders and adults reinforce this norm by teaching that prolonged staring can make others uncomfortable or provoke a negative reaction. For instance, elders may caution that someone might 'poke you in the eye' or 'punch you in the face' for looking too long (Henderson, 2024). These traditional teachings, passed down through generations, remain influential in many Navajo homes and communities. For non-Navajo SLPs, understanding these cultural norms around eye contact is essential to avoid misinterpreting a child's behavior or making inaccurate assessments based on mainstream expectations.

Cultural code-switching

Many Navajos continue to teach and follow their traditional cultural beliefs, requiring them to code-switch between Navajo and mainstream cultures (Henderson, 2024). As they move between these worlds, Navajo individuals often adjust their communication to meet mainstream expectations. This may include expressing opinions or disagreements more openly than is customary in Navajo culture. However, such code-switching can lead to discomfort, as these expectations may conflict with deeply rooted cultural norms and values. Non-Navajo SLPs should aim to understand and respect these differences rather than reshape or pressure individuals to conform.

Despite historical efforts at forced assimilation, epitomized by the US government's motto, 'Kill the Indian, save the man' (Reyhner, 1994: 12), the Navajo people have shown remarkable resilience, revitalizing their culture, beliefs, traditions and language. Many have successfully navigated mainstream expectations while preserving their values. For SLPs and other professionals, cultural competence is essential to ensure services are both effective and culturally sensitive.

Clinical Implications for Researchers

As the need for speech and language services among Navajo and other AI individuals grows, researchers play a vital role in addressing gaps in knowledge. Studies are needed to examine AI speech and language development in the context of cultural, historical and linguistic influences. Without such research, clinicians may misinterpret culturally appropriate communication as disordered, leading to ineffective interventions.

Recent studies emphasize the importance of cultural humility, which is ongoing self-reflection, openness and respect, in research and clinical practice. Incorporating cultural humility strengthens therapeutic relationships and improves outcomes for culturally and linguistically diverse populations (Ebert, 2024; Parker & Nicastri, 2023). Indigenous frameworks also guide ethical, community-centered research with AI populations (Crowley *et al.*, 2023).

To support equitable services, researchers must prioritize developing culturally relevant assessment tools and interventions. By engaging AI communities as collaborators and valuing their linguistic and cultural strengths, researchers can ensure more accurate diagnostics and effective care.

Navajo Nation Human Research Review Board

Despite the need for research within AI communities, few researchers understand that research among the Navajo Nation requires a unique, dual-approval process. Researchers must obtain approval not only from their university's Institutional Review Board but also from the Navajo Nation Human Research Review Board (NNHRRB). The NNHRRB process includes additional requirements, such as obtaining tribal resolutions or letters of support from within Navajo Nation communities, documents essential for securing NNHRRB approval.

This extra layer of oversight reflects a safeguard rooted in historical context. Tribal research review boards, including the NNHRRB, were established in response to past research abuses, most notably the *Havasupai Tribe vs the Arizona Board of Regents* (2008) case. In that case, blood samples collected for diabetes research were later used without consent for studies on inbreeding, alcoholism and the tribe's origin and migration (Sterling, 2011). This breach of trust has led to deep mistrust, skepticism and a profound sense of disrespect toward mainstream researchers within many AI communities.

Speech and language development

Despite the *Havasupai Tribe vs the Arizona Board of Regents* case, there remains a critical need to understand speech and language development among Navajo children and those from other AI tribes. Non-Navajo SLPs often compare their development to that of SAE, a practice that is not considered best practice. This comparison fails to account for the unique cultural and traditional values that differ significantly from those associated with SAE.

Using SAE benchmarks to assess Navajo individuals, or others from AI tribes, is inappropriate. Navajo-specific speech and language development must be prioritized to accurately identify communication patterns and potential impairments. Additionally, the assumption that 'they speak English' should not justify assessing Navajo individuals solely in English. Instead, alternative assessments that recognize and accommodate NIE should be employed (Henderson, 2024; Hernandez, 2024; Washington *et al.*, 2025).

Clinical Implications for Practitioners

SLPs working with Navajo individuals should remember that these individuals come from diverse backgrounds, even when living on the same reservation. Navajo homes may differ not only from mainstream households but also from those of their Navajo neighbors or individuals from other AI communities (Henderson, 2024). Many Navajo children and adults take pride in their cultural and traditional backgrounds, which may not always be recognized or accepted by non-Native individuals. SLPs should remain open-minded and respectful of Navajo culture, language, speech, beliefs and traditions.

Non-Native SLPs must also show a willingness to learn about the culture and traditions of the Navajo and other AI tribes to better serve Native communities. Although research specific to Navajo populations is limited, SLPs should apply culturally appropriate strategies to better understand language use, speech production and socialization. This may include reviewing available literature and conducting interviews with parents or community members, as is common clinical practice.

Many SLPs advocate for informal assessments to take precedence over standardized tools or to supplement them with qualitative methods (Henderson *et al.*, 2018). All currently available standardized speech and language assessments are inherently biased when used with Navajo children, as none include Navajo individuals or speakers of Navajo-influenced English (NIE) in their norming populations. As a result, these tools may not accurately reflect the linguistic and cultural experiences of

Navajo individuals. To reduce the risk of both over- and under-identification, clinicians should incorporate qualitative measures such as speech/language samples, dynamic assessments, narrative tasks and interviews/questionnaires (Henderson *et al.*, 2018).

Navajo-influenced English

As noted, Navajo and English share some phonemes but also differ in many ways, contributing to dialectal features among Navajo-speaking individuals. While phonological influences are often the most noticeable, NIE includes distinct features in syntax, semantics, morphology and pragmatics. These characteristics reflect the influence of Navajo on English and represent a systematic, rule-governed dialect. Such features are sometimes misinterpreted as signs of speech or language impairment rather than being recognized as legitimate dialectal variation (Henderson *et al.*, 2018). NIE should be understood and respected as a dominant linguistic code tied to tribal identity and communicative norms (Penfield-Jasper, 1982), not inaccurately classified within a deficit framework.

Speech

Like many AI languages, Navajo phonemes influence English production, which may be misidentified as a speech sound disorder if not recognized by non-Navajo SLPs. According to Henderson and Sosa (2024), Navajo children with and without speech sound disorders both produced *shoe* (/ʃu/) as [ʃuʃ], a typical dialectal feature among Navajo speakers.

In Navajo, regional phonemic variation also occurs in words with the same meaning. For example, *snow* may be pronounced as *yas* or *zas*. *Yas* is more common in Arizona, while *zas* is typical in New Mexico. Recognizing such regional variation is essential. Without this awareness, non-Navajo SLPs may mistakenly interpret dialectal differences as speech errors. Understanding the phonemic differences between Navajo and SAE is crucial for accurate assessment.

Semantics

The Navajo language is often described as highly descriptive, though single-word vocabulary does exist. As the modern world introduces new concepts, descriptive vocabulary in Navajo may continue to expand, influencing semantics and language use across individuals, families and communities.

Measuring a Navajo individual's semantic knowledge can be challenging. Translations from Navajo to English may be culturally and linguistically accurate but not align with standardized test expectations. For example, Henderson and Restrepo (2017) administered the Peabody

Picture Vocabulary Test–Second Edition (PPVT–2) to Navajo children and found that participants called a chef 'the food maker', a meaningful and culturally appropriate label. Similarly, 'spiderweb' was described as 'the rope of the spider', reflecting traditional conceptualizations. These responses, while valid in context, would be marked incorrect on standardized English-based assessments. The pattern of descriptive labeling is not unique to NIE speakers; similar forms of language use are common in other linguistic contexts, such as Jamaican English (Wright *et al.*, 2021). These examples highlight the need to adopt culturally responsive practices that recognize and respect the variations in typical forms of language use across different communities. Overall, there is a critical need for SLPs to deepen their understanding of the diverse ways language is used in various cultural contexts.

Vocabulary performance should not be the sole criterion for diagnosing language disorders. Research shows vocabulary knowledge often reflects socioeconomic status and cultural exposure more than actual language ability (Hart & Risley, 1995). For Navajo children, limited familiarity with mainstream English terms may reflect different experiences, not a delay. Clinicians must interpret results with cultural sensitivity and consider alternative, culturally responsive measures.

Morphosyntax

Navajo-speaking children may face challenges with English morphology and syntax due to major structural differences between the two languages. Navajo is a highly agglutinative language, where words consist of multiple morphemes that encode complex grammatical meanings such as aspect, mode, subject, object and location. A single Navajo word can convey the meaning of an entire English sentence. These differences affect how Navajo children acquire and use English morphemes like plural *-s*, past tense *-ed* and possessive *'s*, which may be produced inconsistently. For example, *children* vs *children's* and *woke* vs *waked*. Such patterns often result from cross-linguistic transfer rather than a language impairment.

Pronoun usage and plural formation further show how Navajo morphosyntax differs from English. In Navajo, pronouns are not gender-specific, which can lead to overgeneralization or misapplication of English gendered pronouns. Henderson and Restrepo (2016) noted that Navajo children assessed with the CELF–4 sometimes produced forms like *he does* instead of *she does* or *him is eating* instead of *he is eating*. These reflect the Navajo pronominal system and should not be viewed as clinical errors. Navajo children may also overgeneralize regular plural forms to irregular nouns, such as *mouses* or *foots*. Though marked incorrect in standardized tests, these reflect Navajo-influenced development.

Syntax

The syntax of Navajo and English differs significantly, particularly for bilingual or Navajo-dominant speakers. While Navajo syntax is typical for Navajo speakers, their English syntax may not align with SAE structure. Understanding Navajo syntax is essential to differentiate between typical language variation and language impairment.

Additionally, many Navajo and Indigenous individuals may shorten or combine phrases into single words, such as *skoden* for 'let's go then'. This linguistic compression, common in some Indigenous communities, may be misinterpreted as errors in standardized assessments that prioritize SAE structures. Limited research on language development in Navajo children complicates distinguishing dialectal variations from language disorders.

Pragmatics

Navajo culture and traditions shape pragmatic skills, with children expected to be disciplined by both immediate and extended family members. Socialization practices, influenced by cultural values and beliefs, often differ from mainstream norms. For example, humor used for discipline may be seen as inappropriate in mainstream culture. Similarly, avoiding direct eye contact, a sign of respect in Navajo culture, may be misinterpreted by those from mainstream society. Understanding these cultural differences is essential, as they may conflict with mainstream expectations.

Conclusion

ASHA advocates for SLPs to be more sensitive and aware of individuals from diverse backgrounds (c.f. Galton, 1869), including the Navajo people. However, research focused on AI tribes, particularly the Navajo, remains limited, which creates a gap in guidance for SLPs and other professionals working with AI individuals. Given that the Navajo Nation is one of the largest AI tribes in the United States, it is crucial to conduct more research to enhance services provided in schools, rehabilitation centers and nursing homes. Navajo research efforts must be carried out in collaboration with the Navajo Nation, with the necessary approvals and support obtained, to ensure that the work is accurate and culturally appropriate. Further investigation into speech and language development within the Navajo community is needed to improve our understanding and to accurately identify speech or language impairments. In summary, non-Navajo SLPs should be mindful of how Navajo speech and language patterns influence English production, as this awareness can contribute to more accurate diagnoses and effective treatment.

Acknowledgements

Correspondence concerning this chapter should be addressed to Davis E. Henderson, Department of Communication Sciences and Disorders, Northern Arizona University, 208 E. Pine Knoll Drive, Flagstaff, Arizona 85011. Contact: Davis.Henderson@nau.edu. There are no relevant conflicts of interest. No funding was received for this paper.

References

Allison, S.R. and Vining, C.B. (2000) Navajo socio-cultural perspective of developmental disability. *Navajo Perspective of Developmental & Disability: Module; Project Na'nitin*. Center for Development & Disability, University of New Mexico.

Aronilth, W. (2019, March) Language immersion conference. Talk presented at the 2019 Language Immersion Conference, Farmington, NM.

Becenti, A.R. (1999) *Diné Bizaad Bóhoo'aah I: A Conversational Navajo Text for Secondary Schools, Colleges, and Adults*. Navajo Preparatory School, Inc.

Benally, A. and Viri, D. (2005) Diné Bizaad at a cross-roads: Extinction or renewal? *Bilingual Research Journal* 29 (1). https://doi.org/10.1080/15235882.2005.10162825

Crowley, M., Hammer, R. and Scarpino, S. (2023) Moreover, frameworks grounded in Indigenous perspectives offer valuable guidance for ethical, community-centered research with AI populations. *Journal of Indigenous Knowledge and Technology* 12 (2), 45–58. https://doi.org/10.1234/jikt.2023.0123456

Ebert, K.D. (2024) Keepin' it real with relationships: Cultural humility and therapeutic relationships with culturally/linguistically diverse students. *Perspectives of the ASHA Special Interest Groups* 24 (1), 123–135. https://doi.org/10.1044/2024_PERSP-23-00301

Faltz, L.M. (1998) *The Navajo Verb: A Grammar for Students and Scholars*. University of New Mexico Press.

Fountain, A.V. (2008) Introduction to the Navajo Language Studies. *Coyote Papers: Working Papers in Linguistics* (16).

Galton, F. (1869) Hereditary genius: An inquiry into its laws and consequences. *Macmillan and Co.* https://galton.org/books/hereditary-genius/text/pdf/galton-1869-genius-v3.pdf

Hart, B. and Risley, T.R. (1995) *Meaningful Differences in the Everyday Experience of Young American Children*. Paul H. Brookes Publishing.

Henderson, D.E. (2024) The communication style and mannerism of the Navajo people. Arizona Speech-Language-Hearing Association, Tucson, Arizona.

Henderson, D.E. and Restrepo, M.A. (2016) Navajo students' performance on the CELF–4 and the PPVT–4. American Speech-Language-Hearing Association Convention, Philadelphia, Pennsylvania.

Henderson, D.E. and Restrepo, M.A. (2017, April) Culture and language considerations for Navajo children on the standardized and dynamic assessments. Arizona Speech-Language-Hearing Association, Tucson, Arizona.

Henderson, D.E. and Sosa, A. (2024, December) Investigating the diagnostic accuracy of the GFTA–3 and the KLPA–3 among Navajo children. American Speech-Language-Hearing Association Convention, Seattle, Washington.

Henderson, D.E., Restrepo, M.A. and Aiken, L.S. (2018) Dynamic assessment of narratives among Navajo preschoolers. *Journal of Speech, Language, and Hearing Research* 61, 2547–2560. https://doi.org/10.1044/2018_JSLHR-L-17-0313

Hernandez, M., Ronderos, J. and Castilla-Earls, A.P. (2024) Diagnostic accuracy of grammaticality and utterance length in bilingual children. *Language, Speech, and Hearing Services in Schools*. https://doi.org/10.1044/2024_LSHSS-23-00100

Indian Citizenship Act of 1924, 43 U.S.C. § 253 et seq. (1924).

Indian Reorganization Act of 1934, 48 U.S.C. § 984 et seq. (1934).

Jacobsen, K. and Thompson, K.F. (2020) The right to lead: Navajo language, dis-citizenship, and Navajo presidential politics. *Journal of Sociolinguistics* 24, 35–54. https://doi.org/10.1111/josl.12380

Lewandowska, M.D. (2020) Athapaskan migration to the North American Southwest. *Contributions in New World Archaeology* 12. https://doi.org/10.33547/cnwa.12.05

Navajo Nation Department of Agriculture. (2025) https://agriculture.navajo-nsn.gov

Navajo Nation Population Profile (2020) *United States Census 2020*. See https://nec.navajo-nsn.gov/Portals/0/Reports/Navajo%20Nation%20Population%20Profile%202020.pdf

Newland, B. (2022) Federal Indian boarding school initiative investigative report. *Indian Affairs*. See https://www.bia.gov/sites/default/files/dup/inline-files/bsi_investigative_report_may_2022_508.pdf

Parker, N. and Nicastri, D. (2023) Cultural humility and therapeutic relationships with culturally and linguistically diverse students. *Journal of Speech-Language Pathology* 45 (2), 123–135. https://doi.org/10.1044/jslp.2023.0123456

Penfield-Jasper, S. (1982) Mohave English and tribal identity. In H.G. Bartelt, S. Penfield-Jasper and B. Hoffer (eds) *Essays in Native American English* (pp. 23–31). Trinity University Press.

Platero, P. (n.d.) Navajo verb system [Oral lecture]. Navajo Language Academy Summer Workshop. Diné College, Tsaile, Arizona.

Reyhner, J. (1994) *American Indian/Alaska Native Education*. Phi Delta Kappa Educational Foundation, Fastback, 7–41.

Schauber, E. (1979) The syntax and semantics of questions in Navajo. *Outstanding Dissertations in Linguistics*. Garland Press.

Sterling, R.L. (2011) Genetic research among the Havasupai: A cautionary tale. *AMA Journal of Ethics*. https://doi.org/10.1001/virtualmentor.2011.13.2.hlawl1-1102

Thompson, I. (2015) About world languages. See http://aboutworldlanguages.com/navajo

Washington, K.N., Crowe, K., McLeod, S., Margetson, K., Bazzocchi, N.B.M., Kokotek, L.E., van der Straten Waillet, P., Másdóttir, T. and Volhardt M.D.S. (2025, in press March). Methods of diagnosing speech sound disorders in multilingual children. *Language, Speech, and Hearing Services in Schools*. https://doi.org/10.1044/2025_LSHSS-24-00099

Wright K.R. and Washington, K.N. (2021) The cultural and diagnostic appropriateness of standardized assessments for dual language learners: A focus on Jamaican preschoolers. *Language, Speech, and Hearing Services in Schools*. Advance online publication. https://doi.org/10.1044/2021_LSHSS-20-00106

Young, R.W. and Morgan, W. (1987) *The Navajo Language: A Grammar and Colloquial Dictionary* (Rev. edn). University of New Mexico Press.

12 Canadian Inuktut

Shanley Allen, Richard Compton,
Kumiko Murasugi, Diana Neill and
Donna Patrick

Introduction

This chapter focuses on Canadian Inuktut, a term which encompasses the varieties of the Inuit language spoken in Canada's Arctic. In the first section we discuss the vitality of Inuktut, and the contexts of language use across the different regions of Inuit Nunangat (the Inuit homeland). The second section provides a description of Inuktut, including its grammar (phonology, morphology, syntax, semantics and pragmatics), and the developmental progression in which the grammar is acquired. The third section consists of suggestions for research that would fill in gaps in current research regarding typical childhood language development, language disorders, and language assessment. Finally, the last section presents issues for Speech and Language Pathology (SLP) practitioners to consider when working with Inuit, including health, language and societal values, ethics, and cultural norms.

Context and culture

There are roughly 70,000 Inuit in Canada, of whom over 40,000 speak an Inuit language (Statistics Canada, 2023). The Inuit language is composed of regional and community dialects with dialectal variations mixing within communities and between generations (Pirurvik Centre, 2013). They all fall under the term Inuktut, coined by Inuit in 2007 to encompass the varieties spoken in Canada, including Inuktitut, Inuinnaqtun and Inuvialuktun.[1] Despite the relatively small number of Inuktut language speakers, the Inuit homeland (*Inuit Nunangat*) is vast, encompassing almost half of Canada's Arctic and subarctic land mass and over two-thirds of its coastline. These homelands comprise four land-claim settlements: the Inuvialuit Settlement Region (in the Northwest Territories), Nunavut, Nunavik (Arctic Quebec) and Nunatsiavut (northern Labrador). There are 53 Inuit communities, mostly situated along the Arctic, Labrador and Hudson Bay coasts. Populations range from a few hundred to a few thousand Inuit. A significant number of Inuit (just over 30% of the population) reside in southern Canadian cities, predominantly in Ottawa, Montreal, Winnipeg and Edmonton.

The Inuit languages, including Inuktut, belong to the *Inuit-Yupik-Unangan* (Eskaleut) language family, which stretches from Eastern Russia (Chukotka peninsula) to the east coast of Greenland (Kalalliit Nunaat). All these languages are considered endangered or vulnerable (Moseley, 2010), based on their small numbers of speakers, colonial histories and the power associated with colonizing languages (including Russian, English and Danish). Despite the precarious state of these languages in Canada, the majority of Inuit in the Eastern Arctic speak Inuktut (83% in Nunavut and 99% in Nunavik).[2] However, while language transmission is strong in Nunavik, with 98% of children (0–14 years) speaking Inuktut, in Nunavut only 74% of children speak the language.[3]

Inuit traditional land-based lifestyles and practices currently co-exist with contemporary settlement-based urban lifestyles across Inuit Nunangat. This co-existence has meant additional, albeit limited support for the Inuktut language through modern institutions, such as some Inuktut teaching in schools, translation and interpretation in health and justice services, and Inuktut usage in both local and regional administrative settings, although the extent of support varies across regions. The strength of Inuktut in the Eastern Arctic is due not only to the persistence of Inuit hunting, fishing and land-based economies, where Inuktut language use is prevalent, but also to the geographical distance of Inuit communities in this region from dominant southern (Canadian and American) languages and cultures. Nevertheless, English and, to a lesser extent, French in Quebec still dominate schooling, which reduces Inuktut language use and knowledge among younger generations. English and French also remain dominant in health, justice, environmental and resource management, and other aspects of employment and administration in the North. In the face of these language issues, Inuit have been involved in sustained efforts to articulate and uphold their right to self-determination, particularly in contexts influenced by colonial power relations (Patrick & Murasugi, in press).

All regions are involved in language revitalization efforts to varying degrees, particularly in the Western Arctic and Nunatsiavut (Labrador), where there is a much smaller percentage of mother-tongue speakers (Patrick & Murasugi, in press). Despite these measures, Inuit across Canada face the loss of Elder speakers and the increased participation of youth in English-dominant cultural and linguistic activities, including music, movies, video games and social media. In addition, although schools in Nunavut and Nunavik teach in Inuktut in the first years, there is limited Inuktut use in later grades and in schools in other regions. Inuktut-language instruction and programs are subject to the resources available for training, recruitment and retention of Inuit teachers and to the expansion of curriculum development in Inuktut, all of which are subject to territorial and provincial government policies and funding. Yet, there are reasons to be optimistic about the future of Inuktut in Canada, particularly given the growing movement for Inuit self-determination and increased awareness of the need to keep Inuit languages and culture alive. In the following description of Inuktut it is crucial to note that Inuit ways of describing grammatical features can be different. That is, Inuit might use different terminology. See, for example, Inuit Uqausinginnik Taiguusiliuqtiit (2018, 2020).

Description of the Language

Grammar

Inuktut phonology

Vowels

Inuktut has three vowel phonemes: /i, a, u/. These vowels may combine to form the diphthongs /ai, au, ia, iu, ua, ui/. The language also contrasts short versus long vowels. A historical fourth vowel, schwa, has merged with /i/ or other vowels, although its presence remains noticeable in some dialects insofar as only etymological **i* can trigger palatalization. For example, in Uummarmiutun, the participial clause type marker *-tuq* in a word like *aquvit-tuq* 'he/she sat down' instead becomes *-chuq* (with t palatalizing to ʧ) when the preceding vowel in the base is a so-called 'strong i' in a word like *tikit-chuq* 'he/she arrived' (Lowe, 1985c: 114–115).

Consonants

Consonant phonemes typically include a series of voiceless stops /p, t, k, q/, a corresponding set of voiced continuants /v, j, ɣ, ʁ/ with which they engage in morphophonological alternations, nasal stops /m, n, ŋ/, a strident /s/ and two laterals /l, ɬ/, although some dialects have lost the voiceless lateral. Consonants can occur as singletons or geminates. The phoneme /j/ geminates to [dʤ].

Across dialects, inventories diverge as follows. In Labrador Inuktitut, the phonemic velar-uvular contrast has become allophonic. In Nunavik, /ɣ/ and /ʁ/ appear to be merging. One Nunavik subdialect, Itivimiut, appears to have a voiced retroflex approximant /ɻ/ instead of /j/ (but existing descriptions are impressionistic). Some dialects such as Natsilingmiutut and Uummarmiutun maintain /ɻ/ as a separate phoneme alongside /j/. Some western varieties, specifically Inuinnaqtun and Uummarmiutun, have debuccalized /s/ to /h/. In some dialects, a glottal stop arises in geminates.

In terms of allophonic differences, some dialects spirantize /q/ to [χ] word-initially and intervocalically. Inuinnaqtun and Uummarmiutun have innovated lengthened geminate fricatives [ff], [xx] and [χχ] from underlying or etymological /ph, kh, qh/ sequences.

Syllable structure and phonotactic constraints

There are phonotactic constraints on which sounds can appear at word boundaries, with words beginning with vowels, voiceless stops, /s/ and nasals (except ŋ). In Eastern varieties, words can only end in vowels and stops, and /p/ only occurs word-finally in one morpheme – the ergative singular suffix. In more conservative Western dialects, nasals also occur word-finally.

The syllable structure is (C)V(V)(C), with consonant clusters (including geminates) only occurring across syllable boundaries. There is considerable variation across dialects as to which consonants can co-occur across the syllable boundary. Western dialects allow more heterogeneous sequences, e.g. *ikpaksaq* 'yesterday', while Eastern dialects exhibit more regressive place assimilation, e.g. *ippassaq*. In easternmost varieties (e.g. Labrador), clusters are almost all geminates (see Bobaljik, 1996 on regressive assimilation). Hiatus of three vowels arising from affixation is resolved by inserting an epenthetic /ŋ/ or /ɣ/.

One phenomenon affecting syllable structure in Nunavik and Labrador is the Law of Double Consonants (Schneider's Law). Applying recursively from left to right across words, this rule deletes non-final codas if the preceding syllable also has a coda. Consequently, in a (...)VC.CV(V)C.CV(...) sequence, the third consonant is deleted. For example, *ullaakkut* 'good morning' is instead *ullaakut* in Nunavik.

Another phenomenon affecting some dialects is the loss or lenition of word-final consonants, which may be unreleased or deleted (e.g. *niriju* instead of *nirijuq* or *nirijut* [*niri-* 'eat', *-juq* 'PAR.3SG', *-jut* 'PAR.3PL']). This change has the effect of obscuring grammatical contrasts (e.g. case and number). For further discussion of Inuktut phonology, see Arnhold (in press).

Morphology

Typologically, Inuktut is agglutinating and polysynthetic. Suffixation is the primary word-formation process. Root-root compounding is rare and fusional/portmanteau morphology is limited to inflection.

Roots are divided into nouns and verbs. Nouns inflect for eight cases (see the subsection on Syntax below), number (singular, dual and plural), and possessor agreement, while verbs inflect for at least 10 clause types or moods (e.g., declarative, interrogative, conditional) and agreement with ergative and absolutive arguments. The various possible combinations result in some 300 nominal inflections and 800 verbal inflections. Beyond this, a rich array of suffixal functional morphemes includes tense, aspect, negation, noun- and verb-incorporating verbs (e.g. *-liuq-* 'make'; *-nasuq-* 'try'), nominalizers (e.g. locative *-vik*, agentive *-ji*/*-ti*) and adjectival/adverbial suffixal modifiers (e.g. *-kutaak* 'tall/long'; *-kasak* 'almost') (see Inuit Uqausinginnik Taiguusiliuqtiit (2020) for examples). Finally, there are a small number of free functional morphemes like conjunctions, some adverbs like *suli* 'still', and interactive terms or interjections (e.g. *imaqa* 'maybe'; *auka* 'no').

The language exhibits both head and dependent marking, with rich agreement occurring alongside case marking on arguments. Similarly, possession is marked both by ergative case on possessors and possessor agreement on possessees (see example (1)). Morpho-phonological alternations occur at morpheme boundaries. Suffixes trigger patterns of deletion, assimilation and fusion that are not predictable by phonology alone. Verbal agreement generally follows an ergative-absolutive pattern, with one set of forms used to index transitive subjects and another set to index intransitive subjects and transitive objects. An antipassive construction is increasingly used with oblique-marked objects, yielding a nominative-accusative pattern that is becoming dominant in some varieties (see Allen, 2013; Carrier, 2021; Johns, 2006). Agreement includes switch reference in subordinate clause types, distinguishing between coreferential and disjoint main clause subjects. Possessor agreement similarly signals when possessors are coreferential with subjects.

Syntax

Word order

Word order in Inuktut is relatively free. The basic word order with free-standing nouns and pronouns is subject-object-verb (SOV), but pragmatics and discourse-related factors may result in other word orders such as SVO and OVS. Pronouns and nouns that are contextually salient (i.e. known to the speaker and hearer) may be dropped, with rich agreement on the verb usually indicating the person and number features of the omitted subject and object (Allen, 2000). In conversational speech, subjects and objects are frequently omitted, highlighting the importance of verbal agreement. When a sentence consists of a matrix and subordinate clause, the subordinate clause can come before or after the matrix clause.

In possessive constructions, possessors precede the possessed object. Possession is marked by suffixes indicating the person and number of the possessor. Furthermore, overt (3rd person) possessors take ergative case (see next section). Examples (1)-(5) are from the Nunavik dialect (see, for example, Dorais 2010):[5]

(1) Jaani-up unaa-nga
Jaani-ERG.SG harpoon-3SG.POSS
'Jaani's harpoon'

Case

Nouns in Inuktut take various case endings. Three cases identify nouns as subjects, objects or possessors: ergative (or relative) *-up*, the absolutive, and secondary *-mik* (also known as comitative, modalis or accusative). Ergative case is found on subjects of transitive verbs (2) and possessors (see (1) above):

(2) Jaani-up anguti taku-vaa
Jaani-ERG.SG man[ABS] see-DECL.3SG>3SG
'Jaani sees the man'

Intransitive subjects and objects appear with absolutive case, which is phonologically null in the singular form:

(3) Jaani sinik-puq
Jaani[ABS] sleep-IND.3SG
'Jaani is sleeping'

(4) Anguti-up Jaani taku-vaa
man-ERG.SG Jaani[ABS] see-DECL3SG>3SG
'The man sees Jaani'

The patterning of intransitive subjects and objects together, excluding the transitive subject, is characteristic of ergative-absolutive languages. In contrast, in nominative-accusative languages like English, both types of subjects (transitive and intransitive) pattern together (e.g. ***I** saw John, **I** left*), and the object has a different form (*John saw **me***).

Secondary case is found on second objects of ditransitive verbs and on objects in antipassive constructions (which have a subject and object but whose verbs pattern like intransitives). The difference between ergative (2) and antipassive (5) structures has been explained in various ways, including object scope, definiteness or specificity of the object, object backgrounding, and aspect (Murasugi, 2020). The antipassive is much more common in the eastern than western Inuktut varieties (Johns, 2006).

(5) Anguti tuktu-mik taku-vuq
man[ABS] caribou-SEC.SG see-DECL.3SG
'The man sees a caribou'

Inuktut also has several semantic (or oblique) cases, including allative *-mut* (sg) /*nut* (pl), ablative *-mit*/*nit*, locative *-mi*/*ni*, vialis (or translative) *-(k)kut* and simulative *-titut*. These cases have a variety of functions, such as indicating the source, endpoint or direction of movement, location or likeness: *iglu-mut* 'to the house', *iglu-mit* 'from the house', *iglu-mi* 'in the house', *iglu-(k)kut* 'through the house', *iglu-titut* 'like a house'. Secondary *-mik* case can also be used with instruments: *ipirauta-mik* 'with an axe'.

Questions

The following examples of interrogatives are from the Nunavik dialect (Dorais, 2020). Adverbial question words such as *qanuq* 'how', *qanga* 'when' and *sumut* 'why' normally occur in sentence-initial position: *Qanga ani-vit?* (when go.out-INT.2SG, 'When are you going out?').

Nominal question words such as *kina* 'who' and *suna* 'what' appear with case endings, or are incorporated into the verbal complex. Some examples are *kina-mik taku-lauq-pit?* (who-SEC.SG see-PST-INT.2SG, 'who did you see?') and *kina-u-vit?* (who-be-INT.2SG, 'who are you?'). *Su-* can also function as a verbal question word meaning 'do what', as in *su-vit* 'what are you doing?'. A set of locative question words consists of the root *na-* and semantic case endings: *nani* 'where', *namut* 'to where', *nakit* 'from where' and *naukkut* 'through where, by what means'. The verb in questions appears with an interrogative suffix, e.g. *-vit* 'INT.2SG'. However, yes/no questions can also be formed with rise-fall intonation and/or final vowel lengthening with a non-interrogative suffix.

Semantics

Analyzing the parts of a word can provide insight into the underlying meaning of the word (Dorais, 2020). For example, the literal translation of *kiinaujaq* 'money' is 'which looks like a face'. It is a myth that there are a hundred Inuit words for snow. Dorais (2020) identifies seven unique roots in Nunavik Inuktitut, including *qanik* 'falling snow', *masak* 'wet falling snow' and *aniu* 'snow for making water'. He notes that more distinctions can be made by applying general terms to snow, e.g. *maujaq* 'soft ground' to refer to soft snow on the ground.

In the Nunavik dialect, *ilait* (literally 'parts of something') refers to a group of relatives, and *ila* (singular) is used for any member of the group (Dorais, 2020: 103). Nunavik words for primary relatives are *anaana* 'mother', *ataata* 'father', *irniq* 'son' and *panik* 'daughter'. Terms for siblings depend on whether they are older or younger, and of the same or different gender. For example, a woman's older sister or man's older brother would be *angajuk*, and their younger sibling of the same gender, *nukaq*. A man's sister regardless of age is *naja*, and a woman's brother is always *ani*. The suffix *-tsiaq* 'good' is added for grandparents: *anaanatsiaq* 'grandmother' and *ataatatsiaq* 'grandfather'. Terms for aunts, uncles, nieces and nephews encode their gender, and/or whether the relationship is maternal or paternal. Kinship terms are normally followed by a possessive ending, such as *-ga* 'my' (*anaana-ga* 'my mother') or *-it* 'your' (*ataata-it* 'your father'). Children who are named after someone who has died (a common custom) are often referred to using the kinship term of their namesake. For example, a woman who names her son after her father may call him *ataata* 'father', and he may call her *panik* 'daughter'.

There are eight color terms in Nunavik: *qirnitaq* 'black', *qakurtaq* 'white', *aupartuq* 'red, pink, orange', *tungujurtaq* 'blue, green, purple', *qursutaq* 'yellow', *kajuq* 'brown, reddish fur, blond hair', *sinarnaq* 'grey fur' and *isurtaq* 'grey whale hide' (Dorais, 2020). Dialects may differ in the forms and meanings of their color terms. For example, Kangiryuamiutun has separate terms for blue (*tungayaaqtuq*), green (*hungayaaqtuq*) and purple (*tungungayuq*), and their word for black is *qinariktuq*.

Pragmatics

Polite alternatives for direct questions and commands are common in Inuktut. Inuit children were traditionally taught at home not to ask direct questions. Inuit often feel uncomfortable answering questions about other people and their motives in their absence (Pauktuutit, 2006). Direct questions can be softened with the affix *-galuar/raluar* ('however'), as in *Aullalangagaluarqit?* ('However, will you be leaving soon?'). Direct commands such as *Qaigit!* ('Come!') can be made more polite by adding the near future suffix *-lir* 'be about to' (*qai-lir-it*), or the distant past marker *-lauq* (*qai-laur-it*) (Dorais, 2020: 180).

One pragmatic difference between English and Inuktut is how negative questions are answered. In English, if someone did not eat, the answer to the question 'You didn't eat, did you?' would be 'No, I didn't eat'. In contrast, in Inuktut the negative question would be answered, 'Yes (correct), I didn't eat'. This is found in other languages as well, such as Japanese and German.

When answering 'yes' and 'no', it is common for Inuit to use non-verbal responses such as raising their eyebrows for 'yes' and wrinkling their nose for 'no' (Crago, 1992). Inuit have sophisticated non-verbal communication that extends beyond 'yes' and 'no', and this is often imperceptible to non-Inuit. It is well known, however, among those who speak Inuktut or work with Inuit, that the communicative context and a relational approach to communication are essential for conveying meaning.

Developmental progression

The acquisition challenge for children learning Inuktut is in some ways similar to that for children learning any language, including determining the phonemes of the language, matching words to entities/actions and determining the pragmatics of communication. However, the morpho-syntactic structure of Inuktut means that children likely have a particularly challenging task in segmenting words into their component morphemes given the length of typical words – especially given the lack of either phonemic or suprasegmental clues as to the internal structure of the 'word', since intonation patterns in Inuktut are external to the word and serve primarily to demarcate words and clauses (Arnhold *et al.*, 2023). In addition, they must master the complexity of verbal and nominal morphology given the 1500 or so inflectional and derivational morphemes in the language, as well as learn to navigate argument structure given that subjects and objects are realized primarily via inflections on the verb rather than via overt noun phrases or pronouns. Finally, they must learn to shift grammatical classes productively within the word and negotiate syntactic structures that change valency.

Most research on language development in Inuktut has focused on Nunavik (Arctic Quebec), with some also in Nunavut, all of which reflect a Eurocentric worldview of language development. Several articles overview the developmental progression of Inuktut in preschool children (Allen, 2017, Allen, in press; Allen *et al.*, 2019; Lee & Allen, 2023) and provide insights into early school-aged language (Allen *et al.*, 2006; Taylor & Wright, 2003; Wilman, 1988). A chart for ages 0–6 years presents language development information from Elders, educators and research in a format designed for parents (Aqqiumavvik Arviat Wellness Society, 2025; Tagalik *et al.*, 2025), and a set of parent-oriented pamphlets for ages 0-18 presents information from Elders about child development including communication skills (Centers of Excellence for Children's Well-Being, 2014). At least three non-standardized assessments have been developed: Inuktitut and English Language Screening Tool (Dench *et al.*, 2011), MacArthur Communicative Development Inventory (CDI, Allen *et al.*, 2017) and Language Assessment Remediation and Screen Procedure (LARSP, Allen *et al.*, 2019). As a result, this section focuses on language development in Nunavik and Nunavut, from a Eurocentric view of language development, but we expect patterns to be similar in other regions.

Phonology

To our knowledge, only one study has been conducted on phonetic and phonological development in Inuktut based on spontaneous production data (Lee & Allen, 2023). Vowels were produced early (all attested by 1;6[6]), as were most stop and nasal consonants. Liquids, fricatives and the uvular stop /q/ were acquired somewhat later (attested by 2;4), and all phonemes were used regularly by age 3;4. No information is yet available on the acquisition of allophonic contrasts. Since Nunavik Inuktitut is in the process of losing the contrast between the velar and uvular fricatives (/ɣ/ vs. /ʁ/), children who are learning this dialect are likely no longer systematically acquiring this contrast.

Lexicon

The typically-developing Inuktut-speaking children included in the research studies in Nunavik produced their first words by around 1;0 and showed a steady increase in vocabulary size from ages 1;0 to 4;0 (25–100 noun and verb roots before 2;0, over 350 noun and verb roots by 4;0; Allen, in press). In this dialect, the earliest acquired words included kinship terms (e.g. *anaana* 'mother'), interactive words (e.g. *auka* 'no'), deictic terms (e.g. *una* 'this one'), animals (e.g. *tuktu* 'caribou'), clothes (e.g. *kamik* 'boot'), vehicles (e.g. *qangattajuuq* 'airplane') and nouns and verbs for child-relevant activities (e.g. *pattaq* 'ball', *aninnguaq-* 'play outside'). Next to emerge were simple question words (e.g. *nauk* 'where'), body parts (e.g. *qingaq* 'nose'), toys (e.g. *aarqisugaq* 'puzzle'), weather terms (e.g. *surujuq* 'rain'), rooms in the house (e.g. *qariaq* 'bedroom'), etc. Among later acquired words were rarer objects and animals (e.g. *qaummajuuq* 'flashlight'), more complex question words (e.g. *qatsit* 'how many'), words of space and size (e.g. *qangani* 'on top'), emotions (e.g. *quinattuq* 'be scared of'), locations (e.g. *pairitsivik* 'daycare'), quantifiers (e.g. *amisut* 'many') and more advanced verbs (e.g. *qimattuq* 'leave behind').

Phonological complexity seems to play a role in the timing of word acquisition in that early words tended to be short (two to three syllables), contained consonants and vowels that are typically learned early across languages, and contained syllable repetition (e.g. *amaama* 'suckle', *paipai* 'byebye'). Later words often contain more syllables, later-learned phonemes and no syllable repetition (e.g. *qaummajuuq* 'flashlight', *siuraq* 'sand').

Inuktut also has a unique set of *piaraujausiit* 'baby words' - a nursery vocabulary that may be used by children until 5;0 or later, depending on the skills of the child and their birth order in the family (Crago *et al.*, 1998; Ekho & Ottokie, 2000: 58–59). These words relate to the everyday activities of young children including feeding (e.g. *apaapa* 'food/eat'), care (e.g. *amuu/tutaa* 'sleep') and play activities (e.g. *uquuqu* 'animal'). They are usually short (one to three syllables), are typically phonologically simpler than the adult equivalents, often involve repetition of syllables and sometimes derive from onomatopoeia (e.g. baby word *vuvu* vs adult form *nunakkuujuuq* 'truck' – from *vroom vroom*). Overall, baby words behave like typical noun roots and verb roots, and can take affixes and inflectional endings.

Morphology

Inuktut-speaking children's first utterances typically comprise one word (uninflected particle, noun root, or verb root), which is also one morpheme. Mean length of utterance in morphemes (MLUm; Brown, 1973) in Inuktut-speaking children observed in studies in Nunavik and Nunavut increased with age from around 1.0 at 1;0 to around 3.0 at 3;0 and 3.9 at 6;0 (Allen, in press; Allen & Dench, 2015; Wilman, 1988). The mean longest utterance in morphemes was 8.6 at 3;0 (range 5–13) and 22.3 at 6;0 (range 10–39). In contrast, the mean length of utterance in words (MLUw; Arlman-Rupp *et al.*, 1976) did not increase significantly with age (1.0 at 1;0, 1.2 at 3;0, 1.6 at 6;0), which is not surprising given the agglutinative nature of Inuktut. This means that words also increased significantly in length, and children could produce words containing six or seven morphemes by 3;0.

Verbal inflections appeared early, with more than 90% of verb roots inflected in a target-like way by 2;0. Participial (e.g. *-juq/-tuq* 'PAR.3SG') and imperative (e.g. *-guk* 'IMP.2SG>3SG') moods were the earliest to appear, while moods used to mark time coordination between main and subordinate clauses or expressing doubt about the proposition were the latest to appear. Verbal inflection seems to be vulnerable in children with developmental language difficulties (Crago & Allen, 2001). The one Inuktut-speaking child studied so far whose family identified her as having language difficulties showed three different patterns that are ungrammatical in the target language: omitting the verbal inflection, using a filler syllable *-mi* instead of the expected verbal inflection and substituting a full pronoun for the inflection.

Verbal derivational morphemes in the Nunavik dialect representing tense (e.g. *-langa-* 'near future', *-lauq-* 'past'), aspect (e.g. *-si-* 'PRSP'), negation (*-nngit-*) and politeness (e.g. *-lauq-*) started appearing by 2;0. Nominalizer morphemes, which cause a change in word class, started appearing by age 2;6.

Nominal case also emerged early. The first form to appear was the absolutive case first person singular possessive (*-ga*), followed by singular forms of some lexical cases (e.g. locative *-mi*, allative *-mut*), the ergative singular form marking possessors *-up* and the plural absolutive marker *-it* (the singular absolutive marker is null). Nominal inflections marking dual and plural nouns and other persons and numbers for possession gradually appeared as well. Dual inflection showed signs of being vulnerable, especially in situations where more contact with English or French was present (Allen *et al.*, 2006).

The earliest non-inflectional nominal morphology included the emphatic marker *-aluk*, the greeting enclitic *-ai*, and conjunction enclitics *-lu* and *-li*. Other modifiers (e.g. *-apik* 'little', *-nnguaq* 'pretend') and the passive participle *-jaq* came in by 2;6-3;0. Verbalizer morphemes, which cause a change in word class, started appearing by age 2;6; some 23 different verbalizers were present by age 3;6, and children produced words that changed class as many as four times within one word. Other early nominal forms included the absolutive singular demonstrative *una* 'this one' and the locative *maani* 'here'. The first and second person singular pronouns *uvanga* 'I/me' and *ivvit* 'you' (and *mine/yours*, respectively, in some dialects) started appearing by 2;6, as did other demonstratives and locative forms.

In general, Inuktut-speaking children typically become proficient with morphology and master an impressive range of morphemes and morphological processes by an early age.

Syntax

As noted earlier, most of the syntactic 'action' occurs within the word in Inuktut. The typical utterance is only one or two words in length, even by 6;0, with the longest utterances being three or four words. Inuktut-speaking children nonetheless develop in syntactic ability as demonstrated both within words and across words.

In studies of Inuit children learning the Nunavik dialect (e.g. Allen, in press), possession utterances began appearing by about 1;4, with most utterances at this age and older expressing the possessee as the root and the possessor in an inflection (e.g. *anaana-ga* [mother-ABS.1SG.POSS] 'my mother'). Utterances with separate words for possessor and possessee were rare in both child speech and child-directed speech, but started appearing around age 3;0 (e.g. *Saali-up pi-nganik* [Charlie-ERG.SG thing-MOD.3SG.POSS] 'Charlie's thing').

The earliest questions were expressed with single question words. *Suna* 'what' and *nauk* 'where' were the first to emerge around 2;0, followed by *kina* 'who' around 2;6, and more conceptually complex question words like *nani* 'where at' and *sumut* 'why' appearing later. The enclitic *-li* 'where' on nouns was very common for asking about locations, and appeared by around 2;6 (e.g. *Jaiku-li*? 'where is Jacob?'). Yes-no questions expressed by interrogative verbal inflections on any verb root start appearing around 3;0; *-vit* 'INT.2SG' was the first inflection to appear consistently.

Passive and causative structures started appearing by age 2;6, and structures equivalent to complement-taking verbs in English started appearing by age 3;0 except for the desiderative *-guma-* 'want to' which appeared by 2;0. Early uses of these 'syntactic morphemes' often appeared in fixed chunks such as *-ti-lau-nnga* [CAUS-POL-IMP.2SG>1SG] 'cause me to X' suffixed to various verb roots. However, these structures showed increasing signs of productivity by 3;0. Note that the passive was used surprisingly early by the children, in both short and full forms, at least partly due to the frequent use of passive structures in Inuktut (Allen & Crago, 1996). Further, intransitive constructions were much more frequent than transitive constructions because many bivalent propositions are expressed with detransitivizing structures like passive, antipassive, and noun incorporation (Allen, 2013).

Four syntactic constructions in the Nunavik dialect related to the verb clause started appearing by 2;0 to 2;6: subject-complement constructions (6a), subject-verb constructions (6b), object-verb constructions (6c) and adverbial constructions where an adverb is used with another element (6d).

(6) a. *Maaki* *langa-vuq*
Maggie FUT-PAR.3SG
'Maggie will be (coming)' (Jini 1;8; Allen *et al.*, 2019)

b. *Imiq* *pi-jariir-ti-tara*
drink PLEON-already-CAUS-PAR.1SG>3SG
'I finished the drink' (Paul 2;6; Allen *et al.*, 2019)

c. *U-kua-it* *iirqa-it.*
this.one-ABS.PL-ABS.PL pill-ABS.PL
'These are pills' (Tumasi 2;1; Allen *et al.*, 2019)

d. *Aamu-tuq* *ma-ani*
sleep.BW-PAR.3SG here-LOC
'You are sleeping here' (Jini 1;8; Allen *et al.*, 2019)

Three-word verb clause constructions appeared consistently for the first time around age 2;6 or 3;0, although they were quite rare. The most frequent structures were subject-verb-adverb and verb-adverb-adverb (7a), but subject-object-verb and subject-complement-adverb were also seen. The first subordinate clause structures also appeared by around age 3;0 (7b).

(7) a. *Qaupasaaq* *kisiani* *siqinni-laar-tuq.*
day.after.tomorrow only be.sunny-FUT-PAR.3SG
'It's going to be sunny only in two days' (Elijah 2;5; Allen *et al.*, 2019)
b. *Pii-runna-i-lugu* *ani-langa-mmat.*
remove-can-NEG-ICM.XSG>3SG go.out-FUT-CTG.3SG
'It can't be taken off because she's going out' (Lizzie 2;10; Allen *et al.*, 2019)

The target-like expression of multiple clauses in one utterance remains a challenge into the school years. In the sentence in (8) from a narrative, for example, a nine-year-old child produces two subordinate inflections rather than one main and one subordinate inflection.

(8) *Surusi=lu* *qimmi=lu* *tapa-tsuti,* *nirinaujaq* *aju-tsuni.*
boy-and dog-and awake-CTM.4DU frog escape-CTM.4SG
'When the boy and dog woke up, when the frog is escaping' (Allen *et al.*, 2006: 591)
[describing a picture in which the frog has escaped before the boy and dog awake]

Narrative

To our knowledge, only one study of narrative production in Inuktut has been published, looking at narratives in children aged 9 and 15 years as well as adults (Allen *et al.*, 2006). This study asked participants to narrate a wordless picture book about a boy and a dog who look through the forest for their lost frog (Mayer, 1969), a task that has been used in many languages to look at narrative development. Since many of the concepts are culturally alien to most Inuit (e.g. frog, deer, trees, etc.), future studies should use materials that are more culturally relevant, and be done from an Inuit perspective to fully capture Inuit oracy and Inuit Qaujimajatuqanit (see below). In this study, the complexity of narrative structure increased with age: for example, only the 15-year-olds and adults situated their narratives in an overall time frame, using phrases like *ullakut* 'in the morning'. Finally, the level of descriptive detail also increased with age: nine-year-olds tended to include only bare details of the story, 15-year-olds provided more details about the protagonists' thoughts and motives, and adults offered further detail about the physical and emotional setting of the story.

Clinical Implications for Researchers

While there is substantial Eurocentric research about typical preschool development in Inuktut, almost all this research is from Nunavik and based on data collected in the 1980s and 1990s. Inuit worldviews have not been included. Thus, Inuit-led research uplifting Inuit worldviews, respecting Inuit self-determination and Inuit data sovereignty is direly needed (Inuit Tapiriit Kanatami, 2018a). In addition, relatively little academic research on school-aged language development including literacy or narrative development has been published, so this is another area of need. Another topic ripe for research is the effect of bilingualism with English and French on typical development, including the effect of Inuktut-English bilingual vowels in reading/writing. Finally, it would be very useful to study the social determinants of health effects (see below) on language acquisition.

For language disorders, we are only aware of one academic study of developmental language disorder (Crago & Allen, 2001). In some ways, this is very fitting with the cultural norms that children with language (and other) disorders should be accepted for who they are (e.g. Ekho & Ottokie, 2000: 58–59), and that assessments should reflect what children can achieve rather than highlighting their deficits (e.g. YFNED, 2021: 18–19). To further this field, it will be valuable to create opportunities for Inuit to take the lead in identifying the supports they prioritize for children with learning differences.

Relatedly, it is important to support Inuit in determining how they would like Inuktut to be assessed and supported for their children (cf. Inuit Tapirit Kanatami 2018b). Non-Inuit can play a significant role in supporting Inuit self-determination, including the right of Inuit to transmit Inuktut to their children in whatever manner they consider appropriate (United Nations, 2007, Articles 13 & 14; Truth and Reconciliation Commission of Canada, 2015, Calls to action 13 & 14, pp. 156–157). Land-based language programming would be very valuable, as is taking place in other Indigenous communities in North America.

Clinical Implications for Practitioners

This section presents a set of issues that practitioners working with Inuit should keep in mind.

Social determinants of health

Language health is not separate from societal influences on an individual's health. Clean water, adequate housing and food security continue to be challenges for Inuit communities. All aspects of health covered under the scope of practice of Speech Language Pathology (SLP) cannot be addressed separately from the health of the environment, community, family and individual physical and mental health. The SLP scope of practice in the North is broad and includes advocacy for these basic human needs and human rights.

Hearing

Hearing health is a foundation for oral language acquisition. Since Inuit children have high rates of hearing loss, hearing screenings and referrals to audiologists are very important. Clinicians can become familiar with options for Inuit Sign Language (ISL), American Sign Language (ASL), Quebec Sign Language (LSQ), auditory-verbal therapy or even Inuktut augmentative and alternative communication (AAC) in their region. No matter which option is selected by the client, every effort should be made to familiarize children with Inuktut, including reading and writing in the language. See Canadian Deafness Research and Training Institute (2022) for more details.

Language value and preservation

Inuktut is a relatively strong language, though it remains threatened by English (and to some degree French in Nunavik) and due to the ongoing effects of colonization. Non-Inuktut speakers can support language preservation through showing the value of the language and promoting it in every aspect of the SLP process, starting with assessment and throughout therapy. Colonization continues when Inuit identity is ignored. SLPs can learn to pronounce people's names, Inuit place names and basic greetings. Clinicians should advocate for Inuktut-language education, in line with UNESCO's recommendations that children receive at least the first six years of education in their Indigenous language (Ball, 2010).

Societal values

Inuit Qaujimajatuqangit (Inuit Traditional Knowledge) are Inuit societal values that guide all aspects of life and respectful relationships. They are intertwined with child-rearing practices and shine through communication and language (e.g. Crago, 1990; Aqqiumavvik Arviat Wellness Society, 2024). Inuktut is learned and used within a culture and traditional knowledge system. As such, cultural learning is an integral part of SLP professional development and directly applicable to clinical practice.

Bioethics, translators and interpreters

Informed consent is required throughout assessment and treatment. SLP is based on a Eurocentric theoretical approach, and so clinicians need to take extra measures to ensure that their cross-cultural communication truly conveys the SLP process and to ensure both the interpreter and client understand the medical jargon. It is important to note that interpretation and translation should not be understood solely as mechanisms for explaining Eurocentric approaches so that Inuit adapt to Eurocentric worldviews; instead, they can serve to assist SLPs and other practitioners in understanding Inuit ways of expressing concerns, questions, and priorities, and in facilitating informed communication appropriate to the setting (MacLachan, 2022). There can be ethical considerations around using family members to interpret, though sometimes this is the only option. When interpreters are used during an assessment, SLPs should give clear instructions on how to refrain from prompting and providing cues – especially nonverbal cues, as children are very perceptive and quick to follow indirect cueing.

Anonymity

The anonymity that SLPs enjoy elsewhere is not possible in the Arctic where communities are small. Dual relationships (professional and personal) are common, while ethical guidelines for dual relationships are lacking (Lints-Martindale *et al.*, 2025). Clinicians can inform clients that they will wait for the client to initiate greetings or conversation in social settings, in order to respect clients' desire for anonymity or relationship-building in the community setting. On the other hand, SLPs can have clear boundaries for personal and work topics and also participate in community life as a community member.

Community health and education assistants

These professionals are often more permanent than the teachers in the schools or healthcare personnel in health centers. They understand the culture and have likely known your clients long-term from within the community. These healthcare personnel are working within cross-cultural settings and doubling their workload because they need to work in both Inuit and Western language systems. SLPs and other practitioners are encouraged to adapt their practices and to develop an understanding of Inuit cultural communicative practices.

Geography and service delivery models

No matter where an SLP lives in Canada, they are likely to encounter an Inuktut speaker in their practice. Inuktut speakers from remote communities will travel to major centers to receive medical services in hospitals, rehabilitation centers or long-term care facilities. SLP clinicians can be based in regional hospital centers in the North while others may travel to remote communities a couple of times per year.

There are ethical considerations for SLPs providing services to Inuktut speakers. It takes time and effort to become proficient with cross-cultural communication within SLP clinical practice. An in-person language assessment is absolutely required to fully capture the subtle non-verbal communication and full abilities of a child developing language. In other words, to provide virtual-only SLP services to Inuit cross-culturally is unethical and imprudent. Virtual therapy can be supplementary to a minimum of biannual in-person travel clinics.

It is important for SLPs to indicate in their reports which dialects a client has been exposed to, which ones they understand and which they speak, especially given the phonological, lexical and grammatical differences across dialects. Dialects can be named by geographical region and the community they are spoken in, such as South Qikiqtaaluk (South Baffin) or Kimmirut. It is not uncommon for Inuit to have multi-dialectal language knowledge.

Consider cultural norms in assessing pragmatic and language skills

Non-verbal communication, indirect communication and many cultural norms have an impact on communication and language use (e.g. Crago, 1990). SLPs may want to take extra time to establish a rapport with children to get valid verbal responses. Traditionally, children are expected to observe and listen before speaking, and silence is very normal and expected. Cultural norms for eye contact are different from those in English and French cultures, which should be taken into account.

Kinship and Adoption

Kinship and customary naming practices are expressions of culture. Open adoption is very common, so SLPs will want to ask about how caregivers or family members are related.

Vocabulary

Vocabulary development is tied to the environment. The Arctic environment where most Inuktut speakers live affects vocabulary for weather and seasons, transportation, food and animals, people, relationships and occupations, as well as sports and activities. In addition, higher level language, such as figurative language and expressions, is influenced by environmental experiences. SLPs may consider filtering all assessment and therapy materials through these environmental vocabulary lenses, or collaborate with Inuit in the development of appropriate materials.

Assessment for Inuktut speakers

While the Inuit approach to childrearing emphasises that each child develops in their own time, there may be times where assessment is still requested. For children, collaborative assessment is supported by research. The SLP works with parents/caregivers, educators and others familiar with the child's language to determine together their strengths and stage of language development (Ball, 2021).

Analysing an Inuktut language sample is part of an assessment. A language sample can be taken by observing the child play or interact with a familiar family member or friend. For bilingual Inuit, English standardized assessments can be administered but must be interpreted carefully, as the norms are not valid. How the assessment is administered and adapted is hugely important (Ball, 2021). Take note of adaptations and also when standardized administration has ended and informal administration begins. This should be clearly indicated in the assessment report and the results interpreted with caution. Include Inuktut translations of key concepts in the report. Bring Inuit Qaujimajatuqangit into your assessment and recommendations.

Intervention with bilingual Inuktut-English or Inuktut-French speakers

Eurocentric language facilitation methods can be great supports, though they are not always appropriate for Inuit languages or culture. The process itself of a southern clinician guiding a parent on how to talk to their child, even if to use a language supporting strategy, is a delicate action to undertake given the colonial history of Canada. Ideally, Inuit are the ones to provide language supports to Inuit children. When non-Inuktut speakers provide therapy, the line between supporting communication development and more assimilation to English or French language or culture is thin. Inuktut speakers need to see and hear their language being recognized, supported, and valued by Speech-Language and Hearing Professionals.

Conclusion

There are various issues SLP practitioners should take into consideration when working with Inuit. It is important to acknowledge the history of colonization and its effect on the people, their language and their environment, and to include advocating for basic human needs and human rights within the scope of SLP practice. By learning about Inuit methods of communication, societal values, traditional knowledge and cultural norms, SLP practitioners can show their support for and recognition of the value of language to Inuit identity and culture. Finally, given the differences between Inuktut and English in their grammar, usage and social context, SLPs may need to find alternative methods of assessment and therapy that are appropriate for Inuktut speakers.

Notes

(1) The term Inuvialuktun encompasses the three Inuktut language varieties spoken in the Inuvialuit Settlement Region: Sallirmiutun, Kangiyuarmiutun and Uummarmiutun. Linguistically, they belong to different branches of the language family: Sallirmiutun (Siglitun) is a variety of Western Canadian Inuktut, as is Inuinnaqtun; Kangiyuarmiutun is a variety of Inuinnaqtun; and Uummarmiutun belongs to the Alaskan Inupiaq language group (Dorais, 2020: 28).

(2) https://www12.statcan.gc.ca/census-recensement/2021/dp-pd/prof/details/page.cfm?Lang=E&SearchText=Nunavik&DGUIDlist=2021A000262,2022A00072417&GENDERlist=1&STATISTIClist=1&HEADERlist=21,18,16,14

(3) https://www12.statcan.gc.ca/census-recensement/2021/as-sa/98-200-X/2021012/98-200-X2021012-eng.cfm] This is a decline from the 82% of children who could converse in Inuktut in 2016 https://www.gov.nu.ca/sites/default/files/publications/2022-11/statsupdate_inuit_data_2016_census.pdf

(4) Nunavik Inuktitut and Sallirmiutun show evidence of an adjective category (see Compton, 2012).

(5) For reasons of space we abstract away from more fine-grained descriptions of the mood system, but it should be noted that the system is more complex than the systems found in European languages. There is considerable variation across dialects in the inventory and meanings of mood markers, and even the names used for them in the literature.
(6) Age is indicated as years;months, so 1;6 represents the age one year and six months.

References

Allen, S.E.M. (2000) A discourse-pragmatic explanation for argument representation in child Inuktitut. *Linguistics* 38 (3), 483–521.

Allen, S.E.M. (2013) The acquisition of ergativity in Inuktitut. In E.L. Bavin and S. Stoll (eds) *The Acquisition of Ergative Structures* (pp. 71–105). Benjamins.

Allen, S.E.M. (2017) Polysynthesis in the acquisition of Inuit languages. In M.D. Fortescue, M. Mithun and N. Evans (eds) *Handbook of Polysynthesis* (pp. 449–472). Oxford University Press.

Allen, S.E.M. (in press) The acquisition of Inuit languages. In A. Berge, A. Arnhold and N. Trondhjem (eds) *Handbook of Inuit-Yupik-Unangan*. Oxford University Press.

Allen, S.E.M. and Crago, M.B. (1996) Early passive acquisition in Inuktitut. *Journal of Child Language* 23 (1), 129–155.

Allen, S.E.M. and Dench, C. (2015) Calculating mean length of utterance for Eastern Canadian Inuktitut. *First Language* 35, 377–406. https://doi.10.1177/0142723715596648

Allen, S.E.M, Crago, M.B. and Pesco, D. (2006) The effect of majority language exposure on minority language skills: The case of Inuktitut. *International Journal of Bilingual Education and Bilingualism* 9 (5), 578–596.

Allen, S.E.M., Cain, M., Dench, C., Genest, C. and Trudeau, N. (2017) Inuktitut adaptation of the MacArthur-Bates Communicative Development Inventory [Conference poster presentation]. 14th International Congress for the Study of Child Language, Lyon, France.

Allen, S.E.M., Dench, C.B. and Isakson, K. (2019) InuLARSP: An adaptation of the Language Assessment Remediation and Screening Procedure for Inuktitut. In M.J. Ball, P. Fletcher and D. Crystal (eds) *Grammatical Profiles: Further Languages of LARSP* (pp. 270–296). Multilingual Matters.

Aqqiumavvik Arviat Wellness Society (2025) Inuktitut language development chart. Retrieved on April 19, 2026 at: https://www.aqqiumavvik.com/_files/ugd/1f7032_1009787050ff4d79950777f8cb1418b4.pdf

Arlman-Rupp, A.J.L., van Niekerk de Haan, D. and van de Sandt-Koenderman, M. (1976) Brown's early stages: Some evidence from Dutch. *Journal of Child Language* 3, 267–274.

Arnhold, A. (in press) Phonology and phonetics in Inuit, Yupik and Unangan languages. In A. Berge, A. Arnhold and N. Trondhjem (eds) *Handbook of Inuit-Yupik-Unangan*. Oxford University Press.

Arnhold, A., Elfner, E. and Compton, R. (2023) Inuktitut and the concept of word-level prominence. In K. Bogomolets and H. van der Hulst (eds) *Word Prominence in Languages with Complex Morphologies* (pp. 138–177). Oxford University Press.

Ball, J. (2010) Enhancing learning of children from diverse language backgrounds: Mother tongue-based bilingual or multilingual education in the early years. United Nations Educational, Scientific and Cultural Organization (UNESCO).

Ball, J. (2021) Finding fitting solutions to assessment of Indigenous young children's learning and development: Do it in a good way. *Frontiers in Education* 6, 696847. https://doi.org/10.3389/feduc.2021.696847

Bobaljik, J.D. (1996) Assimilation in the Inuit languages and the place of the uvular nasal. *International Journal of American Linguistics* 62 (4), 323–350.

Brown, R. (1973) *A First Language: The Early Stages*. Harvard University Press.

Canadian Deafness Research and Training Institute (2022) Inuit sign language. See https://cdrti.org/en/inuit-sign-language (accessed 25 November 2024).

Carrier, J. (2021) Ergativity on the move (Publication No. 2826349). Doctoral dissertation, University of Toronto. ProQuest Dissertations & Theses Global.

Centers of Excellence for Children's Well-Being (2014) Inunnguiniq: Child rearing advice from Inuit Elders. Retrieved on April 19, 2026 from: https://www.inuuqatigiit.ca/inunnguiniq-child-dev-t-pamphlets

Compton, R. (2012) The syntax and semantics of modification in Inuktitut: Adjectives and adverbs in a polysynthetic language (Publication No. NR79427). Doctoral dissertation, University of Toronto. ProQuest Dissertations & Theses Global.

Crago, M.B. (1990) The development of communicative competence in Inuit children of Northern Quebec: Implications for speech-language pathology. *Journal of Childhood Communication Disorders* 13 (1), 54–71.

Crago, M. B. (1992). Communicating with Inuit: A case study in sociocultural and linguistic c differences. *Inuit Studies* 16 (1/2), 67–94.

Crago, M.B. and Allen, S.E.M. (2001) Early finiteness in Inuktitut: The role of language structure and input. *Language Acquisition* 9 (1), 59–111.

Crago, M.B., Allen, S.E.M. and Pesco, D. (1998) Issues of complexity in Inuktitut and English child directed speech. In E.V. Clark (ed.) *Proceedings of the 29th Annual Stanford Child Language Research Forum* (pp. 37–46). CSLI.

Dench, C., Cleave, P.L., Tagak, J. and Beddard, J. (2011) The development of an Inuktitut and English language screening tool in Nunavut. *Canadian Journal of Speech-Language Pathology and Audiology* 35 (2), 168–176.

Dorais, L.-J. (2010) *The Language of the Inuit: Syntax, Semantics, and Society in the Arctic*. McGill-Queen's University Press.

Ekho, N. and Ottokie, U. (2000) *Childrearing Practices* (Vol. 3 of *Interviewing Inuit Elders*). Nunavut Arctic College.

Inuit Tapiriit Kanatami (2018a) *National Inuit Strategy on Research*. https://www.itk.ca/wp-content/uploads/2018/09/ITK_NISR_Implementation-Plan_Electronic-Version.pdf

Inuit Tapiriit Kanatami (2018b) Indigenous Early Learning and Child Care Framework. Ottawa: Inuit Tapiriit Kanatami https://www.canada.ca/en/employment-social-development/programs/indigenous-early-learning/2018-framework.html#h2.7

Inuit Uqausinginnik Taiguusiliuqtiit (2018a) *Inuktut uqausiup aaqqiksuutingit* / ᐃᓄᒃᑐᑦ ᐅᖃᐅᓯᑉᐅ ᐋᖅᑭᒃᓲᑎᖏᑦ / *Inuktut reference grammar*. Inuit Uqausinginnik Taiguusiliuqtii

Inuit Uqausinginnik Taiguusiliuqtiit (2020) *Inuktut uqausiliurut* / ᐃᓄᒃᑐᑦ ᐅᖃᐅᓯᓕᐅᕈᑦ / *Inuktut Affix Dictionary*. Inuit Uqausinginnik Taiguusiliuqtiit, Iqaluit, Nunavut.

Johns, A. (2006) Ergativity and change in Inuktitut. In A. Johns, D. Massam and J. Ndayiragije (eds) *Ergativity: Emerging Issues* (pp. 293–311). Springer.

Lee, H. and Allen, S.E.M. (2023) An acquisition sketch of Inuktitut. *Language Documentation and Conservation* 28, 135–213.

Lints-Martindale, A., Schroeder, M., Goodwin, S., Dean, M., Hutchings, V.M.M., Carlson, A.M. and McDougall, T.D. (2025, July 17) "But I know you!": Navigating dual relationships in rural, northern and remote psychology practice. *Canadian Psychology / Psychologie canadienne*. Advance online publication. https://dx.doi.org/10.1037/cap0000439

Lowe, R. (1985c) *Uummarmiuit uqalungiha ilihaur̂r̂utikr̂angit: Basic Uummarmiut Eskimo grammar*. Committee for Original Peoples Entitlement, Inuvik, Northwest Territories.

MacLachlan, J. (2022) Engaging Inuit perspectives on Timimut Ikajuqsivik (rehabilitation services): Critical disability and decolonizing analyses (Doctoral dissertation, University of Toronto).

Mayer, M. (1969) *Frog, Where are You?* Dial Books.

Moseley, C. (ed.) (2010) *Atlas of the World's Languages in Danger* (3rd edn). UNESCO Publishing. Online version: https://unesdoc.unesco.org/ark:/48223/pf0000187026?posInSet=3&queryId=8d96e2e4-4ae1-4290-a3ea-0bfed0278830

Murasugi, K. (2020) Antipassives. In M. Barrie, J. Coon, C. Gillon, J. Haugen, E. Mathieu and D. Siddiqi (eds) *Routledge Handbook of North American Languages* (pp. 275–289). Routledge.

Patrick, D. and Murasugi, K. (in press) Language status, maintenance and revitalization. In A. Berge, A. Arnhold and N. Trondhjem (eds) *Handbook of Inuit-Yupik-Unangan*. Oxford University Press.

Pauktuutit Inuit Women of Canada (2006) *The Inuit way: A guide to Inuit culture*. Available from: https://www.relations-inuit.chaire.ulaval.ca/sites/relations-inuit.chaire.ulaval.ca/files/InuitWay_e.pdf

Pirurvik Centre (2013) ᐱᒋᐊᕐᕕᒃ / *Pigiarvik Level 1, 2, 3 Textbook*. Pirurvik Press, Iqaluit.

Statistics Canada (2023) *Census in Brief: Indigenous Languages across Canada, Census of Population, 2021*. Available from: https://www12.statcan.gc.ca/census-recensement/2021/as-sa/98-200-X/2021012/98-200-X2021012-eng.cfm

Tagalik, S., Dench, C.B., Allen, S.E.M., Anoee, N., Karetak, R., Novalinga, A., Putulik, M. and Weetaluktuk, M. (2025) Creating a culturally grounded tool to support Inuktut language development: A collaborative project combining knowledge from Inuit and Western research perspectives. In A. Skilton, R.E. Henke and M.R. Chee (eds) *Bridging Child Language Research to Practice for Indigenous Language Revitalization*. Language Documentation and Conservation Special Publication 30, 187–214. University of Hawai'i Press. http://hdl.handle.net/10125/74827

Taylor, D.M. and Wright, S.C. (2003) Do aboriginal students benefit from education in their heritage language? Results from a ten-year program of research in Nunavik. *Canadian Journal of Native Studies* 23, 1–24.

Truth and Reconciliation Commission of Canada (2015) *Honouring the Truth, Reconciling for the Future: Summary of the Final report of the Truth and Reconciliation Commission of Canada*. Truth and Reconciliation Commission of Canada. https://nctr.ca/publications-and-reports/reports/#trc-reports

United Nations (2007) *United Nations Declaration on the Rights of Indigenous Peoples*. https://www.un.org/en/fight-racism/resources.

Wharram, D. (2003) On the interpretation of (un)certain indefinites in Inuktitut and related languages (Publication No. 3242006). Doctoral dissertation, University of Connecticut. ProQuest Dissertations & Theses Global.

Wilman, D. (1988) The natural language of Inuit children: A key to Inuktitut literacy (Publication No. 8904899). Doctoral dissertation, University of New Mexico. ProQuest Dissertations & Theses Global.

Yukon First Nation Education Directorate (YFNED) (2021) Environmental scan of Indigenous educational and allied health assessments and interventions. See https://static1.squarespace.com/static/5ddc27b50cfd2a79a6da6595/t/61f0c2c0afea78477f9cbb0a/1643168461937/Final_Report_YFNED_EnvironmentalScan_IndigenousAssessment_08JULY21.pdf

Suggested Readings

Berge, A., Arnhold, A. and Trondhjem, N. (eds) (in press) *Handbook of Inuit-Yupik-Unangan Languages*. Oxford University Press.

Dorais, L.-J. (2010) *The Language of the Inuit: Syntax, Semantics, and Society in the Arctic*. McGill-Queen's University Press.

Dorais, L.-J. (2017) *Inuit Languages & Dialects: Inuit uqausiqatigiit* (updated edition). Nunavut Arctic College Media.

Lowe, R. (1985a) *Kangiryuarmiut uqauhingita ilihautdjutikhangit: Basic Kangiryuarmiut Eskimo grammar*. Committee for Original Peoples Entitlement, Inuvik, Northwest Territories.

Lowe, R. (1985b) *Siglit Inuvialuit uqausiita ilisarviksait: Basic Siglit Inuvialuit Eskimo grammar*. Committee for Original Peoples Entitlement, Inuvik, Northwest Territories.

Mallon, M. and Kublu, A. (1996) Inuktitut 115: An introduction to the structure of Inuktitut. Ittukuluuk language programs coursebook. Nunavut Arctic College, Iqaluit.

Palluq Cloutier, J. and McComber, L. (2014) *Uqausivut sivummuagutivut: Our Language, Our Leadership*. Nunavut Arctic College Media.

Pirurvik Centre (2013) ᐱᒋᐊᕐᕕᒃ / *Pigiarvik Level 1 Textbook*. Pirurvik Press.

Pirurvik Centre (2013) ᐊᓪᓗᕐᕕᒃ / *Allurvik Level 2 Textbook*. Pirurvik Press.

Pirurvik Centre (2013) ᐊᑕᖕᒌᕕᒃ / *Atangiivik Level 3 Textbook*. Pirurvik Press.

13 How to Use and Learn an Indigenous Language: Examples from Ishākkoy

Jeffery U. Darensbourg and Baylee Badawy

Introduction

This work shows methods that have been employed by us to learn and use an Indigenous language, one that is a heritage language for one of us (Darensbourg). There are many methods for doing this, and whereas some Indigenous languages have a rich array of materials that a learner can use, others do not enjoy that privilege (yet). We intend this to be a guide to some things that one can do even if one doesn't know a particular Indigenous language well, or at all, even if one doesn't have easy access to someone who does. We must note that we encourage not only Indigenous People but also those working with such populations to seek out those who might be an expert in a particular language, and that is much easier in our present age, even if the ease of doing so doesn't always translate into action.

In this chapter, we will provide a cultural introduction to Ishākkoy and its population of origin, discuss some recent work on the language and its revitalization, and recount a public creative project.

Context and Culture: The Ishak and their Language

The language we are discussing here is most commonly known by its cultural community, Ishak Indigenous People (Darensbourg, 2022a), as *Ishākkoy*, 'the talk of the Ishak.'[1] It is also correctly known as *Yukhíti Kóy*, 'the talk of the sort of people we are' or 'Indigenous talk,' and definitely incorrectly known, especially in older literature, as *Atakapan*, 'the language of the maneaters.' Until recently, Ishākkoy was a sleeping, or at least sleepy language (De Costa, 2021). It is unclear when the last fluent speaker walked on, but the earliest date possible for that would be 1979, based on numerous conversations at tribal events with family members. Some living Ishak People still have Ishākkoy names or nicknames, with a common name being 'Konesh,' a version of the Ishākkoy word for a hackberry tree (*Celtis laevigata*), used exclusively by men. Some Ishākkoy toponyms continue in common use, the most well-known of which is 'Calcasieu,' the name for a Louisiana civil parish, derived from the name of an Ishak leader in the area during the early colonial period, Kátko-shyok, whose name means 'chirping eagle' or 'singing eagle.'[2]

Ishăkkoy is part of a group of languages from present-day Texas and Louisiana known as Ishakkoyan (formerly known as Atakapan for reasons discussed below). It includes languages such as Bidai, Han and Opelousa, with the dialects of the Eastern and Western Ishak combined being known as Ishākkoy now (Kaufman, 2022: xxiii). According to Kaufman, it, 'like many other North American Indigenous languages, is structurally agglutinative and moderately polysynthetic. This means that many grammatical elements are affixed, or attached, to a head word, usually a verb' (2022: xxiv). It also follows a subject-object-verb sentence structure, an example of which is *wísh wi itét hiyanyánháhshat*, which translates into English as 'I did not fear my father,' but whose words, in order, read 'I my father fear-not-did' (Kimball, 2022: 129).

A feature of particular interest in Ishākkoy is 'spatial language that correlates future with "back/behind" and past with "in front/before"' (Kaufman, 2022: xxv). This contrasts with English in which the future is in front of the speaker and the past is behind. While this feature is rare, it isn't unique to Ishākkoy. As such, *hal Yilhiwéw Pétik Yil* in Ishākkoy could be translated as 'next Monday' but a literal translation would be 'the Monday behind.' An example of another Indigenous language of the Americas that shares this feature is Aymara, spoken in the Andes (discussed in Núñez & Sweetser, 2006).

The language is part of the heritage of the Ishak, an Indigenous People from present-day southwest Louisiana and southeast Texas who currently exist in multiple organized groups in Louisiana and Texas, none of which currently enjoys federal recognition (Darensbourg, 2022a). As part of a common history of enslavement and living together during periods of segregation, Ishak People today are generally part of Louisiana's mixed ethnicity Creole population, a population undergoing a major reconsideration based on contemporary scholarship rooted in critical mixed-race studies from scholars within the population itself (e.g. Prud'homme-Cranford *et al.*, 2022). At present, there are perhaps 2000 individuals actively claiming Ishak heritage, mostly in Louisiana and Texas, with quite a few individuals in California as part of a Louisiana Creole exodus there in the late 20th century (Dunn, 2022).

Ishak People are often, and quite incorrectly, known by the exonym *Atakapa* (in various spellings), from a Choctaw word whose denotation is that of cannibalism, 'maneaters,' with a figurative meaning referring to people who might forcefully adopt others, making them full, if unwilling, members of a tribe, in this case the Ishak (Ellis, 2023: 56ff). While both the Ishak and Choctaw have lived in the American Gulf South from time immemorial, the languages and people in question have different cultural and geographic origins. The word *Atakapa* is a slur and it should generally not be used. During a reorganization of Ishak People in the 1990s, there was talk of dropping *Atakapa* from the official name of the largest group, the Atakapa-Ishak Nation of Southwest Louisiana and Southeast Texas, but instead the decision was made to hyphenate exonym and endonym. The best practice is to refer to the Ishak by the proper name of a group, or simply as the Ishak, avoiding notions of cannibalism, whether literally or figuratively. Accordingly, the name for the language preferred by most of those who have a facility with it is Ishākkoy.

Ishãkkoy has undergone a revival based on a number of factors. First, organized populations of Ishak have shown an interest in using the language again, especially since the 1990s. Second, the published works of non-Indigenous linguists David V. Kaufman and Geoffrey Kimball have made accessing the language easier. For nearly a century, the primary work on the language was Albert S. Gatschet and John R. Swanton's 1932 *A Dictionary of the Atakapa Language Accompanied by Text Material*, a poorly organized and ill-thought-out work that has proved difficult to use. As part of Kaufman's research on Indigenous languages of the Lower Mississippi Valley, as reflected in his fascinating volume *Clues to Lower Mississippi Valley Histories* (Kaufman, 2019a), he began working with Ishākkoy, leading eventually to a revised dictionary with an updated orthography (Kaufman, 2019b), with a second expanded edition arriving a few years later, featuring a further updated orthography based on community suggestions as well as contributions to the corpus from Ishak People (Kaufman, 2022). Geoffrey Kimball (2022) brought out a thoroughly researched grammar of the language as well. The grammar has significantly updated the understanding of how the language works and has significantly influenced those who work with it.

The Value of Indigenous Language Use

Indigenous languages are important for preserving and celebrating Indigenous Peoples and cultures. The use of these languages is a decolonial act. Stephen Bagan (2019) draws attention to Anigiduwagi scholar Qwo-Li Driskill's (2015: 58) notion of 'decolonial skillshares,' meaning,

> Indigenous rhetorics, pedagogies, and radical practices that ask us to continue our rhetorical (visual, material, performative, linguistic, etc.) traditions as Indigenous people, to transform cultural memories for both Indigenous and nonindigenous people, and to create spaces for all of us to learn and teach embodied rhetorical practices as a tactic of decolonization.

Colonization's impacts are abated by Indigenous empowerment through connections with Indigenous culture via language. These languages are ties to specific communities, reflecting their histories and wanderings and ideas. As the first author is an Ishak and does extensive work within the community, we must note that one of the most commonly requested types of information from community members involves language, with special mention given to a longing to speak the language of community ancestors.

Using Indigenous Words and Phrases

The vocabulary of Indigenous languages acts as a window into the ways Indigenous Peoples have thought about their respective environments, forming a significant aid in helping Indigenous People to identify with and understand their cultural heritage. One way of encouraging the use of Indigenous languages is to promote the use of greetings and basic phrases, such as expressions of thanks. These are simple and can be used by teachers, therapists, speech pathologists and other professionals working with Indigenous People (whether or not those professionals are Indigenous), as a way of encouraging Indigenous language use and promoting a welcoming environment for Indigenous People.

These words, in our experience, quickly spread to others in the circle of the Indigenous individual, whether the others are Indigenous or not. To use these in Ishākkoy, for example, one would begin by using the greeting *sla* and the word for 'thanks,' *hiwéw*. *Sla* is a loanword from Mobilian Trade Language's greeting *ishla*. Mobilian was the Indigenous lingua franca of the Gulf South. A direct phrase of *thanks* was not mentioned in Gatschet and Swanton's dictionary, but a phrase of *thanks* can be inferred from an adverb, viz., *hiwéw,* meaning 'powerful.'

As examples of pathways into the thinking of the Ishak, in Ishākkoy the word for an American bison (*Bison bison*) is *shokóṇ*, meaning 'grass thing.' Even though the last free bison was killed in Louisiana sometime in the early decades of the 19th century, it shows the importance of the bison for the Ishak, being the primary animal of note to look for in the prairies within Ishak territories (Darensbourg, 2021a). Furthermore, names for human beings can be telling as to Indigenous thinking. The Ishākkoy name for its parent community is often translated as 'the human beings,' but getting more precise, it relates to the verb for birth, *ishāk*, and, as such, the tribal name has a sense of 'those who have been born.' A common term for French or other people of European ancestry in the language is *kíwilsh*, which serves as a general word for white people, is possibly related to the term for an egg, a bit of snark, those who have been born as opposed to the eggs (Darensbourg, 2022b). The word for an enslaved person is *kiwilshké*, 'someone who has a white person.' *Kíwilsh Nuṇ* 'the white village' became the name for the area now known as Lafayette, Louisiana, after colonization (Darensbourg, 2024).

Using Indigenous place names is a ubiquitous part of language revitalization efforts, and it is important to note that every inhabited colonized place has had an Indigenous name, whether that name persists in use or is recorded or not. Learning these when possible is a way of honoring Indigenous Peoples and recognizing their presence and importance in an area. Indigenous place names can be quite telling. In the lands currently known as the United States of America, Indigenous toponymic practice tends to follow a pattern of naming an area after its most noteworthy feature. As Indigenous cartographer Margaret Wickens Pearce notes, these names pick out 'the salient characteristics of a place, those qualities that clarify the situated identity of the place and distinguish it from other places' (2014: 108). Encouraging the use of these Indigenous toponyms can function both as an education in Indigenous culture as well as a feature of a sort of 'single-word activism' (Schmelzer, 2021). A now commonly used Indigenous place name in Louisiana is *Bulbancha*, the precolonial Choctaw name for what is usually referred to as 'New Orleans.' *Bulbancha* means, approximately, 'the place where speakers of other languages are,' which marks the origins of the place as a multinational trading area, a feature continuing to this day (Darensbourg, 2024).

In Ishākkoy, the relationship of the Ishak to 'settler time,' to use Mark Rifkin's term (Rifkin, 2017), is shown in the greeting for January 1. Rather than a simple translation of 'Happy New Year' or a similar phrase, the Ishākkoy greeting for the day is *kiwĺlsh yil hiwėw hec tol*, meaning 'happy great powerful day of the white people.' Rifkin notes that 'Native peoples occupy a double bind within dominant settler reckonings of time. Either they are consigned to the past, or they are inserted into a present defined on non-native terms' (Rifkin, 2017: vii). The Ishākkoy reflects an assertion of a separate temporal identity, in resistance to colonization, and the phrase is a favorite among learners of the language. In fact, on January 1, the first author commonly receives the phrase in both English and Ishākkoy from friends who don't have any facility with Ishākkoy.

Composing Poetry and Narratives in Ishākkoy

The corpus of Ishākkoy is not large, and this was especially true before the publication of the first edition of the revised Ishākkoy dictionary in 2019, which inspired some published writing in the language. The Gatschet and Swanton dictionary from 1932 has 10 pages of narratives dictated by Kishyúc Huntington to Gatschet at Tew Tul ('Lake's Tail,' also known as 'Lake Charles, Louisiana') in 1885 (Gatschet & Swanton, 1932: 9–20). These narratives contain snapshots of Ishak culture, including family relations and foodways. Kaufman's (2019b) overhauling of their work, including better organization, correction of errors and an improved orthography, has led to a resurgence in the use of the language.

Based on the 2019 dictionary, the first author noticed a plethora of example sentences not based on the narratives in the 1932 dictionary and copied them out on notecards, eventually compiling these into a document using Google Drive. These example sentences in the document and notecards were used in two ways originally. First, they were used to help get a feel for the language and to learn some of its grammar by example, and second, to compose poetry.

The cento is a form of found poetry, 'a poetic form composed entirely of secondary (usually poetic) texts' (Malhotra, 2010). Classic centos usually remix lines of famous poets, with a prominent example being the *Cento Nuptialis* of the 3rd century Roman poet Ausonius, composed using lines from the poet Vergil at the request of the emperor Valentinian (Budarangina, 2017: 49). The example sentences, both from the published Ishākkoy narratives and from entries for specific words, were used to compose cento poems that have been published (Darensbourg, 2020, 2021b). Two of these, 'Hoktiwe' and 'The Ears of That Dog Are Torn,' are proper centos and another of the published poems, 'A Studio in the Woods,' used some lines from the example sentences, with other lines composed by taking example sentences and substituting out some of the words, mostly nouns. Two poems, 'Hoktiwe' and 'A Studio in the Woods,' were used as the script for the 2020 pandemic film *Hoktiwe: Two Poems in Ishākkoy* by Fernando López and Jeffery U. Darensbourg, commissioned by the Contemporary Arts Center New Orleans (Darensbourg, 2021c). The first film in Ishākkoy, it has been shown in festivals and art exhibitions, as well as taught in university classes since its creation and it has introduced audiences to the existence of the language. A section from 'Hoktiwe,' the first of these centos to see publication, follows, with the orthography updated to match that used in the 2022 dictionary, though the published version uses the 2019 orthography:

Katkosh koykit:
An eagle is speaking:

Ishak taysh okiăn yukit he mon yalpeyulăt.
Strangers have come and taken our land.

Shokshos shoksho waṇsholkit.
Birds are tearing up the young seed plants.

Cikip tat.
A blue heron is poised there.

Naw taw walwalshtit.
Many feathers are waving.

Iti hihiwalshat.
I dreamt last night.

The significance of the cento form here is that a language user can compose centos as a way of using a language even in the absence of interlocutors. It is a form that allows language learners to use the language even if they barely know it. It also produces something tangible, a work of art. Language professionals can encourage Indigenous Peoples with whom they are working to compose in heritage languages as a way of working with the thoughts and words of their ancestors, interacting with them across time and text.

It must be noted that besides these poems, the 2019 dictionary and its ease of use as well as online language lessons from linguists David V. Kaufman and Justin Southworth have inspired an expansion of the corpus from other Ishak People. Russell Reed has composed narratives based on his work as a park ranger, and some of these have appeared in the second edition of the Kaufman dictionary (Kaufman, 2022: 169–170). Maaliyah Papillion's short film *ISHAK* debuted at the New Orleans Film Festival in October 2024, opening with a narrative in Ishākkoy. Rose Yard, a student in Houston, Texas, has composed as of yet unpublished narratives in Ishākkoy as well.

Getting People to Use Ishākkoy: A Festival Project

In 2021, A Studio in the Woods, an arts residency campus of Tulane University in a rural part of the West Bank of Orleans Parish, Louisiana, commissioned the authors of this essay to create a workshop using Ishākkoy for its annual November event, FORESTival, which features music, woods walks and artist-led workshops in which festival attendees can create their own works. We set up a workshop in which people could use Ishākkoy to create works of art. Over 60 individuals participated in the workshop, and while some of them were Indigenous, none of them were Ishak. The workshop received overwhelmingly positive comments from attendees.

We had two primary projects that workshop goers could participate in. First, the second author made example drawings of animals with Ishākkoy labels. As many children attend this festival, one project was to encourage them to make drawings of animals using pencils, crayons and markers, labeling the drawings with Ishākkoy names for the animals. Animal names were printed on sheets with translations, but multiple copies of the first edition of the Kaufman dictionary were on hand, and many of the children enjoyed thumbing through it, and especially enjoyed using its appendix of names of fauna. In addition to helping the children learn some Indigenous vocabulary, the children were also given lessons in pronouncing the words. As might be expected, the younger participants – the youngest was four years old – excelled at this task, picking up the sounds much quicker than adults. Though this project was aimed at children, some adults also made drawings, and some children, especially older ones, participated in the next project.

The other primary project for festivalgoers was the creation of centos in Ishākkoy. The materials provided were sheets of Ishākkoy sentences produced using the Google Drive document of example sentences, scissors, glue sticks and construction paper. The sentences used

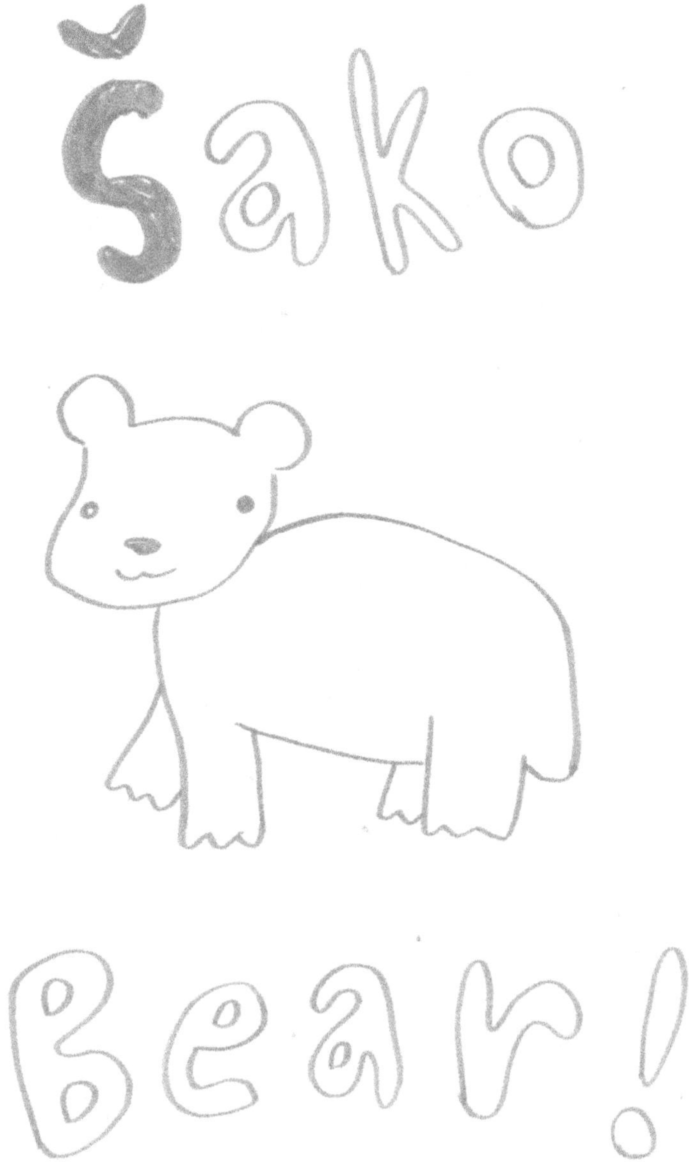

Figure 13.1 Drawing of a bear with labels in Ishākkoy and English by Baylee Badawy

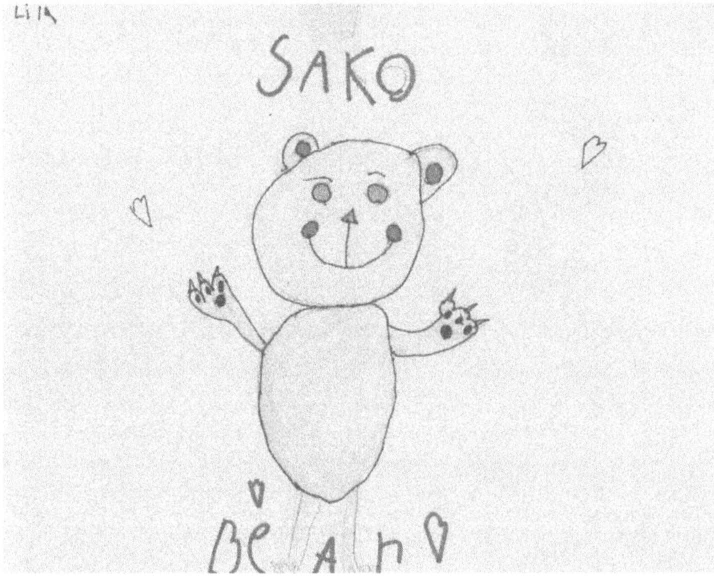

Figure 13.2 Bear drawing by Lisa (last name unknown), a child who attended FORESTival in 2021

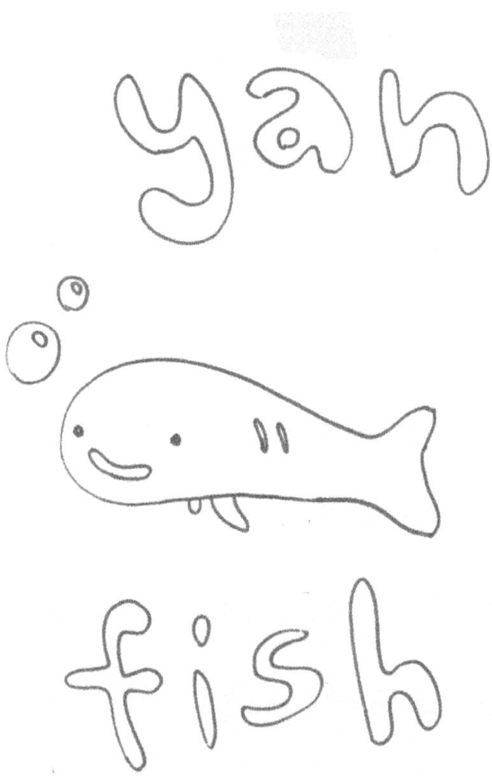

Figure 13.3 Fish drawing by Baylee Badawy with Ishākkoy label

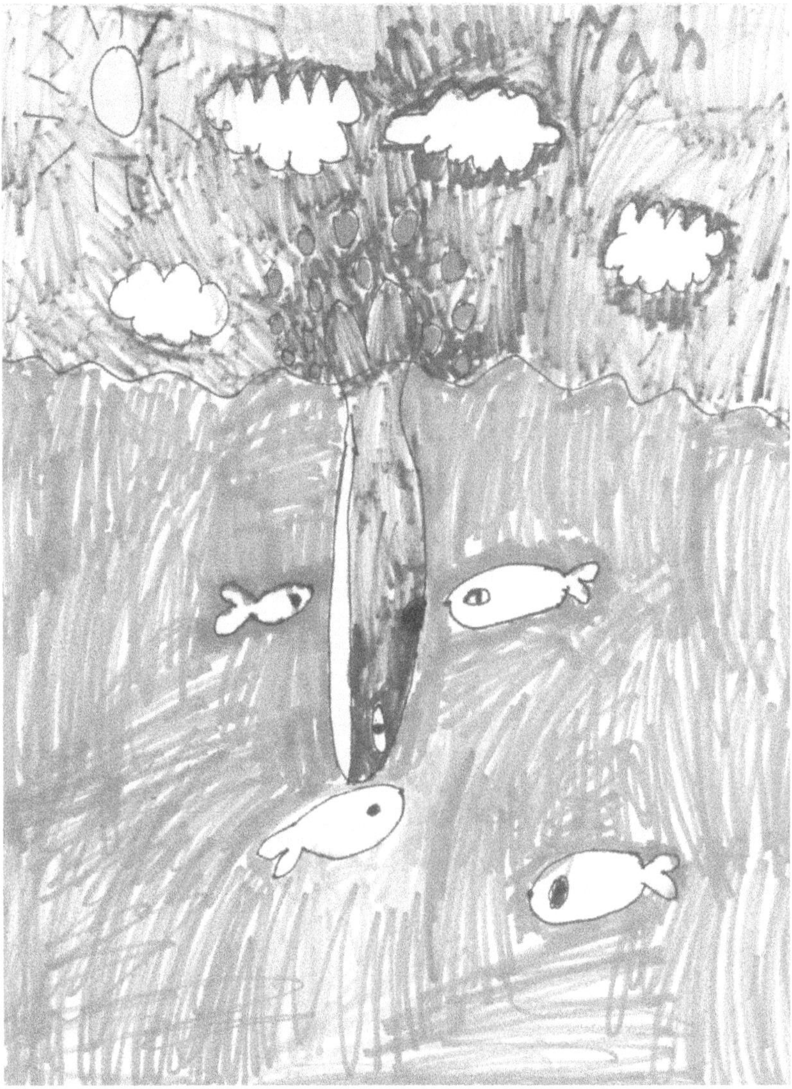

Figure 13.4 Fish drawing by an anonymous child from FORESTival 2021. Note the Ishākkoy word *yan* in the upper right

for composition were given in Kaufman's revised orthography, as well as a version with an English translation below to facilitate pronunciation for the uninitiated. A printout of the poem 'Hoktiwe' was used as an example. Approximately 30 poems were composed, with most being a single page, though some were longer.

Some composers were published writers who were new to both the cento genre and the Ishākkoy language. Both authors were present and helped those who participated to pronounce their poems. One such writer, the poet E. Gross, has published significant works of poetry in

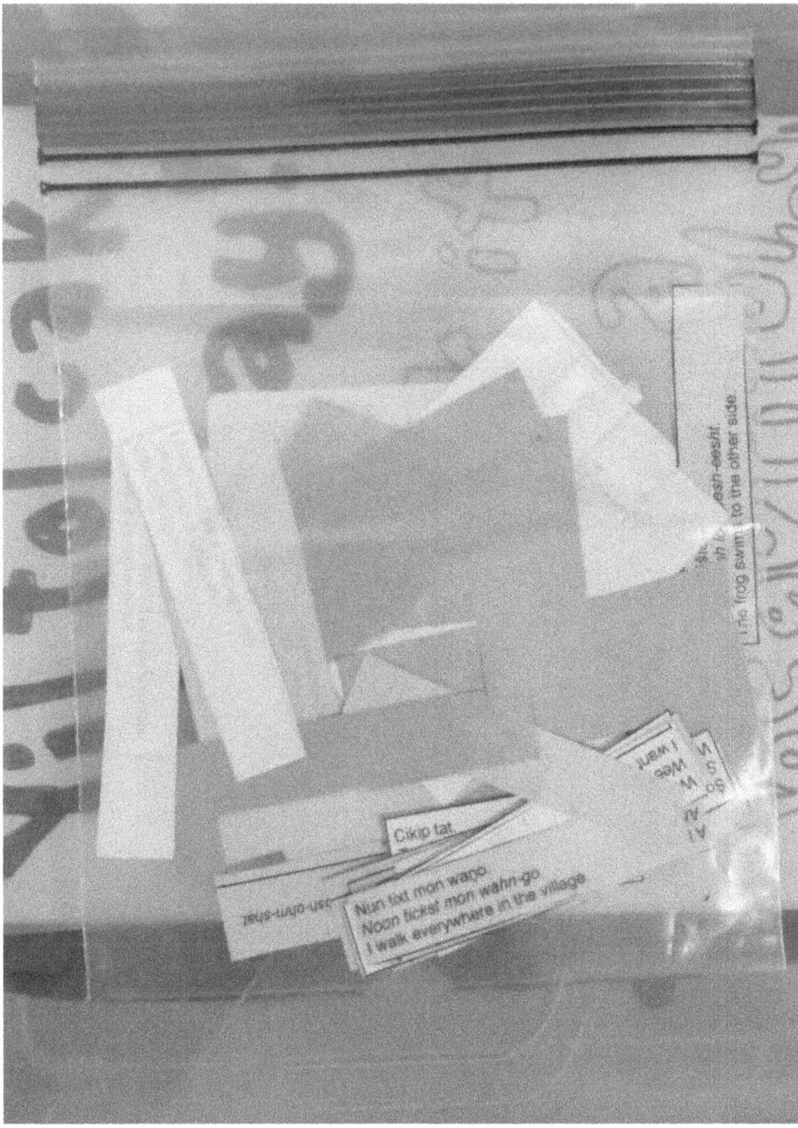

Figure 13.5 An example of materials used at FORESTival for cento composition

English (e.g. Gross, 2019), but had not worked with Ishākkoy or other Indigenous languages before (see Table 13.1). The first four lines from their Ishākkoy poem follow (with updated orthography from the second edition of Kaufman's dictionary).

Most participants posted their works in one of the artist studios at A Studio in the Woods for display during the festival, taking them home afterwards. In addition to the two official projects, we also assisted those who simply wanted to know a few phrases in the language or how to

Table 13.1 Lines of an Ishākkoy poem by E. Gross

Ishākkoy	Simple Pronunciation for Speakers of English	Translation into English
Wi ăm (h)inawsh!	We ahm hee-nowsh!	"Let me drink!"
Kultan oktishat.	Cult-ahn ock-tee-shaht.	"A long time has passed."
Kakaw komi.	Kak-cow koh-mee.	"The rain's heavy."
Wi aŋ ne cakip.	Wee ang nay tsock-kip.	"My house is on dry land."

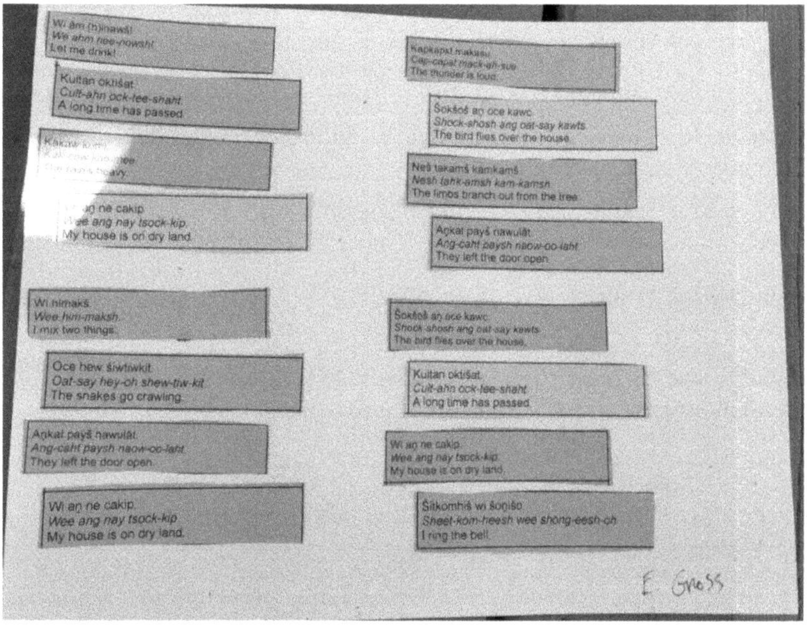

Figure 13.6 An Ishākkoy cento composed by Elizabeth Gross, also known as E. Gross

introduce themselves in it. Importantly, Ishākkoy was used by scores of people who had never used it before, most of whom had never heard of the language. It shows that people can create in a language even if they don't know that language.

Conclusion

Implications for practitioners and researchers

We have attempted to show some ways in which people can familiarize themselves with an Indigenous language, even in the absence of speakers of that language. These methods can also be used by individuals wishing to learn an Indigenous language. We hope this work inspires others to create similar ways of learning Indigenous languages to lift up Indigenous cultures.

Researchers should note that the dormant Indigenous languages of the Americas are understudied, even though some, such as Ishākkoy, have noteworthy features that are ripe for study, such as notions of time. The Ishak have benefited from the work of contemporary linguists. We must also note that these linguists have benefited from working directly with community members to understand the cultural context of the language. Doing outstanding research in a way that both enriches the academic understanding of a language and benefits the language's community represents the best practice in this sort of work.

Language practitioners should note that Indigenous languages are valuable for helping Indigenous populations to connect to their cultural heritages. Even if a practitioner doesn't know a particular Indigenous language, they should still be willing to find resources and contact those involved in language teaching and revitalization. Doing so is easier than ever. Students and clients can benefit even from small efforts in this regard.

Acknowledgements

We are grateful to E. Gross, Pippin Frisbie-Calder, David V. Kaufman, Çaca Yvaire, A Studio in the Woods, FORESTival 2021 attendees and anonymous reviewers for comments and assistance with this work.

Notes

(1) Orthography and references to individual words and phrases follow entries in Kaufman 2022 unless otherwise noted.

(2) One sometimes encounters the name translated as 'screaming eagle,' but that is inaccurate. Americans often want the eagle to sound fiercer in media than it does in reality, with the sound of the red-tailed hawk (*Buteo jamaicensis*) often substituted for that of a bald eagle (*Haliaeetus leucocephalus*). As one birding blogger notes, 'This occurs because producers are lazy, and because a red-tailed hawk sounds much cooler than a bald eagle does. It's as simple as that. Bald eagles have sort of a dopey chuckle for a call, and red-tails have that heart-stopping scream. People making movies want to show the eagle and have an impressive call, so they just put the two together and hope no one notices. Most people don't, but birders do. Learn to laugh, because this happens way more than you realize' (Lund, 2016). Besides birders, Indigenous Peoples of the Americas, for whom eagles are considered sacred, notice as well.

References

Bagan, S. (2019) The power of language: Why Indigenous languages are crucial. *The Cascadian Arc*, blog post, posted 5 May 2019 (accessed 11 October 2024).

Budarangina, O. (2017) Ausonius on the cento technique (*Cento*, Praef. 26–27). *Philologia Classica* 12 (1), 48–53.

Darensbourg, J.U. (2020) Hoktiwe. *Transmotion* 6 (2), 138–141.

Darensbourg, J.U. (2021a) Hunting memories of the grass things: An Indigenous reflection on bison in Louisiana. *Southern Cultures* 27 (1), 14–24.

Darensbourg, J.U. (2021b) A studio in the woods and the ears of that dog are torn. *Yellow Medicine Review*, Spring, 135–139.

Darensbourg, J.U. (2021c) We are together now: Notes on the film *Hoktiwe*: *Two Poems in Ishakkoy*. *Genealogy* 5 (2), 2021. https://www.mdpi.com/2313-5778/5/2/28
Darensbourg, J.U. (2022a) Ishak indigenous people. *64 Parishes Encyclopedia*, 15 August 2022. See https://64parishes.org/entry/ishak-indigenous-people (accessed 24 October 2024).
Darensbourg, J.U. (2022b) Pour la revitalisation de la langue traditionelle dans le district d'Attakapas, en Louisiane, Leçon 1. *Feux Follets: Revue de la création littéraire* 17: *Traces à suivre*, 17–20.
Darensbourg, J.U. (2024) Bulbancha. *64 Parishes Encyclopedia*, 1 May 2024. See https://64parishes.org/entry/bulbancha (accessed 24 October 2024).
De Costa, P.I. (2021) Indigenous language revitalization: How education can help reclaim "sleeping" languages, *Journal of Language, Identity & Education* 20 (5), 355–361.
Driskill, Q.-L. (2015) Decolonial skillshares: Indigenous rhetorics as radical practice. In L. King, R. Gubele and J.R. Anderson (eds) *Survivance, Sovereignty, and Story: Teaching American Indian Rhetorics* (pp. 57–78). University Press of Colorado.
Dunn, C.M. (2022) LA to L.A.: Growing up Louisiana Creole in the Los Angeles diaspora. In R. Prud'homme-Cranford, D. Barthé and A.J. Jolivétte (eds) *Louisiana Creole Peoplehood: Afro-Indigeneity and Community* (pp. 224–239). University of Washington Press.
Ellis, E.N. (2023) *The Great Power of Small Nations: Indigenous Diplomacy in the Gulf South*. University of Pennsylvania Press.
Gatschet, A.S. and Swanton, J.R. (1932) *A Dictionary of the Atakapa Language Accompanied by Text Material*. Smithsonian Institution, Bureau of American Ethnology, bulletin 108. Government Printing Office.
Gross, E. (2019) *This Body/That Lightning Show*. The Word Works Press.
Kaufman, D.V. (2019a) *Clues to Lower Mississippi Valley Histories: Language, Archaeology, and Ethnography*. University of Nebraska Press.
Kaufman, D.V. (2019b) *Atakapa Ishākkoy Dictionary*. Exploration Press.
Kaufman, D.V. (2022) *Atakapa Ishākkoy Dictionary* (2nd edn). Exploration Press.
Kimball, G. (2022) *Yukhíti Kóy: A Reference Grammar of the Atakapa Language*. University of Nebraska Press.
Lund, N. (2016) 'Birdist Rule #50: Learn to live with bird errors in TV and movies. *Audubon*, blog post, posted 29 December 2016 (accessed 1 October 2024).
Malhotra, M. (2010) Weekly prompt: The Cento, semi-Cento, or found poem. *Lantern Review Blog: Asian American Poetry Unbound*, blog post, posted 5 February 2010. See https://www.lanternreview.com/blog/2010/02/05/weekly-prompt-the-cento-semi-cento-or-found-poem/ (accessed 10 October 2024).
Núñez, R.E. and Sweetser, E. (2006) With the future behind them: Convergent evidence from Aymara language and gesture in the crosslinguistic comparison of spatial construals of time. *Cognitive Science* 30, 401–450.
Pearce, M.W. (2014) The last piece is you. *Cartographic Journal* 51 (2), 107–122.
Prud'homme-Cranford, R., Barthé, D. and Jolivétte, A.J. (eds) (2022) *Louisiana Creole Peoplehood: Afro-Indigeneity and Community*. University of Washington Press.
Rifkin, M. (2017) *Beyond Settler Time: Temporal Sovereignty and Indigenous Self-Determination*. Duke University Press.
Schmelzer, P. (2021) Bulbancha forever: From NOLA to Minneapolis, a movement to revitalize Indigenous names grows. *The Ostracon*, 4 January 2021. https://paulschmelzer.com/news/2021/1/5/ostracon-indigenous-naming-bde-maka-ska-bulbancha (accessed 2 June 2026).

14 Koasati in Louisiana

A Native American Language and an English Dialect

Elena Babatsouli and Maria-Sofia Sotiropoulou

Introduction

Aliilamo haslak! Kowassaatilahǫ.
[a.li:.la.mo has.lak! Ko.was.sa:.ti.la.hǫ]
'Welcome! You will become/speak Koasati.'

Kowassatti /ko.was.sa:ti/ 'Koasati' is a Native American language spoken primarily by about 300 people among the 1,000 members of the Coushatta /ko.was.sa:.ti.ha/ Tribe of Louisiana, known as 'lost tribe'. The term *coushatta* is a casual form of *koasati* meaning freely translated as 'those who gather cane'. Koasati in Louisiana is now spoken primarily by adults, as fewer than 5% of Coushatta children (<18 years old) speak it fluently. Most fluent Koasati speakers have Koasati as their first language (L1) or are simultaneous Koasati-English bilinguals (Langley & Langley, 2019). Eli Langley, born to a Coushatta father and a Jewish American mother, is a notable second language (L2) contemporary speaker of Koasati who learned the Koasati language at the age of 18 years. As a student at Harvard University in 2019, he succeeded in changing the university's rules to accept Koasati as a language requirement for bachelor's degrees. No Native American tribal language had previously fulfilled the requirement (Mineo, 2021; Toth, 2019). This is an example of how just a single person can enhance the efforts towards the revitalization and preservation of indigenous and other minority languages in North America.

This chapter is dedicated to Koasati in six sections that look into: (i) context and culture, (ii) the Koasati speech sound system amid American Indian languages, (iii) some American Indian demographics in Louisiana education and speech-language pathology, (iv) implications for practitioners, (v) implications for researchers, and (vi) conclusion. Rather than providing an exhaustive description of Koasati grammar, which is amply and freely available in a plethora of publications cited here, the chapter sets the foundation for the interested practitioner to explore the language/culture, not in isolation but as integral to other Indigenous and non-indigenous languages/dialects in the area. A practitioner, like a *pichi* 'mother' or a *taata* 'father', shows *stimayolikpa* [sti.ma.jo.lik.pa] 'fondness, love, affection' to all *atlawista* 'children', the *aatosi* 'baby', the *ochoski* 'sons', the *tatkasi* 'white child'. While the chapter speaks and writes Koasati, the small language sample highlighted next brings to the forefront two themes that resonate with all who tread the ground of Louisiana: *rainbow* and *tree.*

hanaabitili **'rainbow'**	***itto*** **'tree, wood'**
hommą'red'	*ittosi* 'small tree'
hatka 'white'	*winihkathahi* 'tree struck by lighting'
laana 'yellow, orange, brown'	*ittohissi* 'leaf'
locha [lo.tʃa) 'black'	*thacho* 'acorn'
okchakko [ok.tʃak.ko] 'blue, green'	*ittoinsaawa* 'branch'
	ittoinsaawasi 'twig'
	ittolawista 'sticks'
	ittokchi 'tree sap'
	oak terms:
	baiya 'white oak'
	bosto 'burr oak'
	itto hoomą 'red oak'
	chilaaka 'blackjack oak'
	okwani 'pink oak'

Context and Culture

mikko choba [mik.ko tʃoba] 'head chief'
mikko taiyi [taiji] 'woman chief'
stimmikko 'chief of a group'

Historical setting

The Coushatta people were first encountered by Spanish settlers in Tennessee in the 1500s, and were reported to move subsequently to Alabama, finally settling southwest in Louisiana, Oklahoma and Texas in the 1800s (Gelo & Morales, 1995; Langley & Langley, 2019; Pritzker, 2000; Webb Hodge, 1959). They settled in Louisiana in the 1770s, purchasing their land a century later. The Coushatta people were recognized as an official Tribe by the State in 1972 and, federally, a year later (The Coushatta Tribe of Louisiana, https://coushatta.org). Nowadays, the Coushatta Tribe of Louisiana lives mostly in Allen Parish, just north of Elton and east of Kinder (Figure 14.1). The origins of the Koasati Community of Louisiana are documented by Jacobson (1960).

There are two other federally recognized tribes of the Coushatta people who also speak Koasati: the Alabama-Quassarte Tribal Town with 370 members in Wetumka, Oklahoma (recognized in 1939) and the Alabama-Coushatta Tribe of Texas with 1,100 members in Livingston,

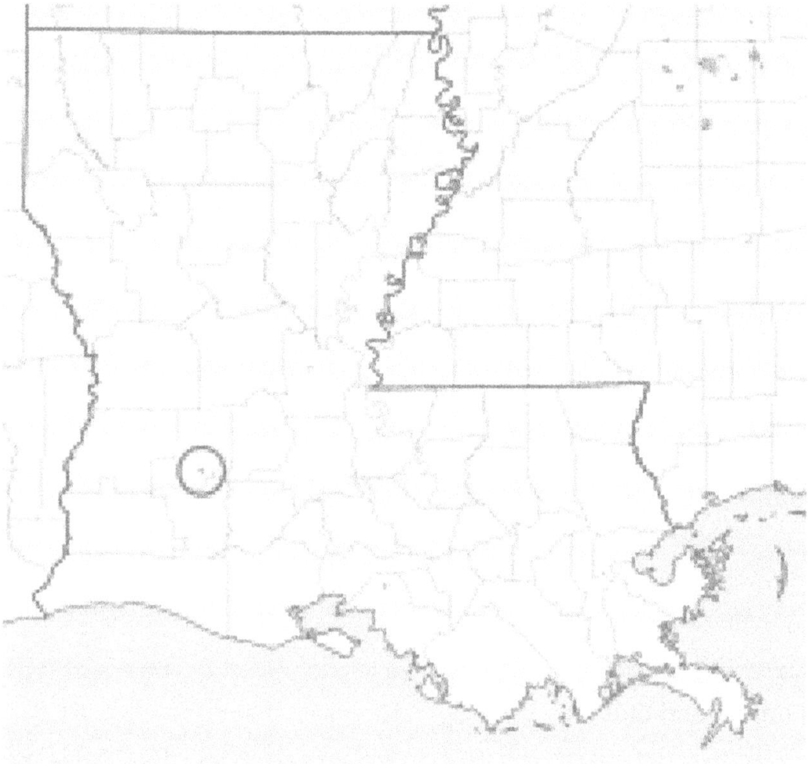

Figure 14.1 The location of the Coushatta Tribe of Louisiana

Texas (federally recognized in 1987). Gelo and Morales (1995) provide an annotated bibliography of the Alabama-Coushatta Indians' history, culture and language up to 1995.

Koasati among other Native American languages

Besides the Muskogean languages, 106 other indigenous languages are spoken in the United States (*Catalogue of Endangered Languages*, n.d.): Navajo (170,000 speakers), Yupik (20,000 speakers), Dakota (18,000), Apache (13,500), Keres (13,200) and Cherokee (11,500) (US Census Bureau, 2013). Among the 26 indigenous language families of the United States, Algic (Algonquin), Athabaskan, Eskimo-Aleut, Iroquoian, Muskogean, Salishan, Siouan and Uto-Aztecan are most widely recognized (Hammarström *et al.*, 2019).

Koasati is a member of the Muskogean language family that also includes Alabama, Apalachee, Chickasaw, Choctaw, Creek (Muskogee) and Mikasuki-Hitchiti. Among these, only Choctaw is also spoken in Louisiana by the Jena Band of Choctaw Indians in

Jena, Louisiana. There are about 10,000 Choctaw speakers in the United States. Besides the Coushatta and Choctaw tribes, Louisiana is the home of two more federally recognized tribes: the Charenton Chitimacha Tribe and the Tunica Biloxi Tribe. While Tunica, Chitimacha and Biloxi are language isolates, Tunica is spoken as an L2 and the other two are languages used by speakers neighboring the Choctaw people, having established the Biloxi-Chitimacha-Choctaw confederation in Schriever. More information on Louisiana native languages and cultures is found in Dajko and Walton (2019). For discussions of Ishākkoy, another Louisiana isolate, see Darensbourg and Badawy (this volume, and 2022a, 2022b).

Loan words

Language contact between North American Indian languages has led to word loans that share morphological and phonological/prosodic features, especially between languages in the same language family, as is the case in Muskogean language examples: Creek *nake*, Choctaw *nata*, Chickasaw *nanta* and Koasati *naasi*, all meaning 'what'. Language contact has created *pidgin* (or trade languages) in Louisiana, namely, the Chinook Jargon (Chinook Wawa) spoken by American Indians in the Northwest and the Mobilian Jargon, spoken among tribes in the Southeast, the Mississippi Valley and the Gulf Coast. Mobilian is primarily based on Muskogean languages and was spoken by the Coushatta and other tribes until the 1950s.

Similarly, contact with other nations internationally resulted in further word borrowing cross-linguistically, e.g. English *hickory*, *moose* from Algonquian languages, Koasati *yon* 'yonder, over there' and Karus *ápus* from English *apples*. Several states carry American Indian names, such as *Oklahoma*, from Choctaw *okla* 'people, tribe, nation' and *homa* 'red', referring to 'Indian Territory' (Bright & Campbell, 2024). Other examples include Koasati *nihta̱* 'tomorrow/day' which is the Greek word *νύχτα* [nixta] 'night' and Creek *abba* 'father', *ishto* 'man', *kora* 'winter' from Hebrew.

Typological neighborhood

American Indian languages in the United States are typologically diverse, even within language families. Mithun (2001) comprehensively discusses such grammatical distinctions, focusing on unusual patterns and speech styles. Typological diversity is also evidenced in phonotactics. For example, while Koasati permits word-final consonant clusters with rising sonority (Gordon *et al.*, 2015b), Alabama (another Muskogean language) does not allow any word-final clusters (Lupardus, 1982). Detailed reports on the morphology and syntax of Muskogean languages can be found in Fitzgerald (2016) and Broadwell (2020), while prosody (tone, stress, intonation) is discussed by Gordon *et al.* (2011, 2015a) and by Gordon (2017) and Gordon and Martin (2023) concerning its relation to morphology. Within the Muskogean language family, there is closer typological similarity between the pairs: Koasati and Alabama, Choctaw and Chickasaw, and Hitchiti and Mikasuki, while Creek is grammatically the most distant of all (Broadwell, 2020; Fitzgerald, 2016; Hardy & Scancarelli, 2005).

Writing system

Unlike the Mesoamerican Indians (Aztecs, Maya, Zapotecs), the North American Indians did not have writing systems, but such systems were developed after Europeans arrived, and often by Europeans. Native American languages spoken in North America use either Latin letters or a syllabary, where symbols represent syllables, similar to ancient Egyptian and Greek scripts, e.g. ᐊᒥᐢᑿᒌᐚᐢᑲᐦᐃᑲᐣ 'Amiskwacîwâskahikan' (Treaty 6 Territory 300, n.d.). For instance, Cherokee, Cree and Inuktut (see Canadian Inuktut, this volume) use modern syllabaries, while Apache and Navajo are written in the Latin alphabet (Syropoulos, 2002). Koasati is also written using the Latin script. Nevertheless, Broadwell (1991) suggested that the Greek alphabet would be more suitable for North American Indian languages, including Muskogean languages to represent the short/long vowel contrasts.

The earliest Koasati dictionaries were written by Gatschet (1885) and Swanton (1911). In these works, Koasati is in Latin script, as was in Haas' (1944) study on Koasati speech. Kimball (1985, 1991, 1994) enhanced the previous attempts at Koasati dictionaries, also documenting Koasati grammar. The Koasati writing system kept changing until, more recently in 2007, the Coushatta Tribe of Louisiana developed and officially approved their Koasati orthographic system, based on field evidence in Hasselbacher (2015a, 2015b). Hasselbacher (2015b) reported that the Koasati Language Committee, comprising 25 fluent Koasati speakers and the scholars Jack Martin, Linda Langley and Susan Penfield devised the writing system by identifying each Koasati phoneme and corresponding to a letter in the Latin alphabet. This orthographic system is similar to Kimball's (1985, 1991, 1994), though not to Haas' (1944) spelling, and it does not encode the Koasati glottal stop and tone. In contexts where vowels are nasalized, the vowel is underlined during spelling.

The Coushatta Tribe of Louisiana, in collaboration with McNeese State University in Louisiana and the College of William and Mary in Virginia (Langley *et al.*, 2018), started a program to revitalize Koasati, which resulted in the *Coushatta Tribe of Louisiana Koasati Digital Dictionary* (Abbey *et al.*, n.d.).

The Koasati Speech Sound System amid American Indian Languages

nathihilka [na:ɬi:hil.ka] ‘language’

This section describes Koasati phonology and compares it with other Indigenous and non-indigenous languages in North America, while also introducing the Native American English (Craig, 1991) dialect as a natural consequence of language change.

Koasati phonology and phonetics

Recent works by Gordon and his colleagues (e.g. Gordon, 2017; Gordon *et al.*, 2011, 2015a, 2015b) have shed new light on the Koasati phonetic and phonological structure in the 21st century, updating previous reports (Haas, 1944; Kimball, 1985, 1991, 1994). This section briefly summarizes Koasati phonology based on these reports and the authors’ observations of transcriptions in *The Coushatta Tribe of Louisiana Koasati Digital Dictionary* (Abbey *et al.*, n.d.). Koasati orthography is mostly transparent, though it is noted that long vowels and nasal vowels are doubled, <*aa*> or underlined, <o̲>, respectively. Also, among the consonants, the voiceless alveolar lateral fricative /ɬ/ <th> is opaque, and the affricate /ʧ/ <ch> less so.

Vowels

Koasati has six vowel phonemes with short/long contrasts /a a: i i: o o:/ in word-initial and word-medial position, e.g. *oki* /oki/ ‘water’, *oolachi* /ˈo:.la.tʃi/ ‘clown’, *Kowassaati* /ko.was.ˈsa:.ti/ ‘Koasati language or person’, *oola* /ˈo:la/ ‘town’. All word-final vowels are short, e.g. *ootooba* /ˈo:to:ba/ ‘dreamer’. Mid-back /o/ distinguishes free allophones [u, ʊ]. Nasal vowels tend to be context-specific, occurring word-finally as part of future tense morpheme *-ho̲* ‘will’, e.g. *onahompanilaho̲* [o.na.hom.pa.ni.la.hõ] ‘will play around something’, in adjectives word-finally, e.g. *takpa̲* ‘bitter’, *koboksi̲* ‘short’, and less commonly in nouns, e.g. *ha̲hka* ‘boogeyman’, and function words, e.g. *aba̲* ‘up’, *nampo̲* ‘how much?’, mostly word-finally.

Consonants

Koasati has 14 consonants: 5 stops: /p b t ʧ k/; 4 fricatives: /f s ɬ h/; 2 nasals: /m n/ and 3 approximants: /l j w/ which appear mostly word-initially and medially. There are few words with word-final singleton consonants, mostly nasals and plosives. So, for instance, among the 240 *a-* words in *The Coushatta Tribe of Louisiana Koasati Digital Dictionary*, only two end in a consonant: akkofon ‘there’, *akkaam* ‘that’s right’. Word-final consonants are also found in numerals, e.g. *chokpi chaffaakan* ‘one hundred’ and onomatopoeia, e.g. *chathathahkaachin* ‘making a rattling sound’.

Syllable structure

CV and CVC are the main syllables of Koasati. However, vowel deletion in word-initial or word-final CV syllables has resulted in CCV and CVCC syllables, respectively, as well. Word-initially, such clusters involve *sC* clusters: /sp sb st sk stʃ sm sn sl sɬ sw sh/, e.g. *stintijapka* 'can opener', *smokafka* 'decorations', *shalathilka* 'handle'. Word-finally, vowel deletion has resulted in word-final consonant clusters that violate the Sonority Sequencing Principle governing many world languages, including English, in that they do not fall but rise in sonority. Examples are: *biitl* 's/he is dancing', *hoofn* 's/he is smelling it'. Other world languages such as Arabic, Russian and Persian (see Taghvafard & Babatsouli, this volume) also have word-final rising sonority clusters.

Prosody

Koasati words are mostly multisyllabic, i.e. longer than three syllables, *paachokokbaski* 'couch', *haipolohkaachilaho̱* 'will keep spinning', but shorter words exist, e.g. *baiba̱* 'heavy'. Koasati is a syllable-timed language, like other American Indian languages. Koasati prosody is complex, distinguishing varying stress, tone and intonation patterns. Lexical stress is predictable, falling on the first syllable. Prosodic tone can have an Accentual Phrase (initial and final high tone that may be superseded by lexical or morphological tone) and an Intonational Phrase (consisting of one or more Accentual Phrases with a terminal boundary tone). Koasati also distinguishes four boundary tones: low, high, high-to-low and low-to-high, and three types of pitch accents: lexical, morphological and phonological (see comprehensive discussion and examples in Gordon *et al.*, 2015a). The tone system of Koasati differs from those of other Muskogean languages, even that of its closest relative, Alabama. Koasati lexical tone rises, primarily occurring in nouns and verbal suffixes. Other American Indian languages distinguish lexical tones, such as Caddo having a falling tone, and Oklahoma Cherokee that has both rising and falling tones.

Prosodic morphology

Like other American Indian languages, Koasati prosody is morphologically determined (Gordon, 2017; Gordon & Martin, 2023). Reduplications are a main characteristic, i.e. doubling (repeating) a morpheme in the word or part of it. In punctual reduplication, <o> is added to the first consonant of the root, e.g. *lapatkin* becomes *lapatlookin* 'to be narrow' adding *lo*, *talasban* becomes *talastooban* 'to be thin', adding *to*. Notably, in the examples of the published works, the reduplicated consonant occurs word-initially, being processed psycho-linguistically in perseveration. In contrast to morphological epenthesis, a subtractive morphological pattern is displayed in Koasati plural formation, e.g. singular forms *lasaplin*, *atakalin* become plural *laplin* 'to lick', *ataklin* 'to hang something', respectively.

Koasati phonology compared to other languages

tiskila foshissi [tis.ki.la fos.his.si] 'blue jay feather'

To facilitate an understanding of Koasati within the context of other Indigenous languages, this section compares phonological structure in terms of consonant inventory, consonant-to-vowel ratio, syllable complexity and tone systems between Koasati and other languages that Koasati speakers have been in contact with, i.e. Alabama, Chickasaw (Muskogean languages), Cherokee, Navajo (other Native American languages) and English, French, Spanish (Romance languages). The data used here for this comparison were drawn from Dryer and Haspelmath's (2013) *World Atlas of Language Structures Online*. Table 14.1 summarizes the terms used to describe comparison metrics for different levels of phonological structure (c.f. Ian Maddieson and other refs in Dryer & Haspelmath, 2013), while Table 14.2 sums the results of comparisons in terms of these metrics.

Table 14.1 Metrics of phonological structure

Consonant inventory	**Small** 6–14	**Moderately small** 15–18	**Average** 19–25	**Moderately large** 26–33	**Large** ≥ 34
Consonant-vowel ratio	**Low** ≤ 2.0	**Moderately low** (2.0, 2.75)	**Average** (2.75, 4.5)	**Moderately high** (4.5, 6.5)	**High** ≥ 6.5
Syllable structure	**Simple** V, CV	**Moderately complex** CVC, CCV	**Complex** CCCV, CVCC, etc.		

Table 14.2 Crosslinguistic comparison of phonological structures

Language	Consonant inventory	Consonant-vowel ratio	Syllable	Tone system
Koasati	Small	Moderately high	Moderately complex	Complex
Alabama	Small	Moderately high	Moderately complex	Simple
Chickasaw	Moderately small	Moderately high	Moderately complex	No tones
Cherokee	Small	Low	Moderately complex	Complex
Navajo	Moderately large	High	Moderately complex	Simple
English	Average	Low	Complex	No tones
French	Average	Low	Complex	No tones
Spanish	Average	Average	Moderately complex	No tones

Overall, Muskogean languages have fewer consonants (small inventory: Alabama, Koasati; moderately small inventory: Chickasaw) and vowels compared to Romance languages. As a result, the consonant-vowel ratio in these languages is moderately high compared to Romance languages. The other American Indian languages show variable consonant-vowel ratios, with Navajo having a higher ratio compared to that of Cherokee. All American languages (Muskogean or not) have moderately complex syllable structures, i.e. V, CV, CVC and CCV.

Tonal systems also vary substantially within and outside a language family. Among Muskogean languages, tone can be simple (Alabama: high and high-falling), complex (Koasati: low, high, mid-level, high-rising, high-falling) or lacking (Chickasaw), similar to Romance languages. Tone also varies among the other Native American Indian languages, being complex (Cherokee) or simple (Navajo) (Gordon, 2017).

Native American English dialect

Native American English is one of 30 major English dialects in the United States, among over 150 English dialects worldwide (e.g. Boyanton, 2024). The Native American English dialect is not to be confused with Native American Pidgin English, a language developed between Europeans and American Indians in the Western United States and Canada for speaking with each other (Leechman & Hall, 1955). Native American English is not a single English dialect but comprises several variants, as a result of the American Indian speakers of English (Leap, 1993). The first American Indian to speak English was Squanto of the Patuxet tribe. After he was taken to Spain as a slave in 1614, he was able to go first to England and then return to what is now Massachusetts. Squanto was an interpreter between the Wampanoag people and the Pilgrims.

Based on Jacobson (1954), the influx of White and Black rice farmers in Southwestern Louisiana in the 1910s forced the Coushatta people of Louisiana to learn English as they worked for the farmers. In 1915, L.L. Simmons went to Elton, LA, where he taught in a public school, staying for twenty years, and introduced the Coushatta people to the white people's ways and the Christian faith. By this time, schooling was compulsory in Louisiana, and the Coushatta children were forced to learn and speak English; speaking English imparted a social and economic advantage (Precht, 2007).

English became the 'lingua franca' in the Coushatta community of Louisiana; families with one parent speaking Koasati use English as the language of communication (Hasselbacher, 2015b). Since the early 1980s, Coushatta toddlers attend English-only preschool on the Coushatta Reservation. As a result, there are three language groups among the Coushatta community of Elton: Koasati speakers, passive bilinguals (they understand English, but do not speak it, e.g. Babatsouli & Ingram, 2018; Babatsouli & Ball, 2020) and English speakers.

Some studies have elaborated on the influence of Koasati on the English speech of the Coushatta people (Hasselbacher, 2015b; Kyzer, 1952), while others describe general American Indian English patterns (e.g. Penfield, 1977; Wolfram, 1984). Arguably, the most striking feature of the American Indian English dialect is prosody (Craig, 1991), influenced by the patterns of the native language (for acoustical studies, see Gordon *et al.* (2011) on Koasati, Martin and Johnson (2002) on Creek, Gordon and Munro (2007) on Chickasaw). Coggshall (2008) compared the prosodic rhythm of Cherokee English and Lumbee English with standard American English, reporting the same syllable duration in the Indigenous varieties of English, indicating the influence of syllable-timed isochrony from the indigenous language to English. Newmark *et al.* (2016) found common prosodic features among American Indian English variants: similar pitch patterns, rhythm and intonation. Interestingly, many of the subjects in their study did not speak their heritage American Indian language. They also found that sentences ended on a middle or light pitch. Additionally, strong evidence of syllable timing surfaced as a common characteristic of American Indian English dialects (Craig, 1991). Last, Coggshall (2015) further elaborated on linguistic and social intersections in the American Indian English variants. Notably, American Indian English speech is commonly known as Rez accent, where 'Rez' abbreviates *reservation*. Newmark *et al.* (2016) attribute the Rez accent to contact between the tribes during the reservation era (1880s) and the relocation era (1950s–1960s), when American Indians were moved to cities. For another resource, see also Hilleary (2022).

The Rez accent is the common thread between culturally and ethnically diverse American Indian groups. Although language ideologies perpetuated social stigmas on ethnic American English dialects for most of the 20th century in the United States, a resurgence of identity and culture among ethnic groups in the late 1900s was reported (Lippi-Green, 2004; Nagel, 1996). Interestingly, one-third of multiracial American Indians and one-sixth of single-race American Indians did not respond to the tribal affiliation question of the US Census 2000 (Liebler & Zacher, 2013), indicating that the American Indian English dialect was more significant to the respondents than their heritage language(s).

White (2006), among others, notes that American Indian English speech has common features with the indigenous language, making it easier for American Indians who are monolingual English speakers to acquire the indigenous language as a second language. These features include narrative form and pauses and appropriate social speech skills such as kinship or elder respect. Further, Hasselbacher (2015b) observed that monolingual English-speaking members of the local Koasati language community had phonetic and social advantages in understanding and speaking Koasati over community outsiders.

Language change

ilimathahkichilahǫ [i.li.ma.ɬah.ki.tʃi.la.hõ] 'change'

Languages undergo a natural change, and Koasati is no exception. Koasati speech has undergone some changes (Hasselbacher, 2015a, 2015b; Kimball, 1987, 1990; Saville-Troike, 1988), since the 1930s (1944). Elder fluent Koasati speakers describe younger speaker usage as 'baby talk', meaning that words are shorter and 'flat' (having improper intonation or lacking tone) (Hasselbacher, 2015a, 2015b). These changes may be attributed to the increasing use of English. Other changes include *h* omission following vowels and vocabulary loss due to lifestyle changes (e.g. the disappearance of the term meaning 'field') or due to generalization (e.g. *toola* is the only term for 'magnolia', instead of three different terms for magnolia types). Even within the Coushatta Reservation, dialectal variations were observed subject to speakers' geographic origin, e.g. *teeth* is pronounced as *innati* in Elton, but *innoti* in the village of Robinson, on the other side of the bayou. Other dialectal variations, evidenced in families, include cluster reduction, e.g. *hachokpalpa*/ *hakchopalpa* 'butterfly', backing or fronting for /s, ʃ/, as per universal substitution patterns in L2 speech (Babatsouli, 2021). With the advent of 20th century technology, new terms appeared in Koasati, e.g. *palki libalti* 'cooks fast' for *microwaves*, and *pitcha-waika* 'flying boat' for *airplane*. Code-switching between Koasati and English is also common, e.g. *Anholikfa iron-kalin* 'let me go iron my clothes' instead of *Anholikfo thimikkochilin*, and the transfer of Koasati suffix *-ka* in English.

A prominent change in Koasati in the last 80 years is gender-based. Haas (1944) reports that spoken Koasati, mostly by middle-aged and elders, was a gender-based language in the 1930s; that is, though women would use women's talk among themselves and shift to men's talk when addressing men, men only used men's talk. This was observed in verb endings in the indicative and imperative, e.g. *ka·hβl* (women) vs *ka·hɑs* (men) 'I am saying'; *v·sk* (women) vs *v·sks* (men) 'you are saying'; and *ka·* (women) vs *kɑ·s* (men) 'he is saying'. By the late 1970s, Kimball (1987, 1990) reports that Koasati was no longer a gender-based language overall, as indicated by deletion and nasalization in word endings, these being mostly genderless. Such observations were further supported by Saville-Troike (1988) who studied her own speech data elicited in the late 1960s (10 years earlier than Kimball's sample). Some Koasati gender terms are: *chika* 'boy', *naani* 'man', *taiyi* 'woman', *taiyosi* 'girl'. The diachronic loss of gender-based distinction in language use has been reported for other world languages, including the Irish Sign Language (Dunn, 2014).

Some American Indian Demographics in Louisiana Education and Speech-Language Pathology

Table 14.3 below shows American Indian/Alaskan Native student enrollment in Louisiana public higher education in the Fall of 2023,

Table 14.3 American Indian/Alaskan native student enrollment (Fall 2023)

Institution/level	Number of students	Percentage to all students (%)
Grambling	9	0.18
LA Tech	38	0.31
LSU Alexandria	151	2.89
LSU A&M	173	0.41
LSU Shreveport	72	0.74
McNeese State	23	0.38
Nicholls State	146	2.33
Northwestern State	108	1.21
Southeastern Louisiana	21	0.15
Southern U A&M	9	0.11
Southern U New Orleans	4	0.19
UL Lafayette	50	0.32
UL Monroe	30	0.35
University of New Orleans	21	0.32
Total: four-year institutions	**853**	**0.57**
LSU HSCN	11	0.41
LSU HSCS	1	0.10
Total: special education	**12**	**0.32**
BPCC	47	0.83
BRCC	43	0.40
CLTCC	7	0.59
Delgado	53	0.44
Fletcher	115	4.74
LDCC	12	0.32
LSU Eunice	25	0.68
NLTCC	9	0.86
NTCC	26	0.45
Nunez	8	0.27
RPCC	3	0.12
SLCC	43	0.73
Sowela	13	0.39
Southern U Shreveport	13	0.41
Total: two-year institutions	**417**	**0.65**
Total: all institutions	**1,282**	**0.59**

Source: Louisiana Public Higher Education.

based on data provided by the Board of Regents of the State of Louisiana (n.d.). The highest percentage of American Indian/Alaskan Native student enrollment in a four-year institution is at Louisiana State University Alexandria, a city started by the Caddo Indians. Although the percentage of American Indian/Alaskan Native student enrollment to all students (undergraduate and graduate) is shown as 2.89% for Fall 2023, LSU Alexandria is a Native American-Serving Nontribal Institution (NASNTI); an institution with a Native American enrollment of not less than 10% of all undergraduates. The number of graduate students is not large enough to shift the percentages, which may be attributed to responses of the American Indians/Alaskan Natives regarding ethnic identity and mixed race. There are 38 NASNTIs in 10 states, nationally, enrolling 12% of American Indian/Alaskan Native undergraduates, conferring 14% and 10% of their associate and bachelor's degrees (Western Interstate Commission for Higher Education, n.d.). In addition, as of 2022, there are 35 Tribal Colleges and Universities in 15 states enrolling 17,110 students, 78% of whom are American Indian/Alaskan Natives (Data USA, n.d.). The highest percentage of American Indian/Alaskan Native student enrollment in a two-year institution is at Fletcher Technical Community College, 4.74%, in Schriever, Louisiana, home of the Biloxi-Chitimacha-Choctaw Confederation. In the same educational service area and Thibodaux, Nicholls State University (a four-year institution) has the second highest percentage, 2.33%, among four-year institutions in Louisiana.

The overall percentage of American Indians/Alaskan Natives in Louisiana public higher education is 0.59%, while the percentage of American Indians/Alaskan Natives to the whole Louisiana population of 4,657,757 is 0.68% as of 2020, the national percentage being 1.1% of 331,656,829 (Louisiana Census, n.d.). In the United States as of 2021, 0.7% of all enrolled in postsecondary education identified themselves as American Indians/Alaskan Natives; among these, 28% of the 18- to 24-year-old American Indians/Alaskan Natives were enrolled compared to 38% of the overall US population. Moreover, as of 2022, 16.8% of American Indians/Alaskan Natives of age 25 or over have a bachelor's degree or higher compared to 35.7% for the whole population in the United States (Postsecondary Public National Institute, n.d.), and compared to 26.8% of the entire Louisiana population (Data USA, n.d.). As of 2022, there are 580 American Indian/Alaskan Native certified speech-language pathologists (SLPs) in the United States and one dual SLP/audiologist, for a cumulative percentage to both certified groups of 0.29%, the second to lowest rate for any race, Native Hawaiian/Pacific Islander being the lowest at 0.13%. In Louisiana, there are 3,136 SLPs and 13 dual SLPs resulting in a cumulative percentage to all certified SLPs in the United States of 1.6% ASHA membership (ASHA, 2022) There is no data on American Indian/Alaskan Native SLPs in Louisiana but, based on national statistics, the number is quite small, estimated at about nine, or 0.29% of the

Table 14.4 American Indian/Alaskan Native demographics

AI/AN number and percentage/control group	Number	Percentage (%)
US population	3,727,135	1.1
US higher education enrollment	121,000	0.7
US bachelor's degree or higher	550,000	0.5
Louisiana population	31,657	0.68
Louisiana public higher education enrollment	1,283	0.59
Louisiana bachelor's degree or higher	5,318	0.46
AI/AN higher education enrollment (age 18–24 years)	121,000	28 of AI/AN (L 33, US 38)
AI/AN bachelor's degree or higher (age 25 years or older)	550,000	16.8 of AI/AN (L 26.8, US 35.7)
US certified SLPs	581	0.29
Louisiana certified SLPs	9 (est.)	0.29 (est.)

3,136 SLPs in Louisiana. The aforementioned demographics of American Indians/Alaskan Natives in education and in speech-language pathology are summarized in Table 14.4.

Implications for Practitioners

As shown, Koasati, like other American Indian languages, differs typologically compared to most widely spoken languages in the United States, English and Spanish. The same holds for the Rez accent. Culture-specific patterns of communication are reported for American Indians, especially in young children. As a result, more published works have recognized that the demographics of SLPs in terms of ethnicity, language and culture are such that the needs of the American Indian communities are either insufficiently served or not served at all (Alison-Burbank & Reid, 2023; Ferris *et al.*, 2021; Gillispie, 2021; Guiberson & Vining, 2023; Meeks, 2023; Vining & Guiberson, 2021). A main challenge in clinical assessment and intervention in the context of American Indian language/speech is to differentiate between impairment and language/dialect difference, and to develop appropriate culturally relevant, as is true for other dialects of English (e.g. Oetting, 2018), and cross-linguistically (e.g. Babatsouli, 2021, 2023). The overwhelming majority (>90%) of SLPs and audiologists (who are ASHA members) are White and Non-Hispanic, both in Louisiana and in the United States, while only 6.5% of practitioners are bilingual compared to 20% of the US population (ASHA, 2022). On the other hand, American Indians/Alaskan Indians are 0.29% of SLPs nationwide and 1.1% of the US population. Across language variation contexts, SLPs who do not speak the client's language rely on culture brokers, typically a client's family or community members; any form or degree of allegiance (e.g. familiarity with) to the clients' language is beneficial to interactions and the SLP's willingness to engage in facilitating communication and interaction, necessary in clinical practicum, instead of referring the client to other professionals (Babatsouli, 2023; Babatsouli & Ingram, 2027). In mostly educational contexts, translanguaging practices are endorsed to allow for clients' affirmation of identity and language practices (Vogel & García, 2017). For guidelines on translanguaging implementation, see Creese and Blackledge (2015).

Implications for Researchers

Efforts to revitalize American Indian languages also take place via academic and cultural programs in higher education. There are 35 Tribal Colleges and Universities and 38 Native American-Serving Nontribal Institutions (NASNTIs) in the nation, one of which is in Louisiana, Louisiana State University Alexandria. Most language revitalization attempts in the Coushatta community began in 2007, together with the new writing system, encouraging non-speakers to learn Koasati. As previously stated, this was an initiative of the Coushatta Tribe of Louisiana in collaboration with McNeese State University in Louisiana and the College of William and Mary in Virginia (Langley *et al.*, 2018). The initiative led to the publication of the Koasati language phrase book, *Iłtooyat Naathiihilka* (Fuseller *et al.*, 2010) and the online *Coushatta Tribe of Louisiana Koasati Digital Dictionary*. Hasselbacher (2015a) reports more revitalization efforts, such as Summer Workshops, Koasati Language Day, Fall Celebration and a revised Koasati curriculum for preschool. In addition, students at the College of William and Mary designed a Koasati language learning program, MEMRISE (MEMRISE, 2015). The ongoing representation of the Koasati language in research and culture/language revitalization serves as a beacon to encourage and motivate new researchers in the field, a line of work that has been discussed before in the context of heritage languages (Lo Bianco & Kreeft Peyton, 2013), and mirrors resilience linguistics (e.g. Bradley, 2011) around the globe. Research outcomes are more reliable when speakers of the minority language actively participate in research teams, not just as study participants. Future research on Koasati can trace demographic and language usage trends, language acquisition/attrition patterns, speech and language disorders in this heritage language context, and assist in creating appropriate clinical batteries that reflect community values.

Conclusion

intihlichilahǫ Koasati 'will support Koasati'

Data from the US Bureau of Labor Statistics (n.d.) indicate that speech-language pathology positions will increase by 29% from 2020 to 2030, outpacing by far the average across all professions. Concomitantly, ASHA members' rising awareness of Native American needs is shown by the establishment of The Native American Caucus of Speech-Language Pathology and Audiology in 1986 (n.d.). Its purpose is 'to increase and improve quality speech, language, and hearing services to Indigenous people who have communication disorders'. Improving the representation of American Indians, including the Coushatta people of Louisiana in the speech-language pathology and audiology profession, as part of increasing cultural awareness and sensitivity for all American Indian communities should result in significant progress in clinical and educational services for these historically important but underrepresented groups in North America. The chapter opens a portal for current practitioners into the Coushatta/Koasati language/culture. The recent language revitalization efforts at all levels of education, including higher education, and the excellent job prospects can also serve as incentives for American Indian youth to step up preparing themselves to contribute to clinical and educational services alongside other practitioners in the communities they live. It is a *topka chokiibǫ* 'small town', but not an *oola tokpa* 'different town'.

References

Abbey R. et al. (eds.) (n.d.) *The Coushatta Tribe of Louisiana Koasati Digital Dictionary*. See https://koasati.azurewebsites.net/ (accessed 30 November 2024).

Allison-Burbank, J.D. and Reid, T. (2023) Prioritizing connectedness and equity in speech-language services for American Indian and Alaska Native children. *Language, Speech, and Hearing Services in Schools* 54 (2), 368–374. https://doi: 10.1044/2022_LSHSS-22-00101

ASHA (2022) American Speech-Language-Hearing Association. See https://asha.org/siteassets/surveys/2022-member-affiliate-profile.pdf (accessed 28 November 2025).

Babatsouli, E. (2021) Diversity considerations in speech and language disorders: A focus on training. In J.S. Damico, N. Müller and M.J. Ball (eds) *Handbook of Language and Speech Disorders* (2nd edn, pp. 33–52). Wiley-Blackwell.

Babatsouli, E. (2023) Ecosystemic clinical assessment of linguistic diversity: Greek-dominant speech. *Perspectives of the ASHA Special Interest Groups* 9 (3), 692–714.

Babatsouli, E. and Ingram, D. (2018) Prologue. In E. Babatsouli and D. Ingram (eds) *Phonology in Protolanguage and Interlanguage* (pp. 1–23). Equinox Publishing. Imprint 2024, University of Toronto Press.

Babatsouli, E. and Ingram, D. (in print, 2027) Multilingual aspects of speech sound disorders in children. In H. Blake, S. McLeod, K. Margetson and B.A. Goldstein (eds) *Multilingual Aspects of Speech Sound Disorders in Children* (2nd edn). Multilingual Matters.

Board of Regents of the State of Louisiana (n.d.) See https://apps.regents.state.la.us (accessed 28 November 2024).

Boyanton, M.U.-L. (2024) A brief history of the United States' accents and dialects: Migration patterns, cultural ties, geographic regions and class differences all shape speaking patterns. *Smithsonian Magazine*, 17 January. See https://smithsonianmag.com/history/a-brief-history-of-the-united-states-accents-and-dialects-180983591/

Bradley, D. (2011) Resilience linguistics, orthography and the Gong. *Language and Education* 25 (4), 349–360. https://doi.org/10.1080/09500782.2011.577222

Bright, W.O. and Campbell, L. (2024) North American Indian languages. *Britannica*. Last updated 7 September.

Broadwell, G.A. (1991) The Myskogean connection of the Guale and Yamasee. *International Journal of American Linguistics* 57 (2), 267–270.

Broadwell, G.A. (2020) Muskogean languages. In D. Siddiqi, M. Barrie, C. Gillon, J.D. Haugen and E. Mathieu (eds) *The Routledge Handbook of North American Languages* (pp. 397–423). Routledge.

Catalogue of Endangered Languages (n.d.) https://endangeredlanguages.com (accessed November 2024).

Coggshall, E.L. (2008) The prosodic rhythm of two varieties of Native American English. In K. Gorman (ed.) *U. Penn Working Papers in Linguistics* 14 (2), Selected Papers from NWAV 36, 1–9. http://repository.upenn.edu/pwpl/vol14/iss2/2

Coggshall, E.L. (2015) American Indian English. In J.P. Williams, E.W. Schneider, P. Trudgill and D. Schreier (eds) *Further Studies in the Lesser-Known Varieties of English* (pp. 99–127). Cambridge University Press.

Craig, B. (1991) American Indian English. *English World-Wide* 12, 2–61.

Creese, A. and Blackledge, A. (2015) Translanguaging and identity in educational settings. *Annual Review of Applied Linguistics* 35 (20–35). https://doi.10.1017/S0267190514000233

Dajko, N. and Walton, S. (eds) (2019) *Language in Louisiana: Community and Culture*. University Press of Mississippi.

Darensbourg, J.U. (2022a) Ishak indigenous people. *64 Parishes Encyclopedia*, 15 August. See https://64parishes.org/entry/ishak-indigenous-people (accessed 24 October 2024).

Darensbourg, J.U. (2022b) Pour la revitalisation de la langue traditionelle dans le district d'Attakapas, en Louisiane, Leçon 1. *Feux Follets: Revue de la Création Littéraire 17: Traces à Suivre*, 17–20.

Data USA (n.d.) See https://datausa.io/profile/university/tribal-colleges) (accessed 30 November 2024).

Dryer, M.S. and Haspelmath, M. (eds) (2013) *World Atlas of Language Structures (Wals) Online* (v2020.3) [Data set] Zenodo. See https://wals.info

Dunn, M. (2014) Gender determined dialect variation. In G.G. Corbett (ed.) *The Expression of Gender* (pp. 39–68). Gruyter Mouton.

Ferris, K.P., Guiberson, M. and Bush, E.J. (2021) Native American caregivers' developmental priorities for young children: Implications for intervention. *Topics in Language Disorders* 41 (2), 170–185. https://doi.10.1097/TLD.0000000000000247

Fitzgerald, C.M. (2016) Morphology in the Muskogean languages. *Language and Linguistics Compass* 10, 681–700. https://doi.10.1111/lnc3.12227

Fuseller, N., Poncho Hill, J., Williams, C. and Williams, H. (2010) *Iłtooyat Naathiihilka*. The Coushatta Tribe of Louisiana.

Gatschet, A.S. (1885) Koasati. *American Anthropological Archives*, ms. 902, Washington, DC.

Gelo, D.J. and Morales, J. (1995) The Alabama-Coushatta Indians: An annotated bibliography. *East Texas Historical Journal* 33 (2), 35–63.

Gillispie, M. (2021) Culturally responsive language and literacy instruction with Native American children. *Topics in Language Disorders* 41 (2), 186–199. https://doi.10.1097/TLD.0000000000000249

Gordon, M.K. (2017) Phonetic and phonological research on Native American languages: Past, presence, and future. *International Journal of American Linguistics* 83 (1), 79–110.

Gordon, M.K. and Munro, P. (2007) A phonetic study of final vowel lengthening in Chickasaw. *International Journal of American Linguistics* 73 (3), 293–330. https://doi.10.1086/521729

Gordon, M.K. and Martin, J.B. (2023) Muskogean prominence. In K. Bogomolets and H. van der Hulst (eds) *Word Prominence in Languages with Complex Morphologies* (pp. 274–307). Oxford University Press.

Gordon, M.K., Langley, L. and Martin, J.B. (2011) The prosodic structure of Koasati. *The Journal of the Acoustical Society of America* 30 (4), 2551. https://doi.10.1121/1.3655212

Gordon, M.K., Martin, J.B. and Langley, L. (2015a) Prosodic structure and intonation in Koasati. *International Congress of Phonetic Sciences*. https://www.internationalphoneticassociation.org/icphs-proceedings /ICPhS2015/Papers/ICPHS0186.pdf

Gordon, M.K., Martin, J.B. and Langley, L. (2015b) Some phonetic structures of Koasati. *International Journal of American Linguistics* 81 (1), 83–118.

Guiberson, M. and Vining, C.B. (2023) Language and literacy strategies for Indigenous children: A scoping review. *Seminars in Speech and Language* 44 (1), 26–41. https://doi.org/10.1055/s-0042-1758802

Haas, M.R. (1944) Men's and women's speech in Koasati. *Language* 20 (3), 142–149.

Hammarström, H., Forkel, R. and Haspelmath, M. (eds) (2019) *Glottolog, 4.1*. Max Planck Institute for the Science of Human History.

Hardy, H.K. and Scancarelli, J. (eds) (2005) *Native Languages of the Southeastern United States*. University of Nebraska Press.

Hasselbachker, S. (2015a) Koasati and 'All the olden talk': Ideologies of linguistic conservatism and the mediation of linguistic authority. *Native South* 8 (1), 31–62. http://doi.10.1353/nso.2015.0001

Hasselbacher, S. (2015b) *'Written in Indian': Creating Legitimized Literacy and Authorized Speakership in Koasati. Dissertations, Theses, and Masters Projects*. William & Mary. Paper 1593092108. https://dx.doi.org/doi:10.21220/m2-j719-kv69

Hilleary, C. (2022) 'The Rez accent': Native Americans are making English their own. *Voice of America*, 14 June. voanews.com/a/6617390.httml

Hodge, W.F. (ed.) (1959) *Handbook of American Indians North of Mexico, 2 Vols*. GPO, 1097, 1010 (2 vols.); rpt. 1959. Pageant.

Jacobson, D. (1954) Koasati culture changes. LSU Historical Dissertations and Theses. 8098. See https://repository.lsu.edu/gradschool_disstheses/8098

Jacobson, D. (1960) Origin of the Koasati Community of Louisiana. *Ethnohistory* 7 (2), 97–120. https://doi.org/10.2307/480751

Kimball, G.D. (1985) A descriptive grammar of Koasati. Unpublished doctoral dissertation. Tulane University. 539 pp.

Kimball, G.D. (1987) Men's and women's speech in Koasati: A reappraisal. *International Journal of American Linguistics* 53 (1), 30–28.

Kimball, G.D. (1990) A further note on Koasati "Men's" Speech. *International Journal of American Linguistics* 56 (1), 158–162.

Kimball, G.D. (1991) *Koasati Grammar*. University of Nebraska Press.

Kimball, G.D. (1994) *Koasati Dictionary*. University of Nebraska Press.

Kyzer, W.M. (1952) A descriptive study of the speech of the Koasati Indians of Louisiana. Master's thesis, Louisiana State University. 172 pp.

Langley, L. and Langley, B. (2019) Kowassaaton Ilhaalos: Let us hear Koasati. In N. Dajko and S. Walton (eds) *Language in Louisiana: Community and Culture* (pp. 28–36). University Press of Mississippi.

Langley, B., Langley, L., Martin, J.B. and Hasselbacher, S. (2018) The Koasati Language Project: A collaborative, community-based language documentation and revitalization model. In S.T. Bischoff and C. Jany (eds) *Insights from Practices in Community-based Research: From Theory to Practice around the Globe*. De Gruyter Mouton.

Leap, W. (1993) *American Indian English*. University of Utah Press.

Leechman, D. and Hall, R.A., Jr. (1955) American Indian Pidgin English: Attestations and grammatical peculiarities. *American Speech* 30 (3), 63–171.

Liebler, C. and Zacher, M. (2013) American Indians without tribes in the 21st century. *Ethnic and Racial Studies* 36 (11), 1910–1934.

Lippi-Green, R. (2004) Language ideology and language prejudice. In E. Finegan and J.R. Rickford (eds) *Language in the United States: Themes for the Twenty-First Century* (pp. 89–304). Cambridge University Press.

Lo Bianco, J. and Kreeft Peyton, J. (2013) Vitality of heritage languages in the United States: The role of capacity, opportunity, and desire. *Heritage Language Journal* 10 (3), i–viii. https://doi.org/10.46538/hlj.10.3.1

Louisiana Census (n.d.) See https://data.census.gov/profile/Louisiana (accessed 4 November 2024).

Lupardus, K.J. (1982) The language of the Alabama Indians. Unpublished doctoral dissertation. University of Kansas.

Martin, J.B. and Johnson, K. (2002) An acoustic study of 'tonal accent' in Creek. *International Journal of American Linguistics* 68 (1), 28–50. https://doi.org/10.1086/466478

Meeks, J.C. (2023) Native American speech-language pathology assistants: Expanding culturally responsive services in reservation schools. *Language, Speech, and Hearing Services in Schools* 54 (2), 395–408. https://doi.10.1044/2022_LSHSS-22-00081.

MEMRISE (2015) See https://koasatiheritage.org/blog/2015/jan/22/koasati-memrise-lessons (accessed 30 November 2024).

Mineo, L. (2021) Blazing trails for others to follow. *The Harvard Gazette*. See https://news.harvard.edu/gazette/story/2021/05/eli-langley-21-preserves-language-of-the-coushatta-tribe%20/

Mithun, M. (2001) *The Languages of Native North America*. Cambridge University Press.

Nagel, J. (1996) *American Indian Ethnic Renewal: Red Power and the Resurgence of Identity and Culture*. Oxford University Press.

Newmark, K., Walker, N. and Sanford, J. (2016) The Rez accent knows no borders: Native American ethnic identity expressed through English prosody. *Language in Society* 45 (5), 633–664.

Oetting, J.B. (2018) Prologue: Toward accurate identification of developmental language disorder within linguistically diverse schools. *Language, Speech, and Hearing Services in Schools* 49 (2), 213–217.

Penfield, S.D. (1977) Some examples of Southwestern Indian English compared. In W. Leap (ed.) *Studies in Southwestern Indian English* (pp. 23–44). Trinity University Press.

Postsecondary National Policy Institute (n.d.) See https://pnpi.org/wp-conent/uploads/2023/11/NativeAmericanFactSheet (accessed 10 November 2024).

Precht, J.H. (2007) 'The lost tribe wanders no more': Indian gaming and the emergence of Coushatta self-determination. Unpublished doctoral dissertation. Arizona State University.

Pritzker, B.M. (2000) *Native American Encyclopedia: History, Culture, and Peoples*. Oxford University Press.

Saville-Troike, M. (1988) A note on men's and women's speech in Koasati. *International Journal of American Linguistics* 54 (2), 158–162. https://doi.org/10.1086/466085

Swanton, J.R. (1911) Koasati texts. *Bureau of American Ethnology, Smithsonian Institution*, ms. 1818. Washington, DC.

Syropoulos, A. (2002) Typesetting Native American languages. *Journal of Electronic Publishing* 8 (1). 'Adding to the sum of accurate information in the world'. https://doi.org/10.3998/3336451.0008.105

The Coushatta Tribe of Louisiana. See https://coushatta.org (accessed 1 December 2024).

The Native American Caucus of Speech-Language Pathology and Audiology (n.d.) See https://sites.google.com/view/nacslpa-org/home) (accessed 3 December 2024).

Toth, K. (2019) First words: Eli Langley speaks Koasati. *CBC radio*. See https://www.cbc.ca/radio/unreserved/first-words-eli-langley-speaks-koasati-1.5018624 (accessed 3 November 2024).

Treaty 6 Territory 300 (n.d.) See https://www.treatysix.org (accessed 3 December 2024).

US Census Bureau (2013) See https://census.gov/hhes/socdemo/language/data/other/detailed-lang-tables.xls (accessed 15 November 2024).

US Bureau of Labor Statistics (n.d.) See https://www.bls.gov (accessed 20 November 2024).

Vining, C.B. and Guiberson, M. (2021) Issue editor foreword: Enhancing language services to Native American children: A look from the inside. *Topics in Language Disorders* 41 (2), 133–139. https://doi.org/10.1097/TLD.0000000000000250

Vogel, S. and García, O. (2017) Translanguaging. In G. Noblit and L. Moll (eds) *Oxford Research Encyclopedia of Education*. Oxford University Press.

Western Interstate Commission for Higher Education (n.d.) See https://wiche.edu/nasnti-institutional-profiles (accessed 20 November 2024).

White, F. (2006) Rethinking Native American language revitalization. *American Indian Quarterly* 30 (1/2), 91–109.

Wolfram, W. (1984) Unmarked tense in American Indian English. *American Speech* 59, 31–50.

15 Assessing Samoan Clients

Elaine Ballard and Ina Fautua

Introduction

Increasing global mobilization has brought demographic changes to Anglosphere countries in the last 20–30 years. With that, speech-language pathologists (SLPs) in countries where English is the dominant language are encountering more clients with a first language other than English and quite different cultural values from those found in Western countries. Included in this group are those of Samoan heritage, who constitute ca. 0.06% (204,640) of the US population (US Census Bureau, 2019)

US-based Samoans have migrated from American Samoa, Samoa or other countries with a sizable Samoan diaspora (e.g. New Zealand). Many are bilingual in Samoan and English, as both languages are official languages in American Samoa and Samoa. However, Samoan is still the language of daily use for many migrants, and their fluency in English is variable (Creevey *et al.*, 2024; Foster, 2024). Samoans are also familiar with Western cultures, as cultural influences from the United States and other Western nations are visible in daily life in the islands. However, traditional *fa'asamoa* (Samoan way of doing things) is preserved in the islands, and migrants to the United States will uphold these values to varying degrees (Creevey *et al.*, 2024).

Despite Samoans being familiar with the English language and Western cultural values, clinicians may still find it challenging to provide them with services. To provide effective therapy to Samoan clients, SLPs should assess skills in all languages spoken and take into consideration cultural values (Scharff Rethfeld *et al.*, 2024). This is difficult when there is a paucity of information on linguistic differences between Samoan and English and/or bilingual language development in speakers of these two languages. The task of differentiating between language disorder and difference (Bedore & Peña, 2008) is compounded by the fact that morpho-syntactic errors from those learning English as a second language are identical to those found with monolingual children with a genuine language disorder (Paradis, 2005). Furthermore, Samoan clients with good English linguistic skills will still not perform as well as English monolinguals on assessments, as indicated in research (Bialystok *et al.*, 2010; Friesen *et al.*, 2022). Linguistic proficiency aside, there is also little information for SLPs on any potential cultural differences.

Our aim in this chapter is to provide information to support SLP engagement with Samoans. We do this by summarizing existing research and then discussing aspects of Samoan language and culture that can facilitate therapy with this population. The linguistic sketch of Samoan below is not a comprehensive description, but it does highlight key differences between this language and English. This is followed by a discussion of cultural considerations when engaging with Samoan clients. Here the focus is once again on differences and core Samoan values are discussed in light of how they can be incorporated into a clinical session.

Previous Research on the Samoan Language and Speakers

Samoan is an Austronesian language. There are descriptive studies on the language ranging from dictionaries (Milner, 1966; Pratt, 1893), to grammatical descriptions (Churchward, 1951; Mosel & Hovdhaugen, 1992; Pawley, 1966; Pratt, 1893). There is also a body of research focused on language socialization and development in children in the islands (Duranti & Ochs, 1986; Hovdhaugen & Simonsen, 1988; Kernan, 1969; Ochs 1982a, 1982b, 1986, 1988).

Research on Samoan speakers within the field of speech language pathology is scarcer. While this research focuses on migrant communities, it is scant, and there have been few Samoan language resources created for SLPs. Given this, there are many projects that can be undertaken with the Samoan population in future research.

Available research on children shows mixed results. Some studies discuss aspects of cross-linguistic transfer between the Samoan and English spoken by children. This has a positive outcome for phonological awareness as children can transfer skills from English into their Samoan (Hamilton & Gillon, 2006). However, the findings for phonological development are more mixed as exposure to English impacts children's Samoan skills (Ballard & Farao, 2008) and leads to children producing error patterns (e.g. initial consonant deletion) deemed atypical in English monolingual contexts (Dodd, 1995). Other studies show that Samoan-speaking children perform more poorly than monolingual English peers on specific language tasks (Hemsley *et al.*, 2006, 2010; Hess *et al.*, 2013). Hemsley *et al.* (2006, 2010) report on school-aged Samoan-speaking children having smaller vocabularies than their peers even when knowledge in both Samoan and English is considered. Hess *et al.* (2013) compare US-based Samoan-speaking children with non-Samoan English-speaking peers and American Samoan peers on a range of speech and language tasks. The island-based children were assessed in Samoan while US-based children were assessed in English. As a group, the non-Samoans performed better than either Samoan group with the US-based children generally scoring better than their island-based peers.

Research on Samoan-speaking adults is even sparser. There are just two published studies, both in bilingual aphasia (Jodache *et al.*, 2015, 2019). Rather than report on language measures, these studies report on the perspectives of participants in the assessment of a Samoan-speaking client. In Jodache *et al.* (2015), the perspectives of the person with aphasia, a family member, two interpreters and an SLP are considered, while the follow-up study (Jodache *et al.*, 2019) focuses on SLPs exclusively. Both studies indicate that language assessment in Samoan is difficult when there are no available formal standardized assessments; there are also concerns regarding the cultural and linguistic appropriateness of existing English language assessments/tasks.

A Linguistic Sketch

The description below is relevant for Samoan speakers from all parts of the Samoan archipelago. According to Mosel and Hovdhaugen (1992) and Pawley (1966) there are comparatively few differences between the dialects spoken by different communities. However, there is a stylistic distinction as Samoan has two registers: a formal (*'o le tautala lelei*, 'the good language') and a colloquial (*'o le tautala leaga*, 'the bad language') (Mosel & Hovdhaugen, 1992; Pawley, 1966). The choice of register depends on social context. *Tautala lelei* is used during formal occasions and ceremonies or prayers; it is also used by speakers of a higher social background in conversation and everyday language (Pawley, 1960). This register is also used in speaking to non-Samoans and is appropriate for public broadcasts, news, educational settings and learning contexts. On all other occasions, speakers use *tautala leaga*, a spoken variant. This variant is used within the home and in daily interactions. The differences between the two registers operate at many levels of grammar and discourse, but are most salient in the phonology (Ochs, 1988).

Phonology

Consonants

The consonants of Samoan are given in Table 15.1. The formal register has 13 consonants and the colloquial has 10. In the table, we have bolded the three additional consonants of the formal register as all other consonants exist in both registers. Of these consonants /h,r/ occur predominantly in loanwords from English (Samoan has a long association with the English language as Christian missionaries from England came to the islands in the 19th century and translated the Bible and many other religious texts into Samoan for the native population (Mosel & Hovdhaugen, 1992)), e.g. *haleluia* 'hallelujah', *rosa* 'rose', and are less

Table 15.1 Consonant phonemes of Samoan

	Bilabial	Labio-Dental	Alveolar	Velar	Glottal
Plosive	p		t	k	ʔ
Nasal	m		n	ŋ	
Fricative		f v	s		h
Approximant			l r		

frequent than other consonants. /h/ is also used with interjections such as *hai* (indicating yawning) and *he* (indicating laughter). Lexical items that have a /t/ in the formal register have a /k/ in the colloquial register. In addition, items with /n/ in the formal register have an /ŋ/ and items with /r/ an /l/. Many lexical items that form minimal pairs in the formal register are homophones in the colloquial register. Lexical items /ti/ 'tea' and /ki/ 'key' in the formal register are both realized as /ki/ in the colloquial, /ana/ 'cave' and /aŋa/ 'conduct' as /aŋa/ and /koko/ 'cocoa' and / toto/ 'blood' as /koko/ (Ballard & Farao, 2008; Ballard & Fautua, 2026; Mosel & Hovdhaugen, 1992). Although /k/ is common in the colloquial register, its frequency in the formal register is restricted to loanwords (e.g. kerisiano 'Christian').

Samoan has three voiceless plosives /p, t, k/ that are generally unaspirated or weakly aspirated (Mosel & Hovdhaugen, 1992). Of the three, /t/ has the greatest degree of aspiration and varies in its place of articulation between dental and alveolar. The three nasals /m, n, ŋ/ are articulated as in English, and all three occur both word-initially and medially. In Samoan, the velar nasal is orthographically represented as <g>, e.g. *gagana* /ŋaŋana/ 'language'.

The fricatives in Samoan are similar to their English counterparts in articulation, with /h/ and /s/ presenting few issues to those acquiring English as a second language. The only fricative that may be challenging is the labio-dental /f/, as this consonant varies somewhat in its articulation from [f] to [ɸ] or [h]. The distinction between /f/ and /p/ is also reported to be the last to develop in a child's speech (Hovdhaugen & Simonsen, 1988). The approximants show some variation, with the lateral /l/ articulated as [l] or the flap [ɾ] intervocalically after back vowels /u, o, a/ and before the vowel /i/ (i.e. /uliuli/ → [uɾiuɾi] 'black') and the rhotic /r/ varying between a trill [r] and approximant [ɹ] articulation (Ballard & Farao, 2008). The glottal stop /ʔ/ occurs frequently in Samoan and is a phoneme and not a regional variant as in English (e.g. Cockney English). It occurs word-initially and medially, and its presence or absence is associated with a difference in meaning: /fai/ 'do' vs /faʔi/ 'banana', /soa/ 'partner' vs /soʔa/ 'hit'. The *'okina* <'>, a reversed apostrophe, is orthographically used for the glottal stop /ʔ/, e.g. *a'oga*, /aʔoŋa/ 'school'. With the exception of the graphemes <g>, <r> and <'> for the velar nasal, rhotic and glottal stop respectively, the graphemes used for the remaining consonants correspond to the consonants represented by the corresponding IPA symbols, i.e. <p, t, k, f, v, s, h, m, n, l> refer to /p, t, k, f, v, s, h, m, n, l/.

Given the smaller consonantal inventory in Samoan, it is not surprising to find children having difficulties in acquiring the consonants of English. Children with little exposure to English before entering the school system will have issues with the greater number of English plosives. Samoan has /p, t, k/ but lacks the voicing contrast found with English /p, b/, /t, d/ and /k, g/. This has consequences for reading and writing as Samoan speakers may find it difficult to associate the appropriate graphemes with the correct consonant. Further difficulties with consonants may be found with English fricatives and affricates /θ, ð, ʃ, ʒ, ʧ, ʤ/ and the approximant /ɹ/. These fricatives do not occur in Samoan and are unfamiliar to speakers learning English. The English rhotic only occurs as a variant of /r/ in Samoan and is often used as an allophone for /l/. Given this, English learners may find clearly differentiating between /l/ and /ɹ/ challenging.

Vowels

The Samoan vocalic inventory consists of ten vowels for both registers (Figure 15.1). There are five monophthongs /i, e, a, o, u/ further phonemically distinguished by length /iː, eː, aː, oː, uː/ (Mosel & Hovdhaugen, 1992). The graphemes <a, e, i, o, u> are used orthographically for vowels /a, e, i, o, u/. Long vowels are indicated orthographically with the *fa'amamafa* (macron), (e.g. *fetū* /fetuː/ 'star', *fa'amālamalama* /faʔamaːlamalama/ 'to explain'). However, the macron is not always consistently produced in literacy materials and it may be omitted in writing

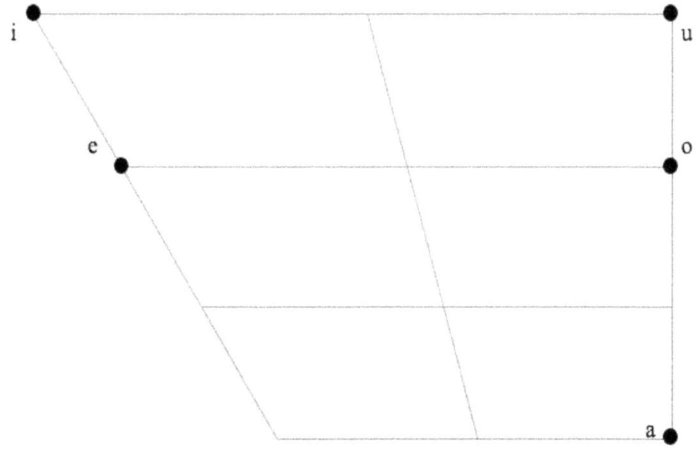

Figure 15.1 Vowel phonemes of Samoan

although long vowels are produced consistently in speaking (Tualaulelei *et al.*, 2015). Minimal pairs are common, e.g. *mama* /mama/ 'ring' and *māma* /maːma/ 'clean', *malu* /malu/ 'shelter' and *mālu* /maːlu/ 'peace'.

The Samoan vowels are similar to their English counterparts. Any articulatory differences are attributed to the fact that the Samoan vowels are closer to the cardinal vowels (Mosel & Hovdhaugen, 1992) than the English equivalents. Samoan /i/ is 'practically identical to cardinal vowel 1' (Mosel & Hovdhaugen, 1992: 25) and this means the tongue is higher and more fronted in Samoan than in English. When this vowel is unstressed and occurs before another vowel word initially, it often is articulated as a glide; e.g. /iato/ 'outrigger' is pronounced as [jato]. Glide formation is also found with /u/, where a word such as /laːuiloa/ 'well-known' is articulated as [laːwiloa]. The Samoan /u/ is higher and further back than English /u/ and is very similar to cardinal vowel 8. The remaining vowels are the mid vowels /e/, /o/ and a low vowel /a/. /e/ is a mid-high front unrounded vowel, articulated somewhere between English /e/ in *bed* and the mid vowel in the first part of our diphthong /ei/ in *bay*. It is identical with cardinal 2. The mid-high back rounded /o/ is very similar to cardinal vowel 7 while the vowel /a/ is a low and central unrounded vowel as in English (Ballard & Farao, 2008; Mosel & Hovdhaugen, 1992).

English has considerably more vowels than Samoan, so it is possible learners of English may find differentiating specific vowels difficult. In English, there is a three-way contrast both front /i,e, æ/ and back /u, ɔ, ɑ/ compared to the two-way contrast in Samoan. Samoan speakers may be able to articulate the differences in any vowel series; the greater issue is being able to associate articulatory differences with separate and distinct phonemes. This is of particular note with vowel pairs such as /i/ and /ɪ/, and /u/ and /ʊ/ that are often described as long-short pairs. While the vowels in each of these pairs do contrast in duration, they also contrast in their vowel quality. Samoan does not have similar contrastive pairs of vowels, and the articulatory qualities of vowels such as /i/ and /ɪ/ are more likely to be interpreted as phonetic variation for one vowel /i/.

Syllable structure

The canonical syllable shape for Samoan is CV *lā* /laː/ 'sun' or V *ie* /ie/ 'cloth material'. The minimal shape of a Samoan word is (C)V where the V is a long vowel or a vowel cluster. There are no words consisting of just a short vowel, although grammatical particles are of this shape (e.g. past tense *na*). Particles are, however, not considered as words since the term 'word' refers here to content-bearing words, e.g. *maile* 'dog'. All consonants in Samoan occur word-initially, but consonantal clusters are not permitted. Therefore, loanwords from English with consonantal clusters are broken up by the insertion of an epenthetic vowel, e.g. *teropika* 'tropics', *pelekifasi* 'breakfast'. Consonantal clusters in English are common, so Samoans learning English may break up clusters in this fashion.

By contrast, clusters of vowels such as [ie, uo, ei, ae] are permitted and occur frequently in Samoan. Pawley (1960) notes all vowel pairs occur, and clusters of up to five vowels are permitted. These vowel clusters are described as 'diphthongs' in many English language descriptions (e.g. Churchward, 1951), but these are not diphthongs phonetically, but rather vowel sequences. The vowels in clusters are distinct in their articulation and do not merge with each other as in English.

Morpho-syntax

Samoan is typologically structured differently from English. In the description below, we highlight some areas where cross-linguistic transfer from Samoan into English may lead to mis- or underdiagnosis of a language disorder.

Word classes

In English there are a series of distinct word classes with clearly defined properties (e.g. verb, noun, adjective). In Samoan, the categorization of word types is not as distinct as the function of a word is defined by its syntactic distribution (Mosel & Hovdhaugen, 1992). As an example, a word such as *selu* can function as either a noun or a verb as shown below.

Noun

se	*selu*
art.	comb

'a comb'

Verb

e	*selu*	*lona*	*lauulu*
pres.	comb	poss.	hair

'she combs her hair'

In English, there are words that belong in more than one category; *comb* above is one such example, but English does not have this to the same extent as Samoan. Unlike English, adjectives, temporal and spatial words, and numbers can all become verbal in nature with the addition of a tense or aspect marker preceding them:

Adjective

sa	*ou*	*fiafia*
pst.	1stps.sg.	happy

'I was happy'

Numeral

e	*lima*	*polo*
pres.	five	ball

'There are five balls'

This fluidity across word classes means that there is no one-to-one classification of word types from Samoan to English. The following example with *lā* 'sun' clearly illustrates this point as the verbal construction with the past tense particle translates in English to a construction with a subject, copula verb and an adjective:

Noun

'o	*le*	*lā*
top.	art.	sun

'the sun'

Verb

sa	*lā*
pst.	sun

'it was sunny'

The English translation highlights clear differences between the two languages. Subjects in Samoan are not obligatory, and copula verbs are not required. Furthermore, a category such as adjective is not clearly defined and changes word class depending on context. All three differences may potentially present as errors in the English spoken by Samoan migrants.

Mosel and Hovdhaugen (1992) note the classification of words into one or another category follows certain patterns but is not entirely predictable. It is acknowledged that certain words seem to belong more to one specific category, but there are no constraints that restrict the same word being identified as a different word class based on its syntactic distribution. In the sections below we give additional details on word classes where there are differences between Samoan and English.

Nouns

One of the biggest differences between Samoan and English is the way grammatical roles are marked on nouns in the respective languages (Ochs, 1982a, 1988). In a language such as English, a nominative-accusative language, nouns functioning as the subject in a clause do not change their form depending on verb type (transitive or intransitive), so the noun phrase *the girl* is the same in both *the girl ran across the bridge* and *the girl is drawing a picture*. By contrast, in Samoan, an ergative-absolutive language, the noun form for the subject of the intransitive verb is different from that for the subject of a transitive verb. In Samoan, the subject of an intransitive verb and the object of the transitive verb (absolutive) are grammatically marked the same, whereas the subject of a transitive (ergative) is marked differently from both of them. Ergative case is formally marked with a particle *e* preceding the noun, and the absolutive has zero case marking. Given the differences morphologically, cross-linguistic transfer may be minimal. However, it is possible for Samoan speakers to omit subjects and objects in their English clauses because they are not always marked overtly in Samoan.

Absolutive Subject

'olo'o	*moe*	*le*	*pusi*
pres. prog.	sleep	art.	cat

'the cat is sleeping'

Ergative Subject

'ua	*fela'u*	*le*	*teine*	*e*	*le*	*pusi*
perf.	scratch	art.	girl	erg.	art.	cat

'the cat has scratched the girl'

Aside from ergative case, Samoan also grammatically marks possession, direction and location with particles preceding the noun phrase. These are equivalent to -s for possessive and prepositions in English.

Another difference is the general lack of grammatical marking for plurality unlike English -s. Samoan does have distinct plural nouns that are formed via vowel lengthening or vowel doubling, but these are reasonably rare, e.g. *tuafāfine,* the plural of *tuafafine* 'brother's sister'. What is more common is to have nouns indicating either singular or plural depending on context. In the example *māile* means either dog or dogs. Plurality is generally unmarked while singularity can be specifically indicated with an article *se* 'a' or *le* 'the'. The lack of plural marking on nouns is therefore potentially an area where Samoans may make errors in English (Mosel & Hovdhaugen, 1992).

Singular			**Plural**	
'o	*le*	*māile*	*'o*	*māile*
top.	art.	dog	top.	dogs
'the dog'			'dogs'	

Pronouns

Mosel and Hovdhaugen (1992) indicate Samoan has three classes of personal pronouns. A distinction is made between singular (one person), dual (two people) and plural (three or more people). First-person dual and plural pronouns also have inclusive and exclusive forms, specifying whether the speaker is including the addressee or not. A distinction that does not occur in Samoan is that of gender in the third-person singular form. Unlike English with 'he', 'she' and 'it', Samoan has *ia* for males and females and uses *lea*, a demonstrative for *it*. Given the lack of a gender distinction in pronouns, there is a possibility that Samoan speakers may indiscriminately use these pronouns and confuse 'he' and 'she' (see Table 15.2).

Articles

There are two articles in Samoan, the specific article *le* and the non-specific *se* (sg) and *ni* (pl). *Le* is often translated as 'the' in English although it is used more widely in Samoan than it is in English and

Table 15.2 Personal pronouns in Samoan

Number	Singular	Dual	Plural
First	a'u	—	—
inclusive	_	('i) tā'ua	('i) tātou
exclusive	_	('i)mā'ua	('i)mātou
Second	'oe	'oulua	'outou
Third	ia	('i)lā'ua	('i)lātou

appears in contexts where English would require an indefinite article (Pratt, 1893). This is because English *the* is restricted to nouns that are known in the discourse while *le* is not restricted in this way. The article *le* refers to a specific item/person that can either be already in the discourse or completely unknown. There is no plural equivalent to *le*.

le	*fa'i*	*fa'i*	
art.	banana	banana	
'a/the banana'		'(the) bananas'	

Non-specific *se* does not refer to any particular person or item and refers to any possible item or person identified by the noun. Its plural form *ni* is often translated as 'some' or 'any'. By contrast *a* in English refers to an item/person that is not already known in the discourse. Like English *the*, it has a more specific use than its counterpart in Samoan.

se	*fa'i*	*ni*	*fai'i*
art.	banana	art.	banana
'a banana'		'(some) bananas'	

There is no one-to-one translation of the articles from English to Samoan or vice versa. As such, this is another area where Samoan learners of English may make errors.

Verbs

English and Samoan differ in their verbal morphology. While auxiliary verbs are used together with non-finite forms of lexical verbs (e.g. past participle) and suffixes are directly added to the verb to mark the past or to indicate the third person present form in English, Samoan uses separate particles to mark those relationships. Particles precede the verb to mark tense (future 'ole'ā, 'ā), aspect (perfect 'ua) and mood (subjunctive 'ia) while preverbal subject pronouns (*na* third person singular) are used to mark person forms (Mosel & Hovdhaugen, 1992). Verbs in Samoan are not conjugated and there is no inflectional marking directly on the verb. Therefore, there is the potential for morpho-syntactic errors on the part of second language learners.

English		**Samoan**		
he	*read-s*	*na*	*te*	*faitau*
3rd ps. sg. pron.	read-3rd ps. pres.	3rd ps. sg.	pres.	read

Samoan does mark plurality on the verb but only for some verbs (Mosel & Hovdhaugen, 1992). The most common strategy for this is with the use of reduplication. Reduplication is either full (entire word) or partial (stressed syllable of the word):

Singular	**Plural**
savali (walk)	*savavali*
una (pinch)	*unauna*

There are also other less common ways of forming plurals; these include adding a prefix such as *fe-* in *fe'aa* (from *'aa* 'kick') or lengthening a vowel as in *fāitau* from *faitau* 'read' (Pratt, 1893).

Word order

As noted in Ochs (1988) Samoan allows several possible word orders in a clause. These include the subject-verb-object order like English.

SV

'o	*le*	*teine*	*'ua*	*sau*
top.	art	girl	perf.	come

'The girl has come'

However, the preferred order is verb-initial with a particle marking tense, aspect or mood preceding the verb and the subject (if expressed) following the verb.

VS

'ua	sau	le	teine
perf.	come	art.	girl

'The girl has come'

Word order may be an issue for a Samoan learning English on two accounts. Word order is much more flexible in Samoan than English, and the preferred Samoan order is the exact opposite of the order preferred in English.

Other differences in word order between Samoan and English are found with the noun phrase. There are some similarities to English in that articles, numerals and quantifiers precede nouns, but there are also differences. Adjectives, for instance, follow the nouns they modify, and demonstratives can vary in their position.

Noun + Article

'o	*le*	*teine*
top.	art.	girl

'the girl'

Noun + Adjective

teine	*fiafia*
girl	happy

'happy girls'

Noun + Demonstrative

le	*teine*	*nei*	
art.	girl	dem.	
'this girl'			

le	*nei*	*teine*
art.	dem.	girl
'this		girl'

le	*teine*	*le*	*nei*
art.	girl	art.	dem
'this girl'			

Clinical Implications for Practitioners

Cultural considerations for working with Samoan clients

Samoan migrants in the United States experience the challenge of adapting and assimilating to American culture despite their familiarity with Western culture from the islands. Research shows that Samoan migrants maintain their cultural values and beliefs (*fa'asamoa*) to some extent (Creevey *et al.*, 2024). One example is White Sunday or *lotu a tamaiti* 'children's service' celebrated annually on the second week of October. This event commemorates children and is especially celebrated by parents and communities in Samoan congregations around the world. The tradition dates back to the 19th century when the London Missionary Society arrived in Samoa.

In contrast to Western cultures where individualism, equal rights and independence are valued, interdependence, collectivism and differentiated rights are valued in Samoan culture (Ballard & Farao, 2010). Key to their values is the relationship individuals hold to their family, village (place) and nation. As His Highness Tui Atua highlights clearly, 'I am not an individual…I belong to my village and my village belongs to me. I belong to my nation and my nation belongs to me. This is the essence of my sense of belonging' (Tui Atua, 2003).

Due to the collectivist nature of their culture, homes are often multigenerational and young children may be looked after by older siblings or adults other than their parents. The family is hierarchical in nature and one's standing depends on age and gender. Children therefore are raised to show respect to elders, not interrupt adult conversations and obey their parents' directives. In contrast to Western middle-class families where caregivers scaffold interactions initiated by their children and focus on developing their children's oral language skills, Samoan children are expected to pay close attention to activities taking place around them (e.g. cleaning, cooking, etc.) and to accommodate the social context

(Ochs, 1988). Children are therefore highly attuned to observe and follow instruction; they are skilled at noticing a variety of communicative cues, but they are expected to be silent, wait and pause. As a consequence, Samoan children may present as silent and unresponsive in a therapy session (Ballard & Farao, 2010). Non-verbal communication, expressed through eye gaze, body and facial gestures, is highly valued and children are not expected to be verbal in front of adults. An important part of Samoan ways of 'speaking' is body language (Tamasese *et al.*, 2005) and body language often gives context and meaning to the verbal message.

A multimodal approach is therefore encouraged when working with Samoan children as communication for Samoans includes both verbal and non-verbal (gestures, facial expressions). Using visual and gestural cues together with verbal ones will provide Samoan clients with more opportunities to understand what is being required in therapy.

Aiga

The values of *alofa* 'love', *faaaloalo* 'respect' and *tautua* 'service' underpin *fa'asamoa* and are centered on *aiga* 'family'. The understanding of family extends beyond the nuclear family to extended and honorary family members, including those without blood relations (Ballard & Farao, 2010; Borrero *et al.*, 2010). The church, as the broadest manifestation of *aiga*, is an important focal part of their community for many because it is a center where Samoan language, identity and culture can be preserved (Duranti *et al.*, 1995).

The concept of *aiga* is also integral to the Samoan view of health and well-being and should undergird any assessments and interventions. A Pacific model commonly used in New Zealand for that purpose is the *Fonofale* framework (Pulotu-Endemann, 2001). This model was originally developed for health practitioners but is now well established in other settings because it provides a Pacific-centered and culturally safe model of service delivery to all Pacific communities. Pulotu-Endemann, a Samoan, uses the metaphor of a Samoan house *fale* to represent the holistic concept of health and well-being. Family in its broadest sense is represented as the foundation of the house while the roof representing cultural beliefs and values provides shelter or protection. The four posts supporting the roof represent the spiritual, mental, physical and other aspects (e.g. gender, age), that bring together the strands connecting family and cultural values (Averill *et al.*, 2020). Surrounding the *fale* are the physical environment, specific time in history and context, all of which may directly or indirectly impact the individual. This is a holistic model that considers all factors that may impact an individual's well-being.

In undertaking therapy with Samoans, SLPs need to step away from exclusively focusing on the communication difficulty and take time to build a relationship with the individual and family. This may mean initially spending time talking about spiritual values, family beliefs, community interests and other aspects that impact their lives, to build rapport before therapy. Developing a relationship of trust with families is a priority and considered culturally responsive. A family-based approach is recommended for working with Samoan families and clients. An approach focused on the collective interests of the family rather than the individual increases the effectiveness of therapy outcomes (Ballard & Fautua, 2026). To build rapport SLPs need to consider both *va* 'space that relates' and *talanoa* 'talk or communicate freely'. *Va* is a core value that threads through Samoan communicative interaction. *Va* is a way of maintaining the sacred space between an individual, God, a fellow person and the physical environment (Clayton, 2007; Simati-Kumar, 2011; Tuagalu, 2009). It is integral to building a respectful relationship. *Talanoa* is a way of communicating that is grounded in the values of respect, honesty, love, forgiving and reciprocity. It gives all the opportunity to share, discuss and nurture good relationships (Vaioleti, 2016). In participating in *talanoa*, SLPs can ensure that family and caregivers are fully engaged in all decision-making, and in respecting *va* gain permission space prior to developing goals or interventions.

Conclusion

In this chapter, we have highlighted the areas in the Samoan language where the greatest differences are found between Samoan and English. Our overview focuses on the aspects of Samoan most likely to have an impact on the English spoken by Samoan second language learners. We have also discussed differences in the cultural values of Samoans and offer suggestions rooted in Samoan values that can lead to better outcomes. The hope is that clinicians will take this content on board when engaging with Samoans.

References

Averill, R., Glasgow, A. and Rimoni, F. (2020) Exploring understandings of Pacific values in New Zealand educational contexts: Similarities and differences among perceptions. *The International Education Journal: Comparative Perspectives* 19 (2), 20–35.

Ballard, E. and Farao, S. (2008) The phonological skills of Samoan speaking 4-year-olds. *International Journal of Speech-Language Pathology* 10 (6), 379–391.

Ballard, E. and Farao, S. (2010) Designing a phonological assessment for Samoan-speaking children: Linguistic/cultural considerations and initial findings. *NZ Journal of Speech language Therapy* 65, 5–14.

Ballard, E. and Fautua, I. (2026) Samoan speech development. In S. McLeod (ed.) *The Oxford Handbook of Speech Development in Languages of the World* (pp. 1047–1057). Oxford University Press.

Bedore, L.M. and Peña, E.D. (2008) Assessment of bilingual children for identification of language impairment: Current findings and implications for practice. *International Journal of Bilingual Education and Bilingualism* 11 (1), 1–29. https://doi.org/10.2167/beb392.0

Bialystok, E., Luk, G., Peets, K.F. and Yang, S. (2010) Receptive vocabulary differences in monolingual and bilingual children. *Bilingualism: Language and Cognition* 13 (4), 525–531. https://doi.org/10.1017/S1366728909990423

Borrero, N.E., Yeh, C.J., Tito, P. and Luavasa, M. (2010) Alone and in between cultural and academic worlds: Voices of Samoan students. *School of Education Faculty Research. Paper 2.* http://repository.usfca.edu/soe_fac/2

Churchward, S. (1951) *A Samoan Grammar.* Methodist Church of Australasia, Samoa District.

Clayton, L. (2007) Patterns and motifs in the va: A Samoan concept of a space between. Master's thesis, Auckland University of Technology.

Creevey, P.R., Wendt, A. and Foster, S. (2024) American Samoa. *Encyclopedia Britannica.* See https://www.britannica.com/place/American-Samoa

Dodd, B. (1995) Procedures for classification of subgroups of speech disorder. In B. Dodd (ed.) *Differential Diagnosis and Treatment of Children with Speech Disorder* (pp. 49–64). Whurr.

Duranti, A. and Ochs, E. (1986) Literacy instruction in a Samoan village. In B. Schieffelin and P. Gilmore (eds) *Acquisition of Literacy: Ethnographic Perspectives* (pp. 213–232). Ablcx.

Duranti, A., Ochs, E. and Ta'asa, E.K. (1995) Change and tradition in literary instruction in a Samoan American community. *Educational Foundations* 9, 57–74.

Foster, S. (2024) Samoa. *Encyclopedia Britannica.* See https://www.britannica.com/place/Samoa-island-nation-Pacific-Ocean

Friesen, D.C., Schmidt, K., Atwal, T. and Celebre, A. (2022) Reading comprehension and strategy use: Comparing bilingual children to their monolingual peers and to bilingual adults. *Frontiers in Psychology* 13, 986937. https://doi.org/10.3389/fpsyg.2022.986937

Hamilton, E. and Gillon, G.T. (2006) The phonological awareness skills of school-aged children who are bilingual in Samoan and English. *Advances in Speech-Language Pathology* 8 (2), 57–68.

Hemsley, G., Holm, A. and Dodd, B. (2006) Diverse but not different: The lexical skills of two primary age bilingual groups in comparison to monolingual peers. *International Journal of Bilingualism* 10 (4), 453–476. https://doi.org/10.1177/13670069060100040040

Hemsley, G., Holm, A. and Dodd, B. (2010) Patterns in diversity: Lexical learning in Samoan-English bilingual children. *International Journal of Speech Language Pathology* 12 (4), 362–374. https://doi.org/10.3109/17549501003721064

Hess, G., Woll, B.H. and Boles, L. (2013) Speech, language, and hearing risk for Samoan children K to 3. *Asia Pacific Journal of Speech, Language and Hearing* 13 (1), 21–40. https://doi.org/10.1179/136132810805335155

Hovdhaugen, E. and Simonsen, H.G. (1988) On the acquisition of the T- and K- languages by Samoan children. In V. Rosen (ed.) *Papers from the Tenth Scandinavian Conference of Linguistics* (vol. 2, pp. 1–15). Bergen, Department of Linguistics and Phonetics, University of Bergen.

Jodache, S., Howe, T. and Siyambalapitiya, S. (2015) Assessment of a Samoan–English speaker with bilingual aphasia: "it's hard." *Aphasiology* 29 (7), 872–888. https://doi.org/10.1080/02687038.2014.1003363

Jodache, S., Howe, T. and Siyambalapitiya, S. (2019) "Are we …providing them with an equal service?": Speech language pathologists' perceptions of bilingual aphasia assessment of Samoan-English speakers. *Clinical Archives of Communication Disorders* 4 (1), 41–51.

Kernan, K.T. (1969) The acquisition of language by Samoan children. PhD dissertation, University of California.

Milner, G.B. (1966) *Samoan Dictionary. Samoan-English, English-Samoan.* OUP.

Mosel, U. and Hovdhaugen, E. (1992) *Samoan Reference Grammar.* Scandinavian University Press.

Ochs, E. (1982a) Ergativity and word order in Samoan child language. *Language* 58, 646–671.

Ochs, E. (1982b) Talking to children in Western Samoa. *Language in Society* 11, 77–104.

Ochs, E. (1986) Variation and error: A sociolinguistic approach to language acquisition in Samoa. In D. Slobin (ed.) *The Cross-Linguistic Study of Language Acquisition* (pp. 783–838). Lawrence Erlbaum.

Ochs, E. (1988) *Culture and Language Development: Language Acquisition and Language Socialization in a Samoan Village*. Cambridge University Press.

Paradis, J. (2005) Grammatical morphology in children learning English as a second language: Implications of similarities with specific language impairment. *Language, Speech and Hearing Services in Schools* 36 (3), 172–187.

Pawley, A. (1960) An outline of Samoan phonology. *Te Reo* 3, 47–50.

Pawley, A. (1966) Samoan phrase structure: The morphology-syntax of a Western Polynesian language. *Anthropological Linguistics* 8(5), 1–63.

Pratt, G. (1893) *A Grammar and Dictionary of the Samoan Language: With English and Samoan Vocabulary*. London Missionary Society.

Pulotu-Endemann, F.K. (2001) *Fonofale Model of Health*. See https://d3n8a8pro7vhmx.cloudfront.net/actionpoint/pages/437/attachments/original/1534408956/Fonofalemodelexplanation.pdf?1534408956

Scharff Rethfeld, W., McNielly, L., Laasonen, M., Meir, N., Abutbul-Oz, H., Smolander, S., Niegia Garcia Goulart, B. and Hunt, E.F. (2024) Assessment of developmental language disorder in multilingual children: Results from an international survey. *Folia Phoniatrica Logopaedica* 76 (2), 127–150. https://doi.org/10.1159/000533139

Simati-Kumar, B. (2011) The potential of Vā: An investigation of how 'Ie Tōga activate the spatial relationships of the Vā, for a Samoan diaspora community. PhD thesis, Auckland University of Technology. http://hdl.handle.net/10292/4431

Tamasese, K., Peteru, C., Waldegrave, C. and Bush, A. (2005) Ole Taeao Afua, The New Morning: A qualitative investigation into Samoan perspectives on mental health and culturally appropriate services. *Australian and New Zealand Journal of Psychiatry* 39, 300–309. https://doi.org/10.1080/j.1440-1614.2005.01572.x

Tuagalu, I. (2009) Heuristics of the Vā. *AlterNative: An International Journal of Indigenous Peoples* 4 (1), 107–126.

Tualaulelei, E.M., Mayer, F.L.J. and Hunkin, G.A. (2015) Diacritical marks and the Samoan language. *The Contemporary Pacific* 27 (1), 184–207.

Tui Atua Tupua Tamasese Taisi Efi (2003) In search of meaning, nuance and metaphor in social policy. *Social Policy Journal of New Zealand* 20, 49–63.

U.S. Census Bureau (2019) Census tables Native Hawaiian and other Pacific Islander alone or in any combination by selected groups. See https://data.census.gov/table/ACSDT1Y2019.B02019?q=pacific&g=050XX00US41051,29095,06045,06001,48439,06081,49035,06075,06097_010XX00US&hidePreview=false&tid=ACSDT1Y2019.B02019

Vaioleti, T.M. (2016) Talanoa research methodology: A developing position on Pacific research. *Waikato Journal of Education* 12 (1). https://doi.org/10.15663/wje.v12i1.296

16 Miami English in Historical, Demographic and Linguistic Perspective: An Overview for Speech and Language Practitioners

Phillip M. Carter

Introduction

Miami: Context and culture

In reality, the term 'Miami English' is a bit of a misnomer, as are all labels that attempt to name language varieties by combining the name of a geographical place or racioethnic group with the name of a language (Erker, 2017). In this respect, the term 'Miami English' is no different than similar such terms – 'Boston English', 'Philadelphia English', 'Charleston English' or 'Chicago English' – in that (1) the speech variety so named is in fact the product of what Weinreich, Labov and Herzog (1968) call 'orderly heterogeneity' – meaning that linguistic variation is built into the system and, as such, no two people speak exactly alike, even those who share the linguistic features that are stereotypic (Labov, 1972) of the place in question; and (2) that within these geographic locations there are people who speak varieties of English in which these stereotypic features, for whatever reason, are not found. Put more simply, there are many ways of speaking English in Miami – and many ways of speaking 'Miami English' – just as there are many ways of speaking the language varieties used in the major metropolises around the world. However, two factors make Miami English, at this stage in its historical development, somewhat different from most of the other regional and ethnic dialects of English in the United States today. The first is the ongoing situation of Spanish/English bilingualism in South Florida, brought about primarily by the political fallout from the Cuban Revolution in 1959, which operates as a force shaping English in Miami not only from some point in the past but also within the present. This is because immigration from Cuba, and then later from countries across Latin America,[1] has continued in the years since the end of the Revolution, reshaping what Miami is in demographic and linguistic terms year after year (Boswell, 1994, 2000; López & Krogstad, 2014).

The second factor that makes the situation somewhat unique is the related issue of the recency of the development of Miami English as a distinctive variety that can be thought of as belonging to Miamians who learn English as their first language or co-first language. That is, compared with the other ethnic-regional dialects associated with major US cities, the situation of Miami English is a relatively new one. Before moving forward, each of these factors deserves further qualification. With respect to the first factor – the influence of Spanish on English[2] – it must be noted that (1) Spanish is a language spoken by some 50–60 million people in the United States (Escobar & Potowski, 2015; Ryan, 2013) today and (2) is a language that has left its mark on the way people speak English in the United States both historically (Lozano, 2018) and in the present (e.g. Fought, 2003; Wolfram *et al.*, 2004; Zentella, 1997) in various regions throughout the country. Miami is but one of many locations where the presence of Spanish has shaped the way people speak English.[3] With respect to the question of time depth, it must be noted that all language varieties – irrespective of how old they are – are subject to the processes of language change, and in fact the major dialect regions in the United States are indeed changing (Labov, 1991; Labov *et al.*, 2005).

Therefore, what makes Miami English unique is not the wholesale distinctiveness of any one of the factors contributing to its development but rather the unique configuration of these factors. At the social level, the historical, political and cultural circumstances that are unique to Miami make English in Miami correspondingly unique. These circumstances give rise to an array of linguistic structures that are influenced by Spanish, some of which are shared with other ethno-regional dialects spoken in the United States that also bear the historical influence of Spanish, and some of which are unique to Miami. It is the unique combination of these features that constitutes the linguistic make-up of Miami English. In this chapter, I seek to provide clarity for readers across the language-related disciplines about what Miami English is, who uses it, where it comes from and how it relates to the other speech varieties and modes of speaking present in South Florida.

The Historical Development of Miami English

Carter and Lynch (2015) describe three kinds of English spoken in Miami: (1) varieties of English spoken in Miami prior to the Cuban Revolution, which they call 'pre-1960 varieties', (2) varieties that emerged among US-born and immigrant Latinos since the 1960s, which they call 'post-1960 varieties', and (3) the immigrant and transplant varieties of English brought to Miami by immigrants from the Anglophone Caribbean and migrants from elsewhere in the United States. They note that the terms 'pre-' and 'post-1960' are used to mark 'the profound influence of the Cuban Revolution on English spoken among Miami-born Latinos in South Florida'. Given this taxonomy and this history, it would be a mistake to collapse all of the English language diversity in Miami to the label 'Miami English' or to attribute the diversification of Miami in linguistic and demographic terms to the Revolution alone. At the turn of the 20th century, about 40% of Miami's population was of African descent, about half of that group being of Bahamian origin (Nijman, 2011: 16). Localized forms of African American English therefore constitute an enduring part of the English language sociolinguistic scene in South Florida (Carter & Lynch, 2018), and may well be some of the oldest, continuously spoken language varieties in the region. Depending on sociocultural factors such as neighborhood, socioeconomic class and social network, speakers of Miami English are thus in contact with a diverse array of Englishes spoken across the metropolitan Miami region.

The variety referred to here as 'Miami English' falls in Carter and Lynch's (2015) second category, 'Post-1960 varieties', and has its roots in the early 1960s when the first refugees from Cuba began arriving in Miami en masse. 1960 is such an important historical cut-off point in the history of Miami language history because it set in motion a double pattern of immigration that first Cubanized and then Hispanicized Miami in less than 50 years (Boswell, 1994). Beginning in 1961, the Cuban Refugee Program, set up by the US federal government, processed as many as 2000 exiles per week in Miami. This program settled most of the earliest Cuban exiles in Miami. Known today as 'the Golden Exiles', (Portes, 1969) this group was comprised primarily of descendants of Spaniards and other European national background groups. The next wave of immigration from the island took place during the 1960s and 1970s, when relatives of the 'Golden exiles' were brought to Miami on flights charted by the US government. This group came to be known as the 'freedom flyers'. Beginning in 1980, Cuban citizens were allowed to leave the island on boats destined for Miami under special permission given by the Castro government. During the first six months, more than 125,000 Cuban nationals arrived. Known as *marielitos,* this group constituted the third major wave of immigration to Miami from Cuba. Throughout the prior three waves, working-class Cuban nationals left the island on boats obtained illegally or on makeshift rafts, known as *balsas*. When legal emigration from Cuba officially ended after Mariel, more people turned to rafts as a means to reach Miami. These people, known as *balseros,* constituted the fourth major wave of immigration from Cuba. Beginning in the 1980s, Miami's Latinx-origin population began to diversify, as Cubans were joined by Nicaraguans, who were fleeing their own political crisis. Later, in the 1990s, Colombians arrived en masse, fleeing violence in Colombia. They were soon followed by Venezuelans following the election of Hugo Chavez in 2000. By 2000 – 41 years after the end of the

Cuban Revolution – 57% of Miami's population was Hispanic/Latino, up from 49% in 1990, 36% in 1980 and 24% in 1970.

Today Miami's population is comprised of a pan-Latinx majority that draws on groups from all across Latin America. Table 16.1 presents US Census data from 2020 (US Census Bureau, 2020), showing the percent Latinx population for eight municipal regions as well as the percent LOTE ('language other than English') used in the home.

The table shows that nearly 70% of Miami-Dade County is ethnically Latinx, as are the major municipalities throughout the county. The use of a LOTE in the home in these neighborhoods ranges from 61% in Coral Gables to 93.5% in Hialeah. While Spanish is not the only non-English language spoken in South Florida, it is safe to presume that the language used in the majority of neighborhoods depicted in this table is Spanish. Across Miami-Dade County, Miami English is spoken alongside diverse dialects of Spanish, learner varieties of English spoken among new and old immigrants, and the dynamic mixing of these languages.

Table 16.1 Percent Latinx population and percent LOTE, by Miami neighborhood

	Latinx (%)	LOTE in the home (%)
Miami-Dade County	69.4	75
City of Miami	72.5	77.6
Hialeah	95.7	93.5
Miami Beach	58	71.9
Kendall	67.5	70.1
Doral	83.7	88.2
Coral Gables	58.4	61
Key Biscayne	73.7	82.8

LOTE: Language other than English

Grammar of the Language

Before turning to an inventory of features of Miami English, I'd like to establish what Miami English is *not* by focusing on three common misperceptions about the variety. First, although the variety referred to as Miami English is influenced historically and contemporaneously by the presence of Spanish through language contact, Miami English is not in and of itself Spanglish. Spanglish is a language variety spoken by US Latinxs that involves the rule-governed alternation between Spanish and English within or between grammatical clauses (Zentella, 2017). Spanish/English code-switching has been studied extensively by linguists in the United States, including Toribio (2001), Poplack (1980) and Zentella (1997).

Second, Miami English as such does not *necessarily* involve the use of Spanish loanwords or borrowings. In theory, it is possible to use the sounds, lexical items and structures of Miami English without ever uttering a word of Spanish. I write 'in theory' because the bilingual situation in Miami, continuous and ongoing as it is, is such that most Miami-born Latinxs who learn Miami English as their home language also fall somewhere on the bilingual continuum (Polinsky & Kagan, 2007; Valdés, 2005), meaning they also have some degree of proficiency in Spanish. Code-switching, Spanglish, Miami English and the many and diverse varieties of Spanish spoken in Miami can be thought of discretely but, in reality, these linguistic varieties are all related linguistic phenomena that very often live in the same homes and speech communities.

Finally, Miami English is also not 'foreign accented speech' or 'immigrant speech'. Although it is true that there are many people in Miami who speak English as a second language and therefore speak 'with an accent', Miami English is not 'a foreign accent'. Miami English is instead an ethno-regional language variety of American English that bears the historical influence of Spanish and is spoken by Miamians of Latinx descent who learned English as their first or co-first language.

The vast majority of linguistic structures that make up Miami English are shared with other varieties that together can be classified as 'American English'. Like these other varieties, the unique structures that make Miami English distinctive are few relative to the overall number of structures that are shared with other dialects of English spoken in the United States. When thinking about what *is* distinctive about English in Miami, it is once again important to recall that Miami is home to a situation of linguistic contact between English and Spanish that is now well into its sixth decade. In these kinds of situations, linguists have observed that the kind of influence languages exert on one another depends on factors such as the intensity of contact (whether the contact between speakers is casual or intense), the duration of contact (whether the contact between speakers is short-lived or long-standing) and the extent to which the speakers of the languages in question are of equal or unequal standing in social, cultural and political terms (Thomason & Kauffman, 1988). In Miami, we can think of the intensity of the contact as being 'high' since levels of bilingualism are high. We can think of the duration of contact as being 'long-term' since the bilingual situation has extended across multiple generations. And although English is clearly the dominant language of prestige in Miami (Lynch, 2022), speakers of Spanish in Miami also enjoy high political, economic and social standing (Carter & Lynch, 2015).

We know that in immigrant situations, children of the immigrant generation have been shown to 'follow the pattern of their peers', meaning they learn the dialect patterns of the peers in their social networks, not from their parents (Chambers, 2003; Labov, 1991, 2008). Sankoff (2002) notes that immigrant influence on local varieties of English is ultimately quite rare, but that 'exceptions tend to be cases in which the immigrant group and its descendants have become the local majority population'.

These factors, coupled with the population ecological factors and ongoing immigration to Miami from Latin America described in the prior section, are key to understanding the kinds of distinctive linguistic structures that have become durable features of English in Miami.

Lexicon, grammar and semantics

In situations of language contact such as the one taking place between Spanish and English in South Florida, the lexicon is important for two reasons. First, linguists agree that of all levels of language, the lexicon moves the most freely from one language to another (Thomason & Kauffman, 1988; Winford, 2003). Second, the sounds, grammatical structures and meaning changes that occur through contact-induced change often travel with lexical borrowings. For this reason, I briefly touch on semantic and grammatical change in this section on the lexicon.

In Miami English we observe lexical influence from Spanish in two ways: (1) camouflaged forms and (2) calque phenomena. Camouflaged forms include words where the orthographic form is the same in Spanish and English, rendering either a Spanish-like pronunciation, or obscuring a unique English pronunciation within the orthography. This is the case of *salmon* which can be pronounced as [sæl-mən] rather than [sæ-mən]. Calques, also known as loan translations, involve translating words from a source language to a target language, while maintaining some linguistic or conceptual aspect of the source language. Carter and D'Alessandro Merii (2023) systematically studied Spanish-origin calques in Miami English and found forms such as those presented in Table 16.2.

These kinds of forms are replete in Miami English. Carter and D'Alesandro Merii (2023) provide explanations for these forms and illustrate the ways in which meaning and grammar are implicated. For

Table 16.2 Spanish-origin calques in Miami English

Local (Miami)	Non-local
Carmen got *married with* Antonio	Carmen got married to Antonio
Maria went to the office and bought a *meat empanada*	Maria went to the office and bought a beef empanada
Thanks god it didn't rain	Thank god
We drove in the garage, *got down from the car,* and went inside	We drove in the garage, got out of the car and went inside
Put me the light, Martin	Turn on the light, Martin
Marco and I went to a bar and he *invited me a beer*	Marco and I went to a bar and he treated me to a beer
After I got my groceries, I *made the line* and paid	After I got my groceries, I waited in line and paid
It's not for anything, but my extended family doesn't talk a lot	For no particular reason, my extended family doesn't talk a lot

example, 'thanks' in the expression *thanks god* is a kind of morphological calque. While 'thank' in the English expression *thank God* is a verb, 'thanks' in the Spanish expression *gracias a Dios* is a plural noun. The expression *he invited me a beer* involves a semantic calque, since the verb *invitar* 'to invite' has a wider semantic range in Spanish than in English, conveying both the English sense of *I invited them to a party* as well as the sense of 'to treat', as in *I'll treat you to dinner.* The semantic transfer involves minor grammatical consequences, in that the local use of *invite* assumes the ditransitivity of the Spanish form, taking both direct ('a beer') and indirect ('me') objects. Another semantic calque is the use of the word *meat* for *beef.* In Spanish *carne* has a wider semantic range than 'beef' does in English and can be translated as either *meat* or *beef* depending on context.

The expression *get down from the car* is a 'literal phrasal calque' and derives from the Spanish expression *bajar del carro* (literally: 'get down from the car'). Carter and D'Alesandro Merii (2023) found these forms to be used not only among the immigrant generation but also among the second generation, indicating that these kinds of calques have become a durable feature in Miami English. In a perception test, they also found that Miami listeners rated local forms more favorably than a group of national listeners not from Miami. This finding also indicates that these lexical items constitute a stable part of the local way of using English. Parkhurst and Carter (2024) found a range of adverbial-semantic calques of Spanish origin in Miami English, including forms such as 'ultimately' for *recently* (from the Spanish *últimamente*) and *already* from the Spanish *ya*. Here again, the Spanish *ya* has a wider semantic range than the English *already* and may occur with events in the future that have not yet taken place. In a perception test, Parkhurst and Carter (2024) found that a sentence such as *He already graduates next year* was rated favorably by Miamians, but less so by nonlocal raters. Just as Pittsburghers may say 'gumband' for *rubber band* and Southerners may say 'lightning bug' for *firefly* (Wolfram & Schilling, 2015), Miamians, too, have their expressions that reflect local demographic, cultural and linguistic history.

In the prior section I wrote that Miami English does not *necessarily* involve direct borrowings from Spanish. In reality, speakers of Miami English – even those who are the most English dominant and rarely use Spanish – will more than likely use direct borrowings from Spanish for specific lexical items. These kinds of direct borrowings include words such as *arepas*, *croquetas*, *maduros*, *lechón*, *chimichurri* and *bistec*, Spanish-origin terms for food items popular in Cuba, Colombia, Venezuela and elsewhere in Latin America. These terms are very frequently – but not always – uttered with Spanish phonology, which makes them difficult to differentiate from single-word code-switches. But whether one classifies them as borrowings or single-word switches, they are common in the English of Miami and thus should be mentioned in this discussion.

Sound system

The dialects of American English are principally differentiated by their sound systems, what sometimes is referred to in popular speech as 'accent'. Pronunciation differences in American English owe to a few different factors, including the 'founder's effect' – or differences in speech traceable to the dialect groups from the British Isles that ended up in particular settings, as well as to geographical boundaries that kept these and other groups in isolation from one another. A third condition producing differences in pronunciation in American English is contact between English and other languages. Many dozens of studies have shown that influences from the non-English immigrant language often persist even if the immigrant language is later lost (Howell, 1993; Purnell *et al.*, 2005; Trudgill, 2010; Winford, 2005). Recent studies of the Miami English vowel system show this kind of influence from Spanish. For example, Carter *et al.* (2020) studied the vowel system of 20 second-generation Cuban American and other Latinx background college students, comparing their speech to that of a non-Latinx white control group. They found significant differences between the groups, with Latinx and non-Latinx participants exhibiting different productions of the vowel sound /u/, as in 'boot'. The Latinx production of /u/ was made more back in the mouth as compared to the non-Latinx production. They also studied the vowel /æ/ as in 'cat', in two kinds of words: (1) before nasal consonants, in words like 'tram', where speakers of American English typically have a fronted and raised pronunciation, and (2) before non-nasal consonants, in words like 'trap', where /æ/ is not raised or fronted in most dialects. They found the Latinx group to produce significantly lower and more backed pronunciations for both classes of /æ/ as compared to the non-Latinx group. Research on Mexican American English (e.g. Thomas, 2019) has shown that some ethnolects where Spanish was historically spoken may merge the /æ/ sound in the two contexts, pre-nasal and non-pre-nasal. Even though Latinxs and non-Latinxs exhibited different productions of /æ/, this merger was not found in Miami. This result confirmed the findings of Rogers and Alvord (2017), who found /æ/-backing among three generations of Cuban Americans in Miami. Hernández (2024) also studied the vowel system in Miami, focusing specifically on Cuban Americans. For the sound /æ/ before nasals (*tram*), she found significantly higher and fronter variants for the second generation as compared to the immigrant generation, but no differences among subsequent generations. This finding points to the stabilizing of this pronunciation in Cuban American speech across generations. For /æ/ before non-nasals, she found a significant difference between the second and third generation, as well as a significant effect for 'English dominance'. This finding shows that certain vowel pronunciations may be acquiring social meaning associated with Cubanness during the third generation.[4] Hernández (2024) also studied the pronunciation of /l/ at the beginning of words, where Cuban Americans have a 'light' /l/ pronunciation that sounds a bit more like Spanish. Here again, she found sociolinguistic variation. In this case, the social meaning was around 'staying' versus 'leaving', with Cuban Americans who had moved away from Miami producing significantly darker /l/ than those who stayed in Miami. Among those who stayed in Miami, a second effect was found: more instances of light /l/ were found in the speech of those with denser Cuban American social networks. All speech communities demonstrate sociolinguistic variation in which linguistic factors co-vary with social factors such as age, level of education, gender and socioeconomic class. The findings reported in Hernández (2024) show this kind of sociolinguistic variation operating in Miami's Cuban American English speaking community.

Prosody

Another feature that likely differentiates the English in Miami from other language varieties is prosodic rhythm. Spanish and English have been theorized as exhibiting different rhythmic patterns. Spanish is commonly described as being 'syllable-timed', characteristic of Italic (Romance) languages, while English is commonly described as being 'stress-timed', characteristic of Germanic languages. According to this system of classification (e.g. Abercrombie, 1967; Pike, 1945), syllable-timed languages are thought to be those in which syllables are of equal or nearly equal duration and recur at regular intervals. Stress-timed languages, in contrast, are thought to be those in which syllables are of varying durations and recur at irregular temporal intervals.

Sociolinguists studying Spanish/English bilingual communities in the United States have documented syllable-timed patterning in the speech of English of Latinx participants in settings across the country (Carter & Wolford, 2016; Robles-Puente, 2014; Shousterman, 2015). In Miami (Carter *et al.*, 2020), we studied the speech of 20 Latinxs (n = 2357) and 5 non-Latinxs (n = 485) born in Miami for prosodic rhythm following the methods set forth in Low and Grabe (1995). We found significantly more stress-timing among the non-Latinx as compared to the Latinx group, who in contrast demonstrated significantly more syllable-timing. This finding also follows Enzinna (2016) who found more syllable-timing in Miami English even among English monolinguals with English monolingual parents.

Clinical Implications for Researchers and Practitioners

In this section I outline four implications for researchers and practitioners working with speakers or language data collected from South Florida. First – for both researchers and practitioners – it is paramount to understand what terms like 'Spanglish', 'code-switching', 'Miami English' and 'Spanish' are and to be sensitive to the nuanced ways they relate to one another. The partition drawn in this chapter between Miami English and everything else may not ring true for all speakers, including those whose English may be classified as 'Miami English', but who may well also speak or understand some variety of Spanish and engage in various kinds of code alternation in bilingual contexts. Thomas's (2019) notion of ethnolects as 'clouds' works well for the multilingual situation in Miami. Thomas (2019: 296) observes that ethnolects are 'dense in some places, thin in others, lacking perceivable boundaries, constantly changing, and often merging or gradating into other clouds'. This is how Miami English works within the broader sociolinguistic milieu of the city. A 30-year-old Cuban American born in Miami with a college degree might exhibit Miami English phonology whenever speaking English, may style-shift to standardized English for business calls, may use more localized forms in English with Latinx coworkers, may use Spanglish when talking to his/her mother, and monolingual Spanish when talking with his/her grandmother.

Implications for researchers

Researchers seeking to collect language data in Miami or collect linguistic information about research participants should avoid discrete and singular categorizations based on monolingual contexts. For example, language background questionnaires and language use surveys should allow participants to select multiple options and even provide space for speakers to describe their patterns of language use in their own words. Researchers working in the field with speakers or with recorded language data should similarly resist making facile categorizations about a speaker's language background based on qualitative interviews or short speech samples.

Second, speakers of Miami English may or may not have metalinguistic awareness of the distinctiveness of their language variety. 'Maria', a 21-year-old Cuban American college student from Miami, remarks on the first time she came to realize that her English is different from the English spoken outside of Miami.

> *I thought I spoke English perfectly, before, like when I was like fourteen, and then I traveled to Tennessee for the first time, yeah like ... someone was like, oh but you're like, you're like you know you're from Miami ... you're like Hispanic. I'm like how can you tell and they're like 'what do you mean your accent is like so strong.' I'm like, 'really?' And they're like 'yeah, like really strong.'*

Maria's story is typical of dialect speakers in many contexts, not only Miami (Wolfram & Schilling, 2015). But in Miami, speakers may have the experience of discovering that their language is 'different' in English and in Spanish. Further, some participants in our research (Carter *et al.*, 2020) reported that when traveling outside of Miami-Dade County, they are habitually asked questions such as 'what country are you from?' An important part of understanding Miami English and language in Miami more broadly is learning about the kinds of experiences speakers have with outsiders as well as speakers' metalinguistic reflections of their own language.

Implications for practitioners

Third, keeping in mind the many documented social, cognitive and psychological benefits of bilingualism, clinicians play a vital role in passing down responsible, linguistically informed perspectives to parents. Research on clinical settings in Miami shows that professionals – including doctors – systematically promote abandoning Spanish in the home. For example, Baralt and Mahoney (2020) studied the role of bilingualism on executive function in preterm-born children. They found that with the preterm-born population, 100% of the parents from the bilingual group in their study reported that their child's pediatric primary care provider advised them to stop speaking Spanish at home. The authors write, 'Clinicians must be made aware of the harm that can be done when they recommend that families switch to English only. Contrarily, when families' home language is supported and maintained, their children may develop bilingually and this may positively modulate their executive function skills'. Baralt *et al.* (2020) document the various ways in which early language environments of low-income Latinx children are negatively affected when their Spanish-speaking caregivers are told to switch to English-only. When assessing the language development or language ability of children in Miami, speech-language practitioners should note that children's developmental patterns may be different from those of both English monolinguals and Spanish monolinguals. It is therefore not appropriate to assess this population with monolingual assessment tools, or give lower scores because of the 'nonstandard' use of the language.

Finally, those working in educational contexts similarly have the opportunity to pass along linguistically informed perspectives to students. Latinx students in primary, secondary and post-secondary settings may face what Carter (2018) refers to as a 'triple-burden' of language ideologies: ideologies that construct Latinx varieties of English negatively, ideologies that construct working-class, Caribbean and non-prestige varieties of Spanish negatively, and ideologies that construct Spanglish and language mixing as problematic. For many decades, sociolinguists have written about how to best approach language arts instruction in primary, secondary and post-secondary educational settings (e.g. García *et al.*, 2017; Hudley *et al.*, 2010; Reaser & Adger, 2007; Rickford & Rickford, 1995; Smitherman, 1977; Wolfram *et al.*, 1999). Strategies include the use of home languages and language varieties in writing assignments, contrastive grammar analysis and translanguaging (a pedagogical strategy that allows students to dynamically incorporate all of their languages into an educational setting). Making space for home languages and language varieties does not have to come at the expense of teaching standardized language, and vice versa.

Conclusion

The purpose of this chapter has been to introduce and describe the ethno-regional variety of American English known as Miami English, to explore its distinctive features, and to outline the historical and demographic conditions that gave rise to it. This work has involved departing from the object of analysis – Miami English – to look more broadly at the sociolinguistic scene of South Florida where diverse varieties of Spanish co-mingle with English in the home and in the community. This is true of many Latinx communities in the United States, where a strict partitioning of English and Spanish does not correspond to how most experience language (Carter *et al.*, 2023). If at some point in the future Spanish were to disappear from the speech community, Miami English would likely live on in some form, joining the many other varieties of American English historically influenced by other languages. But for now, Miami English lives in a bilingual community in which most speakers land somewhere on the bilingual continuum. This means that researchers, clinical practitioners and educators working in South Florida need not only have some understanding of what Miami English is and how it works, but also of how language works more broadly in the lives of Miamians.

Notes

(1) In the wake of the Cuban Revolution, Miami was established as a place welcoming to political exiles, where people could speak Spanish and remain geographically close to Latin America.

(2) For an overview of the inverse, namely, how English shapes Spanish in the United States, see Carter and Varra (2023).

(3) The nature of the influence from Spanish on these varieties depends on a range of factors, including how long Spanish is maintained in the speech community and the size of the Spanish-speaking/bilingual population as compared to the English monolingual population.

(4) In situations of new dialect formation emerging from language contact, social meaning (associations between linguistic forms and aspects of social identity) takes shape in the second and third generations (see Thomas, 2019).

References

Abercrombie, D. (1967) *Elements of General Phonetics*. Edinburgh University Press.

Baralt, M. and Darcy Mahoney, A. (2020) Bilingualism and the executive function advantage in preterm-born children. *Cognitive Development* 55, 100931.

Baralt, M., Darcy Mahoney, A. and Brito, N. (2020) Háblame Bebé: A phone application intervention to support Hispanic children's early language environments and bilingualism. *Child Language Teaching and Therapy* 36, 33–57.

Boswell, T. (1994) *The Cubanization and Hispanicization of Metropolitan Miami*. Cuban American National Council.

Boswell, T. (2000) Demographic changes in Florida and their importance for effective educational policies and practices. In A. Roca (ed.) *Research on Spanish in the United States* (pp. 406–431). Cascadilla Press.

Carter, P.M. (2018) Hispanic-serving institutions and mass media engagement: Implications for sociolinguistic justice. *Journal of English Linguistics* 46 (3), 246–262.

Carter, P.M. and Lynch, A. (2015) Multilingual Miami: Current trends in sociolinguistic research. *Language and Linguistics Compass* 9 (9), 369–385.

Carter, P.M. and Wolford, T. (2016) Cross-generational prosodic convergence in South Texas Spanish. *Spanish in Context* 13 (1), 29–52.

Carter, P.M. and Lynch, A. (2018) On the status of Miami as a southern city: Defining language and region through demography and social history. In J. Reaser, E. Wilbanks, K. Wojcik and W. Wolfram (eds) *Language Variety in the New South: Contemporary Perspectives on Change and Variation* (pp. 375–396). University of North Carolina Press.

Carter, P.M. and D'Allesandro Merii, K. (2023) Spanish influenced lexical phenomena in Miami English: Tracking production and perception. *English World Wide* 44 (2), 219–250.

Carter, P.M. and Varra, R. (2023) Spanish and English contact in the United States. In M. Lopocaro (ed.) *Oxford Encyclopedia of Romance Linguistics* (part of *Oxford Encyclopedia of Linguistics,* ed. M. Aronoff) (pp. 1–29). Oxford University Press.

Carter, P.M., López Valdez, L. and Sims, N. (2020) New dialect formation through language contact: Vocalic and prosodic developments in Miami English. *American Speech* 95 (2), 119–148.

Carter, P.M., Callesano, S. and López-Valdez, L. (2023) Defining Latinx language. *Needed Research in Dialectology. Publication of the American Dialect Society* 108, 52–73.

Chambers, J.K. (2003) *Sociolinguistic Theory* (2nd edn). Polity (imprint of Blackwell Publishers) *Language in Society Series.*

Enzinna, N.R. (2016) Spanish-influenced rhythm in Miami English. *Proceedings of the Linguistic Society of America* 34, 1–15. https://doi.org/10.3765/plsa.v1i0.3733

Erker, D. (2017) The limits of named language varieties and the role of social salience in dialectal contact: The case of Spanish in the United States. *Language and Linguistics Compass* 11, e12232. https://doi.org/10.1111/lnc3.12232

Escobar, A.M. and Potowski, K. (2015) *El Español de los Estados Unidos.* Cambridge University Press.

Fought, C. (2003) *Chicano English in Context.* Palgrave Macmillan.

García, O., Ibarra Johnson, S. and Seltzer, K. (2017) *The Translanguaging Classroom: Leveraging Student Bilingualism for Learning.* Caslon.

Hernández, A. (2024) The role of experience in the cognitive underpinnings of linguistic bias: An interdisciplinary investigation of Miami-based Cuban American speech. Unpublished dissertation, Stanford University.

Howell, R.B. (1993) German immigration and the development of regional variants of American English: Using contact theory to discover our roots. In J. Salmons (ed.) *The German Language in America* (pp. 190–212). Max Kade Institute.

Hudley, C., Anne, H. and Mallinson, C. (2010) *Understanding English Language Variation in U.S. Schools.* Teacher's College Press.

Labov, W. (1972) *Sociolinguistic Patterns.* University of Pennsylvania Press.

Labov, W. (1991) The three dialects of English. In P. Eckert (ed.) *New Ways of Analyzing Sound Change* (pp. 1–44). Academic Press.

Labov, W. (2008) Mysteries of the substrate. In M. Meyerhoff and N. Nagy (eds) *Social Lives in Language — Sociolinguistics and Multilingual Speech Communities* (pp. 315–326). John Benjamins.

Labov, W., Ash, S. and Boberg, C. (2005) *The Atlas of North American English: Phonetics, Phonology and Sound Change.* De Gruyter Mouton. https://doi.org/10.1515/9783110167467

Lopez, M.H. and Krogstad, J.M. (2014) As Cuban American Demographics Change, So Do Views of Cuba. Pew Research Center.

Low, E.L. and Grabe, E. (1995) Prosodic patterns in Singapore English. In K. Elenius and P. Branderud (eds) *Proceedings of the XIIIth International Congress of Phonetic Sciences* (pp. 636–639). KTH & Stockholm University Press.

Lozano, R. (2018) *An American Language: The History of Spanish in the United States.* University of California Press.

Lynch, A. (2022) *Spanish in Miami: Sociolinguistic Dimensions of Postmodernity.* Routledge.

Nijman, J. (2011) *Miami: Mistress of the Americas.* University of Pennsylvania Press.

Parkhurst, B. and Carter, P.M. (2024) Spanish-origin adverbial calques in Miami English: Testing production and perception. Paper presented at: New Ways of Analyzing Variation 52. Miami Beach, FL. November 2024.

Pike, K. (1945) *The Intonation of American English*. University of Michigan Press.
Polinsky, M. and Kagan, O. (2007) Heritage languages: In the 'wild' and in the classroom. *Language and Linguistics Compass* 1 (5), 368–395.
Poplack, S. (1980) Sometimes I'll start a sentence in Spanish Y TERMINO EN ESPAÑOL: Toward a typology of code-switching. *Linguistics* 18 (7–8), 581–618. https://doi.org/10.1515/ling.1980.18.7-8.581
Portes, A. (1969) Dilemmas of a golden exile: Integration of Cuban exile families in Milwaukee. *American Sociological Review* 34, 505–518.
Purnell, T., Salmons, J. and Tepeli, D. (2005) German substrate effects in Wisconsin English: Evidence for final fortition. *American Speech* 80, 135–64.
Reaser, J. and Adger, C. (2007) Developing language awareness materials for nonlinguists: Lessons learned from the Do you speak American? Curriculum development project. *Language and Linguistics Compass* 1 (3), 155–167.
Robles-Puente, S. (2014) Prosody in Contact: Spanish in Los Angeles. PhD Dissertation, University of Southern California.
Rogers, B.M.A. and Alvord, S.M. (2017) Miami Cuban vowels In A. Cuza (ed.) *Cuban Spanish Dialectology: Variation, Contact, and Change* (pp. 3–19). Georgetown University Press.
Ryan, C. (2013) Language Use in the United States: 2011. Retrieved from https://www.census.gov/prod/2013pubs/acs-22.pdf.
Rickford, J.R. and Rickford, A.E. (1995) Dialect readers revisited. *Linguistics and Education* 7, 107–128.
Sankoff, G. (2002) Linguistic outcomes of language contact. In P. Trudgill, J.K. Chambers and N. Schilling (eds) *The Handbook of Sociolinguistics* (pp. 638–68). Basil Blackwell.
Shousterman, C. (2015) Speaking English in Spanish Harlem: Language Change in Puerto Rican English. PhD Dissertation, New York University.
Smitherman G. (1997) Black language and the education of Black children: One mo once. *The Black Scholar* 27 (1), 28–35.
Thomas, E.R. (2019) Mexican American English and dialect genesis. In E.R. Thomas (ed.) *Mexican American English: Substrate Influence and the Birth of an Ethnolect* (pp. 294–311). Cambridge University Press.
Thomason, S.G. and Kaufman, T. (2023) *Language Contact, Creolization, and Genetic Linguistics*. University of California Press.
Toribio, A.J. (2001) On the emergence of bilingual code-switching competence. *Bilingualism: Language and Cognition* 4 (3), 203–231. https://doi:10.1017/S1366728901000414
Trudgill, P. (2010) *Contact and Sociolinguistic Typology. The Handbook of Language Contact*. Wiley.
U.S. Census Bureau (2020) 2020 Census of Population and Housing. U.S. Department of Commerce. Available at https://www.census.gov/programs-surveys/decennial-census/decade/ 2020.html
Valdés, G. (2005) Bilingualism, heritage language learners, and SLA research: Opportunities lost or seized? *The Modern Language Journal* 89 (3), 410–426.
Weinreich, U., Labov, W. and Herzog, M. (1968) Empirical foundations for a theory of language change. In W.P. Lehmann and Y. Malkiel (eds) *Directions for Historical Linguistics* (pp. 95–195). University of Texas Press.
Winford, D. (2003) *An Introduction to Contact Lnguistics*. Blackwell.
Winford, D. (2005) Contact-induced changes: Classification and processes. *Diachronica* 22 (2), 373–427.
Wolfram, W., Adger, C.T. and Christian, D. (1999) *Dialects in Schools and Communities*. Routledge.
Wolfram, W., Carter, P. and Moriello, P. (2004) Emerging Hispanic English: New dialect formation in the American South. *Journal of Sociolinguistics* 8, 339–358.
Wolfram, W. and Schilling, N. (2015) *American English: Dialects and Variation*. John Wiley.
Zentella, A.C. (1997) *Growing Up Bilingual: Puerto Rican Children in New York*. Blackwell.

17 Persian in the Context of North America

Mojtaba Taghvafard and Elena Babatsouli

Introduction

The United States is a multicultural/multilingual community (Rumbaut & Massey, 2013). Among various ethnic groups migrating to North America are Iranians who speak Persian, also known as Farsi. Migration trends from Iran to North America have increased in recent years because of social, economic, political and religious pressures. As a result, an Iranian-English linguistic variety has emerged. Given that the Iranian population in North America is on the rise, it is increasingly important to describe this linguistic variant and the Iranian language/culture as a resource for practitioners engaging in clinical or educational services for children with Persian as a first, heritage or dominant language. Familiarization with the cultural profile of Iranian people can help interested stakeholders make evidence-based decisions. The first part of this chapter briefly reviews demographic and cultural information regarding the Iranian people in North America. The second part briefly describes Persian grammar in terms of syntax, morphology, semantics and pragmatics, focusing on phonology by first illustrating monolingual Persian use with a sample text, and then describing aspects of Persian use in English. We end the chapter with clinical implications for researchers and practitioners.

Context and Culture

Demography

Mid-2019 estimates of the United Nations Population Division indicate that the United States is the first destination for Iranians who live or wish to live abroad (Lai & Batalova, 2023). The Iranian population in the United States is estimated to be around 500,000 (World Population Review, 2024). More than 50% of Iranian immigrants live in California, with one-third residing in Los Angeles. Canada has the second largest Iranian community of 164,000 individuals, most living in Toronto or Vancouver. Compared to other foreign-born populations in North America, Iranians are more likely to hold a college degree, earn higher salaries and have better English language skills (Lai & Batalova, 2023). More than 66% of Iranians speak languages belonging to the Indo-European family; some are closely associated with languages spoken in India, and others with Romance, Germanic and Slavic language branches. Persian is the official and most common language, but Iran also has 66 indigenous languages, and many Iranians speak Azari Turkish, Kurdish, Baluchi or Luri as minority languages. Ethnic groups identified in Iran include Fars, Kurds, Azari and Turks, Lor, Lak, Taleshi, Gilak, Mazani, Turkoman, Sistani, Baluch, Khuzi, Bandari and Bushehri (Shahshahani, 2022).

Culture

Iran has historically experienced political, ideological, economic and environmental controversies that have severely affected its relations with other nations (Nasr, 2010; Radmanesh *et al.*, 2023; Radmanesh & Ahmadi, 2024). Iranian culture stands out for its Persian literature and, more specifically, its poetry, as represented in works by Ferdowsi, Omar Khayyam, Nezami, among others (Yarshater Center, 2023). Iranian handicrafts like tiles, pottery, ceramics, wooden artifacts, woven fabric and prints are as diverse as Iranian literature and are well-known worldwide (Nikouei *et al.*, 2023). Persian literature and handcrafting may serve as resources for teaching and clinical practicum engaging Persian speakers in North America.

Religion and its role in social contact

Iran is an Islamic country (United States Department of State, 2023), with Twelver Ja'afari Shia Islam being specified as the accepted official religion in the country. Statistics show that Muslims account for 99.4% of the population. Between 90 and 95% of this population are Shia, and 5–10% are Sunni. There are three legal religious minorities in the country, including Christians, Jews and Zoroastrians who freely practice their religion. Veiling practices for women in Iran (Fathzadeh, 2022) are part of the constitution, and citizens are expected to observe them. As many Iranian families are religious, practitioners should approach their interactions with cultural sensitivity and respect for the individuals' values. In some families, *hijab* [he.ˈdʒɒb̥] 'body covering' is mandatory for female Iranians when they are outside their homes. Notably, dress code practices (that is, observing or not observing *hijab*) may significantly differ among people of Iranian heritage in North America. Another important point to consider is Muslim practices regarding physical contact which forbids non-related individuals of different genders from touching one another. Therefore, clinicians should be watchful when interacting with people of the opposite sex. Moreover, Muslims observe some special religious laws and prefer not to work or study on those days, such as the nineth and tenth days of *Moharram* (the first month of the lunar calendar), the 28th day of Safar (the second month of the lunar calendar) and the 21st day of *Ramadan* (the fasting month for Muslims during the nineth month of the lunar calendar).

Persian, its Script, Grammar and Some Comparisons with English

This section succinctly summarizes Persian in terms of script, semantics, syntax, morphology and pragmatics. However, its primary focus is on Persian phonology, also highlighting differences with English. Contrastive analysis (CA) (Brown, 2000; Fasold & Connor-Linton, 2006; Yule, 2006) facilitates linguistic comparisons in languages/dialects (e.g. Babatsouli, 2023: Standard and Cypriot Greek with English) and has been extensively utilized cross-linguistically, e.g. English-Indonesian (Suhirman, 2016), English-Korean (Kabak & Idsardi, 2007), English-Pashto (Ali *et al.*, 2016), Greek-English (Babatsouli, 2022), Japanese-English (Anjarningsih & Saraayu, 2016), Russian-Chinese (Doubkova & Zakharova-Sarovskaya, 2018) and Spanish-Dutch (Fraai, 1986). English-Persian CA comparisons are abundantly represented in books (e.g. Keshavarz, 2011; Yarmohammadi, 2002; Ziahosseiny, 2009), book chapters (e.g. Bijankhan, 2018; Falahati, 2020; Kahnemuyipour, 2018; Megerdoomian, 2020; Modarresi Ghavami, 2018; Rafat, 2020) and articles (e.g. Eghlidi, 2016; Hayati, 1996; Joze Tajareh & Khodareza, 2014; Moradi & Chen, 2018; Soltani, 2007).

Script

Persian, and other minority languages in Iran, have developed the Arabic script (26 letters) for use in their context. Persian has four more letters (total: 32), including پ /p/, گ /g/, ژ /ʒ/ and چ /tʃ/. As a result, Persian vocabulary and grammar are influenced to a degree by the Arabic language. Persian scholars find Arabic script usage cumbersome for writing Persian because there is no close alignment between Arabic and Persian consonants as represented in the Arabic script. Also, while Arabic vowels can be mostly predicted with only three vowels included in the Arabic script, this is not true for Persian, which has six distinct vowels and no specific rules for predicting vowel use in words (Daniel & Mahdi, 2006). As a result, learning to read Persian is extremely challenging because of the ambiguity in the script.

Semantics

Like other languages, Persian has content words, like nouns, adjectives, verbs and adverbs, and function words (Jasbi, 2018). The Persian linguistic context is one of diglossia, in that standard Persian, taught in instructional settings, is different from spoken (colloquial) Persian; this creates a major challenge as understanding the spoken (colloquial) Persian of native speakers can be difficult when learning standard Persian as a second language. Persian uses bare nominal (no determiners or morphological markers), as in (1). Persian only distinguishes singular forms for nouns, e.g. سیب [siḇ] 'apple', unlike in English, i.e. *apples*.

(1) من سیب دوست دارم.
[man siḇ dust 'dɒram]
*I apple like.
'I like apples'.

Singular marking is differentiated in standard and colloquial Persian. The nominal suffix *–e* is a marker of definite nouns, like English 'the', appearing in colloquial but not formal Persian, e.g. in (2).

(2) پسره رفت.
['pʰe.sa.re raft]
*boy-e went.
'The boy went'.

Syntax

The basic structure of a sentence in Persian is SOV (subject-object-verb). Therefore, a simple sentence in Persian is as follows (3):

(3) من کتاب میخوانم.
[man kʰe.'tʰɒḇ 'mi.xɒ.nam]
*I book read.
'I read books'.

In standard Persian, it is possible to ask yes-no questions by adding آیا ['ɒ.jɒ] to the beginning of a sentence and having a rising intonation. However, in spoken (colloquial) Persian, it is possible to ask a yes-no question by changing the intonation of an affirmative sentence to a rising one. Persian also has wh-questions with the wh-word starting the sentence, e.g. چرا ['tʃʰe.rɒ] 'why', کجا [kʰo.'dʒɒ] 'where'. One special feature of Persian syntax is scrambling (Karimi, 2018), meaning that phrasal categories can be used in different positions in a clause, as (4a, b):

(4a) من کتاب را خریدم.
[man kʰe.'tʰɒḇ rɒ 'xa.ri.dam]
*I book *ra* bought.
'I bought the book'.

(4b) کتاب را من خریدم.
[kʰe.'tʰɒḇ rɒ man 'xa.ri.dam]
*book *ra* I bought.
'I bought the book'.

Unlike in English, Persian adjectives appear after nouns, e.g. in (5), along with the Ezafe construction, similar to genitive 'of' in English.

(5) کتاب خوب
[kʰe.ˈtʰɒb̥-e xub̥]
*book-e good
'A good book'.

Morphology

Persian distinguishes lexical and functional morphemes that can be free or bound (Mahmoodi-Bakhtiari, 2018). Free lexical morphemes are independent words (contrasted in meaning), while bound morphemes are incomplete in meaning. Free functional morphemes are subdivided into adpositions and conjunctions. The two types of adpositions include the postposition را [rɒ] and nine prepositions: به [be] 'to', در [dar] 'in/into', از [az] 'from', با [bɒ] 'with', تا [tɒ] 'to/until', بجز [ˈbe.dʒoz] 'except', برای [ba.ɹɒ.je] 'for', چون [tʃʰun] 'like' and بر [bar] 'up/over/on'. The first seven prepositions are the most common in daily conversations, but the last two occur mostly in literary texts. The postposition را [rɒ] marks direct objects in accusative cases. Persian conjunctions can be simple or complex. Simple conjunctions are: و [va] 'and', اما [ˈam.mɒ] 'but', زیرا که [ˈzi.ɹɒ.kʰe] and چونکه [ˈtʃʰun.kʰe] 'because', یا [jɒ] 'or', اگر [ˈa.ɟar] 'if', اگر چه [a.ɟar ˈtʃʰe] 'although', هرچند که [ˈhar.tʃʰand̥ kʰe] 'however', تا [tɒ] 'unless/as long as/once/until/to' and که [kʰe] 'that'. Complex conjunctions are هم...هم [ham...ham] 'both...and', نه... نه [na...na] 'neither...nor', یا...یا [jɒ...jɒ] 'either...or' and چه...چه [tʃʰe...tʃʰe] 'whether...or'.

Pragmatics

Pragmatic use in Persian is characterized by politeness, hierarchies and interpersonal communication. Politeness strategies are prominent in Persian communication differentiating, for instance, between polite/formal forms, like شما [ʃo.ˈmɒ] 'you' and casual/informal forms, like تو [tʰo] 'you'. Such usage is subject to context and the level of familiarity, so when young people talk to seniors or when people address strangers, they are expected to use polite constructions. Polite usage extends in written contexts, like when writing a formal letter that requires the use of honorific titles and phrases as an indication of respect. Indirectness is a specific feature of Persian pragmatics mostly seen in requests. When asking for a favor, Persians are more likely to use hints, suggestions or questions to convey their intent rather than directly talking about the main topic first.

Phonology

Several resources compare Persian and English phonologies (e.g. Keshavarz, 2011; Yarmohammadi, 2002; Ziahosseiny, 2009). What follows succinctly summarizes existing literature, also highlighting discrepancies, as well as adding under-represented content that is published in Persian only.

Persian syllable

Yarmohammadi (2002) reports striking differences with English in that Persian only permits six syllable types. Persian syllable types abide by the template $(C_{0\text{-}1})V(C_{1\text{-}2})$ as seen in Table 17.1.

Persian only permits two-member consonant clusters occurring in word-final position (Firouzshahi & Babatsouli, 2020; Shooshtaryzadeh, 2016a, 2016b, 2017; Zarifian *et al.*, 2015). The possible word final clusters are as follows: qd, bz, sb, sk, ʃt, xt, fʃ, mp, mb, mt, md, mn, mq, mʔ, nd, nd͡ʒ, ng, mz, mʃ, nf, bn, zm, zn, ʃm, xm, lm, rm, rn, jm, jn, jb, jf, jt, jd, js, jz, jʃ, jʔ, jl, jr, bl, fl, tl, lb, lf, lv, lt, ld, ls, lz, lk, lx, lq, rb, rf, rv, rt, rd, rs, rz, rʃ, rt͡ʃ, rd͡ʒ, rk, rg, rq, br, tr.

Persian segments

This section describes Persian vowels and consonants, comparing them with English as necessary. English has 26 letters, while Persian has 32 letters. Persian segmental inventories consist of 23 consonants, 6 vowels and 2 diphthongs (Yarmohammadi, 1969), overall, a small inventory compared to General American English (GAE) with 21 consonants, 13 monophthongs, 8 diphthongs and 5 triphthongs (Roach, 1983). In Persian, all consonants can occur word-initially, word-medially or word-finally. Tables 17.2–17.4 contrast segmental inventories of consonants (phonemes/allophones) and vowels in the languages. While Persian does not have /w/, /ou/ is glided to [w] word-finally. Persian consonantal allophones are under-represented in the literature, so special attention is given here in Table 17.3 and a following section below.

Table 17.1 Persian syllables

Syllables	Example
V	او [u] 'he/she'
VC	آب [ɒb] 'water'
VCC	عکس [aks] 'picture'
CV	پا [pʰɒ] 'foot'
CVC	بد [bad] 'bad'
CVCC	پشت [pʰoʃ t̚] 'back'

Table 17.2 Persian and English consonant phonemes

	Shared consonants	Persian-specific	English-specific
Consonant phonemes	p, b, t, d, k, g, m, n, f, v, s, z, ʃ, ʒ, h, tʃ, dʒ, l, r, j	q, x, ʔ	θ, ð, ŋ

Table 17.3 Persian and English consonant allophones

	Shared allophones	Persian-specific	English-specific
Consonant allophones	pʰ, kʰ, tʰ, qʰ p̚, t̚, k̚, ɹ, t͡ʃʰ, ɱ, ŋ	β, ç, c, ɟ, χ, ɣ, ɴ, ʁ, r, ɾ, ɽ	ɫ, ŋ̍, m̩, l̩, ɹ̩, ɾ

Table 17.4 Persian and English Vowels

	Shared vowels	Persian-specific	English-specific
Monophthongs	i, u, e,	a, o, ɒ	ɪ, ə, ɔ, ɑ, ʊ, ʌ, æ, ɜ, ɛ
Diphthongs		ei, ou [ou~w]	eɪ, aɪ, ɔɪ, oʊ, aʊ, ɪə, ea, ʊə,
Triphthongs			eɪə, aɪə, ɔɪə, oʊə, aʊə
Rhotic monophthongs			ɜ, ə
Rhotic diphthongs			ɪə, ɛə, ʊə, ɔə, ɑə
Rhotic triphthongs			aɪə, aʊə, eɪə, ɔɪə, oʊə

Persian consonant allophones

This section comprehensively describes consonant allophones providing examples (see recently: Taghvafard & Babatsouli, 2025). The description of Persian allophones is well-represented in Persian resources (Bijankhan, 2018; Falahati, 2020; Kahnemuyipour, 2018; Keshavarz, 2011; Megerdoomian, 2020; Modarresi Ghavami, 2018; Rafat, 2020; Yarmohammadi, 1985, 2002; Ziahosseiny, 2009), but not so comprehensively in the Western literature (e.g. Firouzshahi & Babatsouli, 2020).

(1) Velar palatalization. When /k, g/ occur word-initially before front vowels [i, e, a], they are palatalized to [c, ɟ], respectively, e.g. کر [car] 'deaf', گر [ɟaɹ] 'bald'. The same holds word-finally but in this context irrespective of the preceding vowel, e.g. درک [daɹc] 'understanding', سگ [saɟ̊] 'dog'.

(2) Uvular plosive/fricative. The Persian uvular plosive is a voiceless segment, /q/, though typically represented in the literature with [ɢ]. Example words include: قند [qʰand̥] 'sugar cube', فقط [fa.ˈqʰat̚] 'only' and وفق [vefq] 'adaptation'. Phoneme /q/ has a voiced uvular fricative allophone, [ʁ], that occurs intervocalically in spoken Persian, e.g. آقا [ɒ.ˈqʰɒ] 'Mr' or [ɒ.ˈʁɒ] 'Mr' or باغچه [bɒq.ˈt͡ʃʰe] or [bɒʁ.ˈt͡ʃʰe] 'garden'. The two allophones, [q] and [ɣ], are mostly used in free variation, thus, not contrasting the meaning, similar to Arabic (Shariq, 2015). Persian uses these contrastively subject to geographical variation. As an example, most Persian speakers pronounce غذا [ɣa.ˈzɒ] as [qʰa.ˈzɒ] 'food', but those who live near the south and southwest of the country consider these two words to be different, غذا [ɣa.ˈzɒ] 'food' and قضا [qʰa.ˈzɒ] 'fate'. Further, phoneme /q/ has a voiceless velar fricative allophone, [x], in intervocalic contexts, e.g. باغچه [bɒq.ˈt͡ʃʰe] or [bɒx.ˈt͡ʃʰe] 'garden', یقه [ja.ˈqʰe] or [ja.ˈxe] 'collar'.

(3) Glottal deletions. In Persian, the glottal stop and fricative are typically not pronounced syllable finally, and as a result the preceding vowel is lengthened, e.g. بعضی [baʔˈzi] 'some' becomes [baː.ˈzi] and بهترین [beh.tʰa.ˈrin] 'the best' becomes [beː.tʰa.ˈrin].
(4) Devoicing of plosives. Voiced stops become voiceless when adjacent to voiceless consonants or when word-finally, e.g. سگ [saɟ̊] 'dog', حدس [had̥s] 'guess', قصد [qʰasd̥] 'intention' and زود [zud̥] 'soon'.
(5) Backing of /x/. When fricative /x/ occurs in clusters word-finally, it is backed to post-velar or uvular, e.g. تلخ [tʰalχ] 'bitter', or فسخ [fasχ] 'revocation', or مسخ [masχ] 'metamorphosis'.
(6) Glottal fricative, /h/, whisper. While /h/ is voiceless, it is voiced when used intervocalically, e.g. بهار [ba.ˈhɒɹ] 'spring', or چهار [t͡ʃʰɒ.ˈhɒɹ] 'four'.
(7) /t͡ʃ/ aspiration. /t͡ʃ/ is heavily aspirated in word-initial contexts, e.g. چوب [t͡ʃʰub] 'wood'.
(8) Labiodentalization of /m/. /m/ occurring before /f, v/, assimilates to [ɱ], e.g. اموات /am.ˈvɒt/ [aɱ.ˈvɒt̚] 'dead people', or سمفونی /sam.ˈfo.ni/ [saɱ.ˈfo.ni] 'symphony'.
(9) /n/ assimilations. The alveolar nasal is assimilated to the place of articulation of following labial and velar consonants, e.g. من بودم /man bu.dam/ [ma**m** bu.dam] 'I was', or شنبه /ʃan.ˈbe/ [ʃa**m**.ˈbe] 'Saturday', or انواع /an.ˈvɒʔ/ [aɱ.ˈvɒʔ] 'types', or پنکه /pan.ˈce/ [pʰaŋ.ˈcʰe] 'fan', or انگار /en.ˈgɒr/ [eŋ.ˈgɒr] 'as if'.
(10) Uvularization of /n/. When /n/ precedes /q/, it is nasalized to uvular [ɴ], e.g. منقار /men .ˈqɒr/ [meɴ.ˈqʰɑr] 'beak', or منقل /man.ˈqal/ [maɴ.ˈqʰal] 'barbecue'.
(11) Rhotic variation. The trill has several allophones: word-initially and word-finally it is always [r], e.g. رفتم [raf.ˈtʰam] 'I went', کار [kʰɒr] 'work'; however, word-medially it is either [ɹ] or [ɾ], e.g. برد [boɾd̥] or [boɹd̥] 'he took'.
(12) Aspiration of voiceless plosives/. Word-initial /p, t, k/, are aspirated, e.g. کار [kʰɒr] 'work', تند [tʰond̥] 'fast' or پر [pʰor] 'full', but not word medially, e.g. فکر [fekr̥] 'thought' or word-finally, e.g. کارت [kʰɒɹt̚] 'card'.
(13) Devoicing of nasals and liquids. Word-final /m, n, l, r/ following voiceless consonants are devoiced, e.g. اسم [esm̥] 'name' or دفن [dafn̥] 'burial', وصل [vasl̥] 'connected', فکر [fekr̥] 'thought'.
(14) Archaic [β] loss. In old Persian, [β] was an allophone of /b/, not used in modern Persian anymore, like زفان [za.ˈβɒn] 'language'. However, in everyday speech, people sometimes use [β] instead of [b], for example باز [βɒz] instead of [bɒz] 'open'.

Persian stress

Persian has fixed lexical stress that falls on the final syllable of words (Yarmohammadi, 2002) and in phrases (Yarmohammadi, 1996), although this applies only to uninflected forms of words (Ferguson, 1957). Persian nominal compounds carry primary stress on the last member of the compound, similar to non-compound words. When considering compounds, the following points are worth noting.

(1) If a compound comprises two or more simple or complex elements, the stress falls on the last syllable, e.g. کتابفروش [kʰe.tʰɒb.fo.ˈruʃ] 'bookseller'.
(2) If there is a conjoined nominal expression or a nominalized sentence, stress falls on the last syllable, e.g. رفت و آمد [raftʰ-o-ɒˈmad] 'coming/going', زمین خوردن علی [zamiɴ xordaɴ-e ˈali] 'Ali is falling down'.
(3) When there is a numeric compound, stress falls on the last syllable, e.g. بیست و پنج [bistʰ-o-ˈpʰaɲdʒ] 'twenty-five'.
(4) However, if a word is used in a vocative manner, stress falls on the first syllable, e.g. کتابفروش! [ˈkʰetʰɒbforuʃ] 'You bookseller!'

Persian Sample Text

This section introduces a sample Persian text, a literary short story, as an example of the Persian language in use. While the full text is provided in the Appendix, the title of the story is shown here in (5) to exemplify Persian script, with phonemic and phonetic transcriptions in the International Phonetic Alphabet (IPA), followed by an English translation. The phonetic transcription includes allophones in bold. Note that the Persian script is read from right to left.

(5) دزد و خورجینش
/dozd va xor.ˈʤi.naʃ/
[dozd̥ va xoɹ.ˈʤi.naʃ]
'The thief and his saddlebag'.

Distinction between adult versus child Persian

Research on child Persian developmental speech has mostly focused on monolinguals in typical and atypical development (e.g. Bayat *et al.*, 2021; Firouzshahi & Babatsouli, 2020; Kazemi *et al.*, 2015; Mohamadi *et al.*, 2019; Sheibani *et al.*, 2020; Zarifian *et al.*, 2020; Zarifian & Fotuhi, 2020), including speech sound disorders and communication disorders affecting speech (e.g. Nikrah & Babatsouli, 2024a, 2024b, 2026; Zarifian *et al.*, 2015), but there is less work done in multilingual contexts (e.g. Farangi & Naami, 2024; Payesteh *et al.*, 2021). On the other hand, developmental research in the context of Persian as a first language in speakers learning English as a second language (e.g. Farangi & Naami, 2024; Namazi & Salehomoum, 2023) or third language (e.g. Sharifian, 2010), or with other languages as additional languages (e.g. Arabic, Khezri *et al.*, 2021; French, Torabi & Jabbari, 2018) has been less well explored.

Persian L2 English Speech Sounds

Persian speakers' speech production patterns are represented in the literature (Keshavarz, 2011; Yarmohammadi, 2002; Ziahosseiny, 2009). 'Interlanguage blueprints' (Babatsouli, 2022, 2023, 2024b) have been proposed as useful guides that help bridge the gap between theory and practice. Towards this goal, a basic Persian-English Interlanguage Blueprint is advanced next.

(1) Learners may aspirate /p, k, t/ in all positions, especially when these phonemes are followed by /s/, or when they are used words-finally.
(2) Persian palatal allophones of /k, g/ before front vowels and word-finally may be transferred in L2 English.
(3) As English-specific interdental fricatives, /θ, ð/ are absent in Persian, learners tend to substitute them with [t, d, s, z]. Most Persian learners achieve native-like production of English interdentals following instruction.
(4) Persian speakers who learn English are accurate in producing target-like English /ŋ/ as a velarized or palatalized nasal in words ending in *-ing*, such as *reading*, *working*, *dancing*.
(5) Learners tend to pronounce the English-specific lateral allophones, i.e. the dark lateral, [ɫ], e.g. *ball* and syllabic lateral, [l̩], e.g. *buckle*, as clear laterals, [l].
(6) The production of General American English /ɹ/ as a flap, [ɾ], intervocalically, or as a trill, [r] in other contexts is common in Persian-speaking learners.
(7) English syllabic consonants [m̩, n̩, l̩, ɹ̩] are difficult for Persian speakers who typically add a vowel before the coda consonant in that context.
(8) Persian /w/ is not allowed word-initially, which results in learners typically substituting English /w/ with [v]. Target-like accuracy may be achieved following phonological awareness drills during instruction.
(9) Persian lacks a tense-lax phonemic contrast in vowels for /i-ɪ/, /u-ʊ/. This leads to the loss of contrast in minimal pairs, like *SHIP/SHEEP*, *LIVE/LEAVE*, *BIT/BEAT*, *SIT/SEAT*, *FULL/FOOL* or *LOOK/LUKE*, as produced by Persian learners of L2 English.
(10) Because Persian only permits clusters word-finally, English-specific prosodic contexts involving clusters are simplified in L2 English by adding a vowel either between cluster members, e.g. *traffic* [tʰeræfɪk̚] or before the cluster, e.g. *school* [esku:ɫ̚].

Clinical Implications for Researchers

Despite the increasing migration of Iranians to North America, little is known about Persian-speaking children's language development and adults' language proficiency in this context. Persian-English bilingualism is represented in studies that investigate an aspect of children's speech or language (e.g. Arab Moghaddam & Sénéchal, 2001; Boudaoud, 2008; Farsi & Zarei, 2013; Foroodi-Nejad & Paradis, 2009). Such research is important to provide the backdrop for practitioners to engage in evidence-based practice. Implications for researchers with a direct impact on clinical and educational procedures relate to identifying aspects of research that are currently under-represented. Specifically, research on Persian-English usage in North America ought to include a variety of methodological contexts and participant groups with variable bilingual exposure and usage patterns. Bilingualism research should also include children and adults who have presented with speech/language impairments to investigate the manifestation of their disorder, disentangling it from speech-language differences resulting from bilingual processing or bidialectal influences (e.g. Babatsouli, 2023; Oetting, 2018). Reliable, valid and practical assessment tools to identify struggling bilinguals early on are also currently missing. Such tools will need to be ecological in perspective, thus, considering a wide range of speaker-internal and speaker-external factors, such as bilingual typologies, ages of acquisition and arrival, socioeconomic situations of their families, learner background, input and usage distribution frequencies, cognitive and affective factors etc. (Babatsouli, 2024a, 2024b). Further, research on cultural aspects such as Persian literature, Iranian handicrafts and religious matters may provide information and resources to clinicians in North America for more culturally sensitive clinical practices.

Clinical Implications for Practitioners

Approximately 5% of any population group has speech/language difficulties, while 15% of the human population shows disability which may also affect functioning (Babatsouli, 2021 and refs. therein for discussion). The 2020 US Census estimates a new immigrant every 34 seconds. Such estimates indicate increasing cultural and linguistic diversity in North America, making it increasingly harder for clinicians and educators to address related challenges in their professions. Given that the American Speech-Language-Hearing Association (ASHA), among other advocates internationally, highlights the significance of cultural/linguistic training in non-English and non-Western cultures, the present chapter has aimed to address the gap in the representation of Persian speakers in North America. Some research has been done on monolingual Persian-speaking children's language development (e.g. Foroodi-Nejad, 2011; Keshavarz & Safa, 2010). Targeted information on navigating the Persian-specific context in typical and atypical child phonologies during development, including a summary of speech assessment tools, is reviewed in Firouzshahi and Babatsouli (2020). The same resource provides additional information on specifics of Iranian culture not discussed here, such as non-verbal communication (gestures/body language), family practices (e.g. child-rearing, collectivity, group orientation, compliments) and education. Multitasking speech and culture in first and additional language contexts is a bare minimum when dealing with clients/students from minority groups within a societal majority. The step-by-step ecosystemic Action Plan with 10 Knowledge parameters, proposed by Babatsouli (2023) to guide clinical and educational assessment in bilinguals, is also relevant for Persian-English children in North America. This hands-on approach encourages practitioners to think holistically and view individuals, and their multilingual/multicultural acquisition/learning as an ecosystem (Babatsouli, 2024a). Being abreast of such cross-disciplinary developments in the field is vital for understanding and interacting with minority populations leading to efficient service provision.

References

Ali, A., Khan, B. and Awan, N. (2016) Contrastive analysis of the English and Pashto adjectives. *Global Language Review* 1 (1), 74–84.

Anjarningsih, H.Y. and Saraayu, A. (2016) A phonetic contrastive analysis of English words in three Japanese songs by akb48. *Jurnal Humaniora* 27 (3), 350.

Arab-Moghaddam, N. and Sénéchal, M. (2001) Orthographic and phonological processing skills in reading and spelling in Persian/English bilinguals. *International Journal of Behavioral Development* 25 (2), 140–147. https://doi.org/10.1080/01650250042000320

Babatsouli, E. (2021) Diversity considerations in speech and language disorders: A focus on training. In J.S. Damico, N. Müller and M.J. Ball (eds) *Handbook of Language and Speech Disorders* (2nd edn, pp. 33–52). Wiley-Blackwell.

Babatsouli, E. (2022) Speech errors Greeks make in English: A tutorial. In E. Kkese (ed.) *Speech Perception and Production in L2* (pp. 78–104). Cambridge Scholars Publishing.

Babatsouli, E. (2023) Ecosystemic clinical assessment of linguistic diversity: Greek-dominant speech. *Perspectives of the ASHA Special Interest Groups* 9 (3), 692–714. https://doi.org/10.1044/2023_PERSP-23-00088

Babatsouli, E. (2024a) Remarks on an ecosystemic view of multilingual acquisition and learning. In E. Babatsouli (ed.) *Multilingual Acquisition and Learning: An Ecosystemic View to Diversity* (pp. 1–35). John Benjamins.

Babatsouli, E. (2024b) Phonological disorders in child bilingualism. In M. Amengual (ed.) *The Cambridge Handbook of Bilingual Phonetics and Phonology* (pp. 309–337). Cambridge University Press.

Bayat, N., Ashtari, A. and Vahedi, M. (2021) The early prelinguistic skills in Iranian infants and toddlers. *Iranian Rehabilitation Journal* 19 (4), 441–454.

Bijankhan, M. (2018) Phonology. In A. Sedighi and P. Shabani-Jadidi (eds) *The Oxford Handbook of Persian Linguistics* (pp. 111–141). Oxford University Press.

Boudaoud, M. (2008) The variable development of /s/ + consonant onset clusters in Farsi-English interlanguage. Master's thesis, Concordia University. https://spectrum.library.concordia.ca/id/eprint/976394/1/MR63169.pdf

Brown, H.D. (2000) *Principles of Language Learning and Teaching* (4th edn). Longman.

Daniel, E.L. and Mahdi, A.A. (2006) *Culture and Customs of Iran*. Greenwood Press.

Doubkova, O.V. and Zakharova-Sarovskaya, M.V. (2018) Contrastive analysis of multicomponent neologisms in modern Russian and Chinese: Enological ergonomics. *Bulletin of Kemerovo State University* 2, 170–175.

Eghlidi, M. (2016) Contrastive analysis of English and Persian intonation patterns: An error analysis study on Iranian undergraduate EFL students. *Journal of Applied Linguistics and Language Research* 3 (4), 88–102.

Falahati, R. (2020) The acquisition of segmental and suprasegmental features in second language Persian. In P. Shabani-Jadidi (ed.) *The Routledge Handbook of Second Language Acquisition and Pedagogy of Persian* (pp. 9–35). Routledge.

Farangi, M.R. and Naami, A. (2024) A study of early multilingualism in Iran: The effects of mother tongue literacy, socio-economic status and foreground TV exposure. *Acta Psychologica* 243, 104167.

Farsi, M. and Zarei, L. (2013) Practical contrastive analysis of English and Persian with special emphasis on relative clauses. *Time Journals of Arts and Education Research* 1 (2), 7–9.

Fasold, R.W. and Connor-Linton, J. (2006) *An Introduction to Language*. Cambridge University Press.

Fathzadeh, F. (2022) Swapping the veil for casual clothing: A study of Iranian immigrant women living in Norway. *Women S Studies International Forum* 92, 102577.

Ferguson, C.A. (1957) Word stress in Persian. *Language* 33 (2), 123.

Firouzshahi, N. and Babatsouli, E. (2020) Iranian Persian: A guide to speech and culture for the international clinician. *Journal of Monolingual and Bilingual Speech* 2 (1), 137–164.

Fraai, G. (1986) Spaanse Si en Cuando zinnen en hun equivalenten in het Nederlands een contrastieve en foutenanalyse. *Toegepaste Taalwetenschap in Artikelen* 26, 51–69.

Foroodi Nejad, F. (2011) Towards the identification of linguistic characteristics of specific language impairment in Persian. Doctoral Dissertation, University of Alberta. See https://era.library.ualberta.ca/items/71305aaa-8ef2-426b-8fc3-40480932308c

Foroodi-Nejad, F. and Paradis, J. (2009) Crosslinguistic transfer in the acquisition of compound words in Persian–English bilinguals. *Bilingualism Language and Cognition* 12 (4), 411–427.

Hayati, A.M. (1996) A contrastive analysis of English and Persian intonation patterns. *Journal and Proceedings of the Royal Society of New South Wales* 129 (1–2), 85–86.

Jasbi, M. (2018) Some unique semantic properties of Persian. In A. Sedighi and P. Shabani-Jadidi (eds) *The Oxford Handbook of Persian Linguistics* (pp. 134–146). Oxford University Press.

Joze Tajareh, M. and Khodareza, M. (2014) The contrastive analysis of Persian and English adjective knowledge. *Journal of Teaching English Language Studies* 3 (2), 7–18.

Kabak, B. and Idsardi, W.J. (2007) Perceptual distortions in the adaptation of English consonant clusters: Syllable structure or consonantal contact constraints? *Language and Speech* 50 (1), 23–52.

Kahnemuyipour, A. (2018) Prosody. In A. Sedighi and P. Shabani-Jadidi (eds) *The Oxford Handbook of Persian Linguistics* (pp. 142–158). Oxford University Press.

Karimi, S. (2018) Generative approaches to syntax. In A. Sedighi and P. Shabani-Jadidi (eds) *The Oxford Handbook of Persian Linguistics* (pp. 161–204). Oxford University Press.

Kazemi, Y., Stringer, H. and Klee, T. (2015) Study of child language development and disorders in Iran: A systematic review of the literature. *Journal of Research in Medical Sciences: The Official Journal of Isfahan University of Medical Sciences* 20 (1), 66–77.

Keshavarz, M.H. (2011) *Contrastive Analysis and Error Analysis*. Rahnama Press.

Keshavarz, M.H. and Ahmadi Safa, M. (2010) Early phonological and lexical development of a Farsi speaking child: A longitudinal case study. *The Journal of English Language Pedagogy and Practice* 3 (6), 131–161.

Khezri, F., Jabbari, A.A., Fazilatfar, A.M. and Jamshidi, F. (2021) Persian and Arabic Students' L3 acquisition of English plural marking: language of contact instruction matters for cross-linguistic onfluence. *Journal of Language Horizons* 6 (3), 65–85.

Lai, T. and Batalova, J. (2023) Immigrants from Iran in the United States. *migrationpolicy .org*, 14 February. See https://www.migrationpolicy.org/article/iranian-immigrants -united-states-2021

Mahmoodi-Bakhtiari, B. (2018) Morphology. In A. Sedighi and P. Shabani-Jadidi (eds) *The Oxford Handbook of Persian Linguistics* (pp. 273–299). Oxford University Press.

Megerdoomian, K. (2020) Linguistic competence of Persian heritage versus second language speakers. In P. Shabani-Jadidi (ed.) *The Routledge Handbook of Second Language Acquisition and Pedagogy of Persian* (pp. 53–99). Routledge.

Modarresi Ghavami, G. (2018) Phonetics. In A. Sedighi and P. Shabani-Jadidi (eds) *The Oxford Handbook of Persian Linguistics* (pp. 91–110). Oxford University Press.

Mohamadi, R., Ahmadi, A., Kazemi, M.D., Minaei, A. and Damarchi, Z. (2019) Development of the Persian syntax comprehension test. *International Journal of Pediatric Otorhinolaryngology* 124, 22–29.

Moradi, H. and Chen, J. (2018) A contrastive analysis of Persian and English vowels and consonants. *Lege Artis Language Yesterday Today Tomorrow* 3 (2), 105–131.

Namazi, M. and Salehomoum, M. (2023) Assessment in Farsi–English emerging bilingual children: A tutorial. *Perspectives of the ASHA Special Interest Groups* 9 (3), 738–753.

Nasr, S.H. (2010) *A Journey Through Persian History and Culture* (Series 10, pp. 1–89). Iqbal Academy Pakistan.

Nikouei, A., Khanpour, A., Grami, M., Feizi Rad, M. and Mirmobin, R. (2023) *Iranian Handicrafts & Traditional Arts*. https://doi.10.13140/RG.2.2.10886.96323

Nikrah, P. and Babatsouli, E. (2024a) Cluster reductions in atypically developing children's speech in Persian. *American Speech-Language-Hearing Association (ASHA 2024) Convention*. Boston, MA, United States.

Nikrah, P. and Babatsouli, E. (2024b) Enhancing phonological skills in Persian-speaking children with social communication disorder through narrative intervention. *Early Childhood Voices 2024 (ECV 2024)*. Charles Sturt University, Bathurst, Australia.

Nikrah, P. and Babatsouli, E. (2026) Phonological skills of Persian monolinguals with social communication disorder (SCD): A comparison with typically developing (TD) peers and effects of narrative intervention. *Clinical Linguistics and Phonetics*. https://doi.org/10.1080/02699206.2025.2568041

Oetting, J.B. (2018) Prologue: Toward accurate identification of developmental language disorder within linguistically diverse schools. *Language, Speech, and Hearing Services in Schools* 49 (2), 213–217. https://doi.org/10.1044/2018_LSHSS-CLSLD-17-0156

Payesteh, B. and Finestack, L.H. (2021) Narrative language development of Persian-English bilingual children attending an immersion preschool. *Clinical Archives of Communication Disorders* 6 (3), 149–159.

Radmanesh, M. and Ahmadi, S.H. (2024) Surge irrigation modeling and scenario analyses for the best furrow irrigation management practices. *Journal of Hydrology* 629, 130618.

Radmanesh, M., Ahmadi, S.H. and Sepaskhah, A.R. (2023) Measurement and simulation of irrigation performance in continuous and surge furrow irrigation using WinSRFR and SIRMOD models. *Scientific Reports* 13 (1), 5768.

Rafat, Y. (2020) Heritage versus second language phonology. In P. Shabani-Jadidi (ed.) *The Routledge Handbook of Second Language Acquisition and Pedagogy of Persian* (pp. 36–52). Routledge.

Roach, J. (1983) *English Phonetics and Phonology: A Practical Course* (4th edn). Cambridge University Press.

Rumbaut, R.G. and Massey, D.S. (2013) Immigration & language diversity in the United States. *Daedalus* 142 (3), 141–154.

Shahshahani, S. (2022 Anthropology and ethnic studies, Iran. *International Journal of Anthropology and Ethnology* 6 (17), 140–154.

Sharifian, F. (2010) Glocalization of English in world Englishes: An emerging variety among Persian speakers of English. In M. Saxena and T. Ominiyi (eds) *Contending with Globalization in World Englishes* (pp. 137–158). Multilingual Matters.

Shariq, M. (2015) Arabic and English consonants: A phonetic and phonological investigation. *Advances in Language and Literary Studies* 6 (6). https://doi.org/10.7575/aiac.alls.v.6n.6p.146

Sheibani, F., Ghoreishi, Z.S., Nilipour, R., Pourshahbaz, A. and Zamani, S.M. (2020) Validity and reliability of a language development scale for Persian-speaking children aged 2–6 years. *Iranian Journal of Medical Sciences* 45 (4), 259–268.

Shooshtaryzadeh, F. (2016a) Nonlinear phonological scan analysis for intervention planning: Farsi. See https://phonodevelopment.sites.olt.ubc.ca/practice-units/farsi

Shooshtaryzadeh, F. (2016b) Sonority and cluster reduction in typical and atypical phonological development in Farsi. In M.J. Ball and N. Müller (eds) *Challenging Sonority: Crosslinguistic Evidence* (pp. 376–396). Equinox Publishing.

Shooshtaryzadeh, F. (2017) Local assimilation in children acquiring Farsi: A study of typical vs. atypical phonological development. In E. Babatsouli, D. Ingram and N. Müller (eds) *Crosslinguistic Encounters in Language Acquisition: Typical and Atypical Development* (pp. 249–276). Multilingual Matters.

Soltani, A.M. (2007) *Contrastive Analysis of English and Persian Intonation.* Iran University Press.

Suhirman, L. (2016) Nuance in simple and past tense patterns by Indonesian EFL learners: A contrastive analysis. *IJOLTL: Indonesian Journal of Language Teaching and Linguistics* 1 (3), 219.

Torabi, F.S. and Jabbari, A.A. (2018) The acquisition of French (L3) Orthography by Persian (L1) Speakers Learning English (L2). *The Journal of Applied Linguistics and Applied Literature: Dynamics and Advances* 6 (2), 29–47.

Taghvafard, M. and Babatsouli, E. (2025) Allophones in the spotlight: Clinical and pedagogical implications. Paper presented at the American Speech-Language-Hearing Association (ASHA) 2025 Convention. Washington, DC, USA

United States Department of State (2023) United States Department of State. 7 December. See https://www.state.gov/reports/2022-report-on-international-religious-freedom/iran/

World Population Review (2024) See https://worldpopulationreview.com/state-rankings/iranian-population-by-state

Yarmohammadi, L. (1969) English consonants and learning problems for Iranians: A contrastive sketch. *TESOL Quarterly* 3 (3), 231–236.

Yarmohammadi, L. (2002) *A Contrastive Analysis of Persian and English (Grammar, Vocabulary, and Phonology).* Payam-e Noor University Press.

Yarshater Center. (2023) *A History of Persian Literature.* Yarshater Center. See https://yarshater.ucla.edu/a-history-of-persian-literature/

Yarmohammadi, L. (1985) *A Contrastive Analysis of Modern Persian and Modern English.* Indiana University Press.

Yule, G. (2006) *The Study of Language* (3rd edn). Cambridge University Press.

Zarifian, T. and Fotuhi, M. (2020) Phonological development in Persian-speaking children: A cross-sectional study. *International Journal of Speech-Language Pathology* 22 (6), 614–625.

Zarifian, T., Modarresi, Y., Tehrani, L.G. and Kazemi, M.D. (2015) Phonetic and phonological acquisition in Persian speaking children. In E. Babatsouli and D. Ingram (eds) *Proceedings of the International Symposium on Monolingual and Bilingual Speech* (pp. 430–438). ISMBS.

Zarifian, T., Ahmadi, A. and Ebadi, A. (2020) Development and measurement of psychometric properties of the Persian test of speech consistency in children with typical development. *Applied Neuropsychology: Child* 11 (3), 226–234.

Ziahosseiny, S.M. (2009) *Contrastive Analysis of Persian and English & Error Analysis.* Rahnama Press.

Appendix

Notes: Persian script is read from right to left. Phonemic transcription is shown with // and phonetic transcription with []; consonant allophones are highlighted in bold.

Source: The Persian text was retrieved from https://dostegolam.blogfa.com/post/53 on November 10, 2024.

دزد و خورجینش
/dozd va xor.ˈʤi.naʃ/
[dozd̥ va xoɹ.ˈʤi.naʃ]
The thief and his saddlebag

دزدی نیمه شبی به خانه ای رفت.
/ˈdoz.di ni.ˈme ˈʃa.bi be xa.ˈne-i raft/
[ˈdoz.di ni.ˈme ˈʃa.bi be xa.ˈne-i raft̚]
‘A thief went to a house in the middle of the night.’

صاحب خانه در گوشه اتاق خوابیده بود.
/sɒ.ˈheb xɒ.ˈne dar gu.ˈʃe-je o.ˈtɒq xɒ.bi.ˈde bud/
[sɒ.ˈheb̥ xɒ.ˈne dar gu.ˈʃe-je o.ˈ**tʰ**ɒq xɒ.bi.ˈde bud̥]
‘The owner of the house was sleeping in the corner of the room.’

دزد خورجینی را که با خود داشت روی زمین انداخت تا اثاثیه ی خانه را در آن بگذارد و ببرد.
/dozd xor.ˈʤi.ni rɒ ke bɒ xod dɒʃt ru-je za.ˈmin an.ˈdɒxt tɒ a.sɒ.si.ˈje-je xɒ.ˈne rɒ dar ɒn bog.zɒ.ˈrad va be.ba.ˈrad/
[doz**d̥** xoɹ.ˈʤi.ni rɒ **cʰ**e bɒ xod̥ dɒʃt̚ ru-je za.ˈmin an.ˈdɒxt̚ **tʰ**ɒ a.sɒ.si.ˈje-je xɒ.ˈne rɒ dar ɒn boɟ.zɒ.ˈra**d̥** va be.ba.ˈra**d̥**]
‘The thief threw the saddlebag he had with him on the ground to put the fittings and furnishings in it and take it.’

امّا هر چه در اتاق گشت چیزی پیدا نکرد.
/am.ˈmɒ har.ˈʧe dar o.ˈtɒq gaʃt t͜ʃi.ˈzi pei.ˈdɒ na.ˈkard/
[am.ˈmɒ har. ˈ**ʧʰ**e dar o.ˈ**tʰ**ɒq ɟaʃt̚ **tʃʰ**i.ˈzi **pʰ**ei.ˈdɒ na.ˈ**cʰ**aɹ**d̥**]
‘However, he did not find anything in the room after searching a lot.’

دزد که ناامید شده بود به سوی خورجین برگشت تا آن را بردارد و برود.
/dozd ke nɒ.o.ˈmid ʃo.ˈde bud be su-je xor.ˈʤin bar.ˈgaʃt tɒ ɒn rɒ bar.dɒ.ˈrad va be.ra.ˈvad/
[doz**d̥** **cʰ**e nɒ.o.ˈmi**d̥** ʃo.ˈde bu**d̥** be suˈje xoɹ.ˈʤin baɹ.ˈɟaʃt **tʰ**ɒ ɒn rɒ baɹ.dɒ.ˈra**d̥** va be.ra.ˈva**d̥**]
‘The thief, who was disappointed, turned to his saddlebag to take it and leave.’

در همین موقع صاحب خانه غلتی زد و روی خورجین او خوابید!
/dær ˈha.min mo.ˈqeʔ sɒ.ˈheb xɒ.ˈne ɣal.ˈti zad va ru-ˈje xor.ˈʤin-e u xɒ.ˈbid/
[dar ˈha.min mo.ˈ qʰeʔ sɒ.ˈheb̥ xɒ.ˈne ɣal.ˈ**t**ʰi zad̥ va ru.ˈje xoɹ.ˈʤin-e u xɒ.ˈbi**d̥**]
'At the same time, the owner of the house rolled over and slept on his saddlebag!'

دزد که خیلی ناراحت شده بود با صدای بلند و عصبانی گفت:
/dozd ke xei.ˈli nɒ.rɒ.ˈhat͜ʃo.ˈde bud bɒ se.dɒ-ˈje bo.ˈland va a.sa.bɒ.ˈni goft:/
[Doz**d̥** cʰe xei.ˈli nɒ.rɒ.ˈhat͡ʃo.ˈde bud̥ bɒ se.dɒˈje bo.ˈlan**d̥** va a.sa.bɒ.ˈni: gof͡t:]
'The thief, who was very upset, said in a loud and angry voice:'

"عجب بخت و اقبالی دارم من! چیزی به دست نیاوردم، خورجینم را هم از دست دادم !"
/a.ˈdʒab baxt va eq.ˈbɒ.li dɒ.ˈram man! tʃi.ˈzi be dast na.jɒ.var.ˈdam, xor.ˈʤi.nam‿rɒ ham az dast dɒ.ˈdam/
[a.ˈdʒab̥ bax͡t va eq.ˈbɒ.li d̥ɒ.ˈram man! **tʃ**ʰi.ˈzi be das͡t na.jɒ.vaɹ.ˈdam, xoɹ.ˈʤi.nam rɒ ham az das͡t dɒ.ˈdam!]
'How unlucky I am! I didn't get anything, and I have also lost my saddlebag!'

سپس راه افتاد تا برود.
/se.ˈpas rɒh of.ˈtɒd tɒ be.ra.ˈvad/
[se.ˈ**p**ʰas rɒh of.ˈ**t**ʰɒ**d̥** **t**ʰɒ be.ra.ˈva**d̥**.]
'Then he started to leave.'

صاحب خانه با صدای بلند گفت:
/sɒ.ˈheb xɒ.ˈne bɒ se.ˈdɒ-je bo.ˈland goft:/
[sɒ.ˈheb̥ xɒ.ˈne bɒ se.dɒˈje bo.ˈlan**d̥** gof͡t:]
'The owner of the house said in a loud voice:'

"آهای دزد، وقتی از خانه بیرون رفتی در را ببند تا دزد دیگری به خانه نیاید."
/ɒ.ˈhɒj dozd, vaq.ˈti az xɒ.ˈne bi.ˈrun raf.ˈti dar rɒ be.ˈband tɒ dozd-e di.ˈga.ri be xɒ.ˈne na.jɒ.ˈjad/
[ɒ.ˈhɒj doz**d̥**, vaq.ˈ**t**ʰi az xɒ.ˈne bi.ˈrun raf.ˈ**t**ʰi dar rɒ be.ˈban**d̥** **t**ʰɒ dozd-e di.ˈɟa.ri be xɒ.ˈne na.jɒ.ˈja**d̥**]
'"Hey, thief! Close the door when you leave the house so that no other thief will come to the house."'

دزد ایستاد و به صاحب خانه گفت:
/dozd is.ˈtɒd va be sɒ.ˈheb xɒ.ˈne goft:/
[Doz**d̥** is.ˈtʰɒd va be sɒ.ˈheb̥ xɒ.ˈne gof͡t:]
'The thief stopped and said to the owner of the house:'

"من زیرانداز را برای تو آوردم و حالا در را باز می گذارم شاید دیگری روانداز ترا هم بیاوردتو از
باز بودن در ضرر نکردی و نخواهی کرد!"

/man zir.an.ˈdɒz rɒ ba.rɒ.ˈje to ɒ.var.ˈdam va hɒ.ˈlɒ dar rɒ bɒz mi.go.zɒ.ˈram ʃɒ. jad di.ga.ˈri ru.an.dɒ.ˈzat rɒ ham bi.jɒ.va.ˈrad! to az bɒz bu.ˈdan-e dar za.ˈrar na.kar.ˈdi va na.xɒ.ˈhi kard/

[man ziɹ.an.ˈdɒz rɒ ba.rɒ.ˈje **tʰ**o ɒ.vaɹ̣.ˈdæm va hɒ.ˈlɒ dar rɒ bɒz mi.go.zɒ.ˈram ʃɒ.ˈja**d̥** di.ɟa.ˈri: ru.an.dɒ.ˈzat̚ rɒ ham bi.jɒ.va.ˈra**d̥**! **tʰ**o az bɒz bu.ˈdan-e dar za.ˈrar na.cʰaɹ.ˈdi va na.xɒ.ˈhi **cʰ**aɹ**d̥**]

'"I brought you the mattress, and now I will leave the door open. Maybe someone else will bring your quilt, too! You did not and will not suffer from the door being open!"'

18 Basic Characteristics of Native Speakers of Korean Learning English

Sea Hee Choi

Introduction

Context and culture

The United States is home to immigrants from many different countries, and among them are Korean immigrants. As of 2023, the estimated number of Korean Americans (including Korean immigrants) living in the United States is approximately 1.9 million. Regardless of whether they are born in the United States or not, many immigrants exhibit specific characteristics in their use of English, and these characteristics are often heavily influenced by their native language. In this context, these linguistic patterns form one of the many varieties of English in North America. For speech and language practitioners, it is crucial to distinguish the L1-influenced patterns made by second language (L2) learners from pathological symptoms.

Although Korean Americans form one of the more visible groups in the United States, it is also worth noting that Korean speakers have established communities in Canada, where Korean is spoken by a smaller but still significant population; in the 2021 Census, 203,885 people reported knowledge of Korean (Statistics Canada, 2022). In both countries, many of the same transfer-based phenomena occur, though the specific sociolinguistic contexts may differ slightly. For instance, Korean communities in certain Canadian provinces might have different levels of institutional support (e.g. heritage language schools or bilingual programs) compared to those in the United States, potentially influencing the extent and type of L1-transfer effects. A thorough comparison of Korean usage in Canada versus the United States is beyond the scope of this chapter, but the discussion below largely applies to both contexts, acknowledging that regional policies and community structures can shape language acquisition outcomes.

In this chapter, I focus on native Korean speakers learning English (hereafter, L1 Korean-L2 English learners) and highlight their linguistic characteristics by discussing the most typical and noticeable non-target-like forms they make due to the influence of their first language (L1). This chapter focuses primarily on speakers whose first language is Korean and who acquire English as a second language, rather than on all Korean Americans or Korean heritage speakers in North America. To better understand L1 Korean-L2 English learners, it is important to grasp basic concepts in second language acquisition (SLA), such as L1-transfer and fossilization. L1-transfer, also known as language transfer or cross-linguistic influence, refers to the impact that a learner's first language (L1) has on the acquisition of a second language (L2). In the field of SLA, it is well established that the use of target constructions in L2 is strongly influenced by the learner's native language (Gass & Selinker, 2008; Lightbown & Spada, 2013; Ortega, 2014).

There are two types of L1-transfer: positive and negative. Positive transfer occurs when structures or rules from L1 are similar to those in L2, facilitating the learning process (Odlin, 1989). This type of transfer is more likely to occur between languages that share similarities, such as English and German or Korean and Japanese. For example, if both L1 and L2 have a similar word order (e.g. subject–verb–object), this similarity can make it easier for learners to construct sentences correctly in L2. On the other hand, negative transfer, often referred to as interference, occurs when L1 structures are applied inappropriately to L2, leading to non-target-like forms. A speaker of Japanese, whose language typically follows a subject–object–verb (SOV) structure, might incorrectly apply this word order when speaking English, which follows a subject–verb–object (SVO) structure, causing syntactic errors.

Another critical aspect of L2 acquisition is the concept of interlanguage. Interlanguage refers to the unique linguistic system that learners develop as they progress from their native language (L1) to the target language (L2) (Selinker, 1972). This intermediate system often involves the application of L1 structures or rules to L2, which can lead to non-target-like forms but also facilitates learning. Additionally, interlanguage is closely related to the phenomenon of fossilization. What has traditionally been termed 'fossilization' refers to the persistence of certain non-native forms despite continued exposure to the target language (Selinker, 1972; Long, 2003). However, recent scholarship has increasingly re-characterized such persistence as stabilization rather than permanent fixation (Han, 2004; Ortega, 2014), reflecting a view that non-target-like forms may be resistant to change without being entirely irremovable. Such persistent patterns are commonly observed after learners have reached a certain level of proficiency, at which point progress may plateau and non-target-like forms become resistant to change despite continued exposure. It can be attributed to various factors, including lack of motivation, insufficient corrective feedback or the learner's reliance on communication strategies that are sufficient for conveying meaning, even if they are not entirely accurate. Fossilization is commonly observed in many L2 learners in the United States and Canada, including L1 Korean-L2-English learners, and can be considered a form of linguistic variation in North America. In some cases, learners may not even perceive these stabilized non-target-like forms as errors, especially if their communicative needs are largely met, further reinforcing these persistent linguistic patterns. When similar L1-influenced patterns are shared across communities, they may contribute to stable features of contact varieties. And such community-level variation should be distinguished from individual interlanguage development.

In SLA research, the effects of L1-transfer are typically explored by comparing specific features of the target language (L2) with those of the native language (L1). When comparing Korean and English, significant differences are evident. According to the Foreign Service Institute (FSI) language difficulty rankings (n.d.), Korean is classified in the highest difficulty category along with Arabic, Chinese and Japanese. The differences encompass vocabulary, pronunciation, grammar, the writing system, as well as underlying cultural and societal norms. Such typological differences can make acquisition more challenging when the two languages differ substantially. As a result, extensive research has been conducted on these challenges and the characteristics of language use by L2 learners, including L1 Korean-L2 English learners, thanks to the efforts of many scholars in the field of SLA (e.g. Kim & Kim, 2013; Schwartz & Sprouse, 1996).

It is also noteworthy that the learning environment plays a major role in how quickly or effectively L1 Korean speakers acquire English. Learners who receive formal instruction in an English-speaking country may show different patterns of development compared to those learning English as a foreign language in Korea. Additionally, sociocultural factors, such as the attitudes of local communities toward immigrants, the availability of bilingual resources and the presence of heritage language programs, can all shape how L1 Korean learners navigate the acquisition process. In some cases, older immigrants might rely heavily on Korean-dominant social networks, resulting in less exposure to authentic English input, whereas younger immigrants who attend local schools may adapt more readily to English-dominant contexts.

Given the breadth of this topic, it is not possible to cover all the characteristics of L1 Korean-L2 English learners in a single chapter. Instead, I will focus on the phonetic and grammatical characteristics, as these are the most easily noticeable and often lead to significant misunderstandings in communication. The first section will examine the factors that contribute to distinctive pronunciation errors in English, comparing the sound patterns of Korean and English. The second section will review specific aspects of Korean grammar that can lead to incorrect grammar usage in English. By focusing on these two areas, this chapter aims to provide a clear understanding of the challenges faced by L1 Korean-L2 English learners and how these challenges can affect their communication in English. Understanding these specific characteristics will not only help in distinguishing between typical language acquisition errors and potential speech or language disorders but will also provide insights into effective strategies for language instruction and intervention tailored to the needs of Korean speakers learning English.

Phonological System

One of the most noticeable characteristics of English spoken by L1 Korean-L2 English learners is their distinct, non-native-like pronunciation. This arises from significant differences between Korean and English speech sound patterns, as Korean speech sounds and their combinations differ greatly from those of English. To fully understand such pronunciation variations and transfer-influenced pronunciations, it is crucial to have a basic understanding of the fundamental differences between the two languages. By grasping these distinctions, we can better comprehend the pronunciation challenges faced by L1-Korean speakers learning and using English.

Consonants

First, voicing is not considered a distinctive feature of Korean consonants. Instead, the pronunciation of each consonant changes depending on its position within a word. For example, in the initial position, singleton consonants such as plosives are voiceless, while between vowels, they become voiced, as shown in (1). However, in English, voicing is a distinctive feature for consonants, and the mental representations of voiced and voiceless consonants differ significantly. Additionally, voicing in English consonants is contrastive, changing the meaning of words, as demonstrated in (2).

(1) 발 [**p**al] 'foot'
바보[pa**b**o] 'a fool'

(2) *Pat* [**p**ʰæt] (voiceless)
bat [**b**æt] (voiced)

On the other hand, aspiration in English is generally predictable (e.g. [pʰ] in word-initial position), whereas in Korean it is a distinctive feature. Compare (3) and (4):

(3) *pin* [**p**ʰ ɪn]
spin [s**p**ɪn]

(4) 바다 [**p**ɑdɑ] 'sea'
파다 [**p**ʰɑdɑ] 'to dig'

Furthermore, Korean also distinguishes tense consonants. Tense consonants are produced with greater laryngeal constriction and are typically voiceless and unaspirated. This contrast does not exist in English in the same way. Based on these articulatory properties, Korean has a three-way laryngeal contrast in stops, commonly described as plain (or lax), aspirated, and tense (Kim & Duanmu, 2004; Lee *et al.*, 2015), as shown in (5). In English, by contrast, the primary contrast is between voiced and voiceless stops, while the difference between [p] and [pʰ] is largely allophonic rather than phonemic.

(5) Aspirated [pʰ] ㅍ
Plain [p] ㅂ
Unaspirated (tense) [p'] ㅃ

As a result, L1 Korean-L2 English learners often struggle to distinguish between voiced and voiceless plosives in English. They might also use tense consonants, which do not exist in English, leading to non-native-like pronunciation. This can manifest in the form of overemphasized or 'tight' stops that English speakers might perceive as unusual or even 'double-articulated'.

A major challenge for L1 Korean-L2 English learners stems from consonants that exist in English but not in Korean. Tables 18.1 and 18.2 illustrate the consonants in Korean and English, respectively. Korean has 19 consonants in the traditional inventory, and if the glides /w/ and /j/ are included as consonantal segments, the inventory contains 21 segments. English has 24 consonants. The most noticeable difficulties often involve English consonants that lack straightforward phonemic counterparts in Korean, especially /f/, /v/, /θ/, /ð/, /z/, and /ʒ/. As a result, for example, the English sound /f/ is absent in Korean, so L1 Korean-L2 English learners often struggle to pronounce words like coffee [kɔfi] correctly, sometimes saying [kʌpi]. Korean has a single liquid phoneme realized as a lateral [l] in syllable-final position and a flap [ɾ] intervocalically (Lee *et al.*, 2015), neither of which corresponds directly to the English approximant /ɹ/. As a result, L1 Korean-L2 English learners frequently map both English /l/ and /ɹ/ onto the Korean liquid, leading to well-documented pronunciation difficulties (Ha *et al.*, 2009). This /l/–/ɹ/ challenge is not unique to Korean learners; it is also observed in learners from other East Asian linguistic backgrounds, but the specific phonetic contexts in Korean can exacerbate it.

In general, when it is difficult to accurately pronounce the consonants of the target language, L2 learners often substitute them with consonants from their native language (Flege, 1995). L1 Korean-L2 English learners employ this strategy by substituting non-existing English consonants with similar sounds from Korean. Table 18.3 provides a summary of such examples:

As shown in Table 18.1, Korean lacks the English [ɹ], so L1 Korean-L2 English learners substitute it with the Korean liquid /l/, as in robin [ɹɑbɪn] → [lobin] (Table 18.3). For other English consonants missing in Korean, L1 Korean-L2 English learners apply similar substitution strategies.

Although Korean does not have a phonemic /s/ -/ʃ/ contrast comparable to that of English, an [ɕ]- or [ʃ]-like realization occurs before high front vowels or glides in Korean. For this reason, English /ʃ/ is generally less problematic for L1 Korean-L2 English learners. While learners may struggle with the voiced palato-alveolar affricate [ʤ], this pronunciation issue is usually more acceptable than other missing consonants listed in

Table 18.1 Korean consonant chart

		Bilabial	Alveo-dental	Alveolo-palatal	Palatal	Velar	Glottal
Stop	lax	p	t			k	
	aspirated	p^{h}	t^{h}			k^{h}	
	tense	P'	t'			k'	
Affricate	lax			ʨ			
	aspirated			$ʨ^{h}$			
	tense			ʨ'			
Fricative	lax		s				h
	tense		s'				
Nasal		m	n			ŋ	
Liquid			l				
Glides		W			j		

(Lee *et al.*, 2015)

Table 18.2 English consonant chart

		Bilabial	Labiodental	Dental	Alveolar	Palatal	Velar	Glottal
Stop	voiceless	p			t		k	
	voiced	b			d		g	
Fricative	voiceless		f	θ	s	ʃ		h
	voiced		v	ð	z	ʒ		
Affricative	voiceless					ʧ		
	voiced					ʤ		
Nasal		m			n		ŋ	
Liquid					l	r		
Glides		w				j		

(Henton, 1987)

Table 18.3 Common pronunciation patterns of L1 Korean-L2 English learners

Original consonant	Consonant substitution	Example
[f]	[f]→[p]	*coffee* [kɔfi]→[kʌpi]
[v]	[v]→[b], [p]	*vase* [veɪs]→[beis]
[ɹ]	[ɹ]→[l]	*robin* [ɹɑbɪn]→[lobin]
[z]	[z]→[ʨ]	*zoo* [zu]→[ʨu]
[θ]	[θ]→[s]	*math* [mæθ]→[mes]
[ð]	[ð]→[d]	*father* [fɑðər]→[pɑdʌ]
[ʤ]	[ʤ]→[ʨ]	*judge* [ʤʌʤ]→[ʨʌʨi]

Table 18.1 because it can be more easily substituted with the Korean alveolo-palatal affricate [tɕ]. Non-target-like forms in pronunciation among L1 Korean-L2 English learners tend to follow surprisingly similar patterns, which can lead to misunderstandings or miscommunications. However, it is important to remember that these pronunciation characteristics are heavily influenced by proficiency level, and there are individual differences as well. At lower proficiency levels, most L1 Korean-L2 English learners exhibit similar pronunciation patterns, but as their proficiency improves, these L1-influenced patterns often diminish, and their pronunciation becomes more native-like. Additionally, due to varying life experiences, some learners may perform better with certain consonants while still exhibiting typical transfer in others, even at higher proficiency levels. Understanding these nuances is crucial for effectively addressing pronunciation challenges in L1 Korean-L2 English learners

Vowels

In Korean, there are 8 simple vowels[1] and 11 diphthongs, whereas English has 12 monophthong vowels and 8 diphthongs. Table 18.4 and Table 18.5 illustrate the comparison between Korean and English simple vowels. As shown in Table 18.4 and Table 18.5, there are significant differences between the two vowel systems, but one of the most prominent differences is the lack of a distinction between short and long vowels in Korean. In the past, vowel length was a distinctive feature in Korean, but in modern standard Korean, it is gradually disappearing, although this

Table 18.4 Korean vowel chart

	Front		Central		Back	
	unrounded	**rounded**	**unrounded**	**rounded**	**unrounded**	**rounded**
high	i (ㅣ)		ɨ (ㅡ)			u(ㅜ)
mid	e/ɛ (ㅔ/ㅐ)				ʌ (ㅓ)	o(ㅗ)
low			a (ㅏ)			

Note. The realization and contrast between ㅔ and ㅐ vary across speakers; for many contemporary Seoul Korean speakers, the contrast has largely merged. (Adapted from Lee *et al.*, 2015)

Table 18.5 English vowel chart

	Front		Central		Back	
	unrounded	**rounded**	**unrounded**	**rounded**	**unrounded**	**rounded**
high	i ɪ					u ʊ
mid	e ɛ		ə ʌ			o ɔ
low	æ a					

topic remains controversial. In contemporary Korean language classes, vowel length is no longer taught, and even among native Korean speakers, only some older individuals distinguish vowel length (Lee *et al.*, 2015).

As a result, many native Korean speakers are not sensitive to vowel length, which impacts their use of English vowels when learning English as a second language (L2). For instance, L1 Korean-L2 English learners may struggle to differentiate between the front high long vowel [i] and the front high short vowel [ɪ], as well as the back high long vowel [u] and the back high short vowel [ʊ]. Since even advanced L1 Korean-L2 English learners often cannot distinguish between [i] and [ɪ], they are likely to pronounce both vowels in the same way they pronounce the Korean front high vowel [i] (ㅣ). Similarly, both /u/ and /ʊ/ are often pronounced as the Korean back high vowel [u] (ㅜ) (Lee & Cho, 2018).

Furthermore, L1 Korean-L2 English learners may struggle to distinguish the English mid-central vowels [ə] and [ʌ] because the distinction of these sounds does not exist in the Korean vowel system. For example, L1 Korean-L2 English learners might pronounce *away* [əˈweɪ] and *us* [ʌs] using the same Korean mid-back vowel [ʌ] (ㅓ), resulting in not differentiating between two different sounds, which can lead to confusion in communication.

Additionally, the English low vowel [ɑ] is likely to be pronounced more centrally, similar to the Korean low central vowel [a]. The English front low vowel [æ], which is not present in Korean, is often pronounced as the Korean mid-front vowel [e]. For example, the word *cat* [kæt] might be pronounced as [ket] by L1 Korean-L2 English learners. This lack of distinction between [æ] and [ɛ], as in the minimal pair *bat* [bæt] and *bet* [bɛt], can lead to misunderstandings and miscommunications (Lee & Cho, 2018).

These pronunciation challenges reflect the influence of the native Korean vowel system on the acquisition and use of English vowels, often resulting in non-native-like pronunciation and potential communication difficulties for L1 Korean-L2 English learners. Understanding these differences is crucial for addressing these challenges in language instruction and clinical service provision in the context of speech disorders.

Syllables and phonotactic constraints

Syllables are units in the prosodic organization of sounds of a language usually considered to affect speech sound patterns because of a language's phonotactic constraints (referring to sequences of possible sound combinations). Languages vary in terms of the richness of syllable structures and phonotactics.

In Korean, the basic syllable structure is outlined in (6), where parentheses stand for optional appearance and the dot (.) stands for the syllable boundary. As shown in (6), a syllable requires at least a vowel; other elements are optional. (7) shows examples of syllables in Korean.

(6) .(C)V(C) [.(consonant) (semivowel)VOWEL (consonant)]

(7) i (이) *this*
yel (열) 'ten'
ku (그) 'that'
os (옷) 'clothes'
pyel (별) 'star'

(Cho *et al.*, 2019)

There are several phonotactic constraints that play a role. For example, consonants [l] and [ŋ] and the flap [ɾ] principally cannot occur in the syllable-initial position. In syllable-final position, all obstruent consonants (stop/fricative/affricate) are neutralized into three stop consonants: [p], [t] and [k]. As a result, only seven consonants [m, n, ŋ, l, p, t, k] can occupy the coda of a syllable in Korean.

More importantly, only singleton consonants are allowed in the syllable-initial and syllable-final positions. No consonant clusters are allowed in the syllable-initial position. However, English allows up to three consonants in syllable-initial and syllable-final positions (e.g. 'str' in *street* and 'sks' in *tasks*). Because of this difference, when L1 Korean-L2 English learners pronounce an English word with consonant clusters, they tend to add/epenthesize a vowel after each consonant, which turns a monosyllabic English word, like *street* into a four-syllable word, roughly, [sɯ.tɯ.ɾi.tɯ]. This type of vowel epenthesis is a well-documented feature of Korean-accented English pronunciation and may cause intelligibility problems, especially in words containing consonant clusters (Seo, 2021).

Intonation

Korean, particularly Seoul/Standard Korean, does not have lexical stress or lexical pitch accent in the way English has lexical stress. Its prosodic structure is organized at the phrasal level, with boundary tones and phrasal accents signaling sentence type, discourse structure, and speaker attitude (Jun, 2005). For example, Korean uses rising intonation in *yes-no* questions and falling intonation for statements (Kim & Tremblay, 2021). The same sentence can have two different meanings based on the intonation in oral communication as in (8).

(8) pap mek-ess-eyo?
meal eat-Pst-Decl?
'Did you have a meal?'

pap mek-ess-eyo.
meal eat-Pst-Decl.
'I had a meal'.

However, English has lexical stress that is contrastive for meaning as in (9). Such lexical stresses do not exist in Korean and do not make any meaning changes either.

(9) *REcord* (noun): I listened to the *record.*
reCORD (verb): Please *record* the meeting.

Due to such differences, when L1 Korean-L2 English learners speak English, their speech can sound monotonous without any lexical stress and even sound like mumbling sometimes. Failing to use lexical stress also leads to frequent miscommunications. Furthermore, lower-proficiency L1 Korean-L2 English learners form questions using only rising intonation, without altering the sentence structure, such as in *You ate your lunch?*. This is influenced by the patterns of their native language. In such cases, even though the intention is to ask a neutral question, it may sound like a confirmation question or it may even convey disbelief. Such subtle meaning differences influenced by Korean speakers' native language can also hinder communication.

Grammatical Characteristics

There are many grammatical characteristics that can pose challenges in the use of English for L1 Korean-L2 English learners, but I will introduce here only those more likely to impact intelligibility or cause significant misunderstandings.

Word order differences

Korean is called a verb-final or adjective-final language, which means that the verb or adjective usually comes at the end of the sentence or clause while other elements such as the subject and the object come before the verb or the adjective. The basic word order in Korean is SOV (subject-object-verb), while English follows SVO (subject-verb-object) as shown in (10).

(10A) Jake plays tennis at school (SVO)
(10B) Ceyikhu-ka hakkyo-eyse theynisu-lul chin-ta. (SOV)
Jake-Nom school-Loc tennis-Acc play-Decl.
'Jake plays tennis at school.'

One thing to be noticed in (10B) is the use of particles. Korean particles refer to suffixes attached to words to indicate the word's role or relationship within a sentence, such as the nominative particle *-ka* in *Ceyikhu-ka* and the accusative particle *-lul* in *theynisu-lul.* They function similarly to prepositions, conjunctions or case markers in English but are more versatile. Using the particles, native speakers of Korean can easily distinguish the part of speech of a word. This is one of the reasons why Korean is often called a 'free word order' language allowing 'word scrambling'; it allows the elements such as the subject and the object before the verb or the adjective to be randomly assigned for emphasis or other purposes, as long as the verb or adjective remains in the final position. Thus (11A), (11B) and (11C) carry the same meaning even though they have different word orders.

(11A) *Ceyikhu-ka hakkyo-eyse theynisu-lul chin-ta.*
Jake-Nom school- Loc tennis-Acc play-Decl.

(11B) *hakkyo-eyse Ceyikhu-ka theynisu-lul chin-ta.*
school-Loc Jake-Nom tennis-Acc play-Decl.

(11C) *theynisu-lul hakkyo-eyse Ceyikhu-ka chin-ta.*
tennis-Acc school- Loc Jake-Nom play-Decl.
'Jake plays tennis at school.'

In contrast, English lacks the kind of overt case-particle system found in Korean and relies much more heavily on rigid word order to signal grammatical relations; as a result, changing word order in English can alter sentence meaning or render a sentence ungrammatical. For instance, *The cat chased the mouse* is different from *The mouse chased the cat.* Interestingly, although overt word order errors in simple declarative sentences are relatively less frequent among L1 Korean-L2 English learners, possibly due to the early salience of English SVO order in instructional contexts, subtle L1 transfer effects may nonetheless emerge in more complex syntactic environments such as relative clauses and embedded clauses (Schachter, 1974).

Discourse- and context-dependent omission of arguments

Korean allows extensive omission of contextually recoverable arguments, with many elements left unspecified when they can be inferred from discourse or situational context. In many cases, the known information such as the second-mentioned or the contextually or situationally given information is often omitted even though it is the subject or the object of the sentence. For example, if one wants to say 'where are you going?' in Korean, one can say it as in (12).

(12) Etika-sey-yo?
Wherego-Hon-Decl?
'Where are you going?'

As shown in (12), Korean allows the subject to be omitted in this question, yielding an expression roughly corresponding to 'where go?' because the subject is recoverable from the one-on-one conversational context.

In contrast, in English, the omission of parts of speech is strictly restricted, and the omission of the subject or the object of the sentence can lead to ungrammaticality. Due to such differences, L1 Korean-L2

English learners can make errors by omitting either the subject or the object when they are the known information. In this case, it can cause ungrammaticality.

Korean demonstratives and the use of articles in English

In English, there are definite, *the*, and indefinite articles, *a/an*. The definite article *the* is used to mark definiteness while the indefinite article *a/an* is used to mark indefiniteness. In English, definiteness is defined as uniqueness and familiarity (see Abbott, 2003, for an overview). For example, a definite noun phrase such as *the book* presupposes the existence of a unique book in the relevant discourse. (13) shows such examples. As shown in (13), in the definite contexts, the definite article *the* and a demonstrative *that* can be used while the indefinite article *a/an* cannot be used.

(13A) Mary got a book from the library. She read the/that/*a book in a single evening.
(13B) Mary can no longer drive her car. Someone stole the/#that/*a steering wheel.[2]

Similarly, the English indefinite article *a/an* is used in indefinite contexts: when the existence of a particular referent is indicated (14A) and when such existence is not asserted (14B). In (14A), a book refers to a specific book that exists in the actual world, while in (14B), a pen does not refer to any specific pen. But in both cases, the indefinite article *a/an* is needed.

(14A) Jane is reading a book.
(14B) Jane needs to buy a pen.

In Korean, however, there are no indefinite and definite articles. Instead of definite articles, Korean marks definiteness using three demonstratives, *i* 'this', *ce* 'that over there' and *ku* 'that' (Sohn, 1999) while it marks indefiniteness using the numeral *one* + classifier. Unlike English articles, however, they are not used obligatorily: as shown in (15), lexical marking is always optional, and a bare noun is always grammatical with both definite and indefinite contexts.

(15A) *Con-un say monithe-lul sa-ss-ta.*
John-Top new monitor-Acc buy-Pst-Decl
Onul *achim ku-nun(ku) monithe-lul chen-ulo takka-ss-ta.*
Today morning he-Top that monitor-Acc cloth-Iinst clean-Pst-Decl.
'John bought a new monitor. This morning, he cleaned that/the monitor with a cloth.'

(15B) *Makhu-nun eceyspam nwunpola-lul ttwulh-ko ilha-le keleka-ya hay-ss-ta.*
Mark-Top last night snowstorm-Acc through-Comp work-to walk-have to-Pst-Decl
Mark had to walk to work through a snowstorm last night.
Kulayse *ku-nun hyenmyenghakey (han-kay-uy) moca-lul sse-ss-ta.*
So he-Top wisely (one-Cl-Gen) hat-Acc wear-Pst-Decl.
So he wisely wore a hat.

(Adapted from Ionin *et al.*, 2022)

Since Korean lacks articles, the acquisition of English articles is notoriously difficult for L1 Korean-L2 English learners. In the use of definite and indefinite articles, L1 Korean-L2 English learners show several types of non-target-like forms. The first type is omission. Especially lower-level proficiency L1 Korean-L2 English learners frequently omit articles due to the absence of articles in their native language. For example, previous studies such as Ionin *et al.* (2004) found that these learners often omitted articles, especially in contexts where native English speakers would use *the* or *a*. This omission is typically attributed to the direct transfer of Korean language structures, which do not use articles, into English.

The second type of L1-influenced patterns in the use of English articles is overuse of *the*. L1 Korean-L2 English learners do not understand when to use the definite article, *the*, properly, so they use the definite article in situations where the article is unnecessary or where an indefinite article *a*/*an* would be more appropriate (e.g. 'The water is necessary for life' instead of 'Water is necessary for life' when referring to water in general and 'She is a doctor in the hospital' instead of 'She is a doctor in a hospital') when referring to someone's occupation without identifying a specific hospital. This is due to the learners' reliance on the definite article to convey specificity[3] or emphasis, as their L1 (Korean) uses demonstratives like 그 [ku] to convey similar meanings, leading to L1-transfer errors.

The third type of errors is confusion between *the* and *a*. L1 Korean-L2 English learners struggle to distinguish when to use *the* versus *a*, often using them interchangeably inappropriately. For example, L1 Korean-L2 English learners may say 'Can you pass me a book on the table?' instead of 'Can you pass me the book on the table?', since they do not understand 'on the table' specifies which book is being referred to, making it clear and definite. Such errors are also due to the lack of understanding of when to use English articles properly and can be considered as evidence of negative L1-transfer from their native language.

Pluralization

English has the obligatory plural marker *-s*, and count nouns can take an indefinite article and plural marking (e.g. *a desk, desks*) while mass nouns cannot (e.g. **an oil*, **oils*). And only mass nouns can occur in bare form without an article (e.g. *I bought water* vs **I bought desk*) while count nouns can be directly combined with numbers (e.g. two desks, *two oils, *two oil).

In Korean, there is no obligatory morphological marker, such as the plural *-s* in English. And nouns cannot be directly combined with numbers as shown in (16A) and (16B); instead, to be counted, all nouns should be combined with classifiers as in (17A) and (17B).

(16A) *twu chayksang
Two desk
'two desks'
(16B) *sey mwul
Three water
'*three water'
(17A) *han can-uy mwul*
One Cl-Gen water
'one cup of water'
(17B) han kay-uy chayksang
One Cl-Gen desk
'a desk'

Even though there is no obligatory plural marker, interestingly, Korean has an optional plural marker *-tul*. It can be combined with count nouns but not with mass nouns as in (18).

(18A) haksayng-tul
'students'
(18B) *kilum-tul
'*oils'

Furthermore, in Korean bare nouns are unspecified in terms of number, so bare nouns can be either singular or plural as in (19).

(19) saja (*lion/lions*) and saja-*tul* (*lion-Pl*)

Due to such differences between Korean and English in terms of the count/mass distinction, the use of English plural marking is challenging for L1 Korean-L2 English learners. Previous studies (e.g. Choi & Ionin, 2021) show that when L1 Korean-L2 English learners acquire the count/mass distinction in English, they rely on universal concepts of boundedness[4] rather than the count/mass distinction morphosyntax in English and make systematic errors when the concepts of boundedness and the English count/mass morphosyntax have discrepancies, such as furniture (furniture has a boundary but is mass in English). It can be partially considered as L1-transfer as well because *kakwu* 'furniture' in Korean can be combined with the Korean plural marker *-tul* even though it is optional (see Choi *et al.*, 2018 and Choi & Ionin, 2021 for more information).

Implications for Practitioners

For language teachers, speech-language pathologists and other practitioners, understanding L1-influenced patterns proves crucial for effective instruction and intervention. A primary consideration involves differentiating between typical L1 transfer patterns and potential language disorders, requiring practitioners to develop and implement assessment protocols that consider the developmental sequences typical of Korean learners of English. This understanding enables more accurate diagnosis and more effective intervention strategies.

In instructional settings, practitioners should focus particularly on areas where Korean and English differ significantly. While explicit instruction in problematic features remains important, such instruction should be integrated into meaningful communication activities rather than treated in isolation. Practitioners should also recognize that some features may require extended periods of exposure and practice before improvement becomes evident, necessitating both patience and systematic long-term instructional planning.

Implications for Researchers

The systematic patterns observed in L1 Korean-L2 English learners' language use provide valuable insights for theoretical and applied research in second language acquisition. These patterns offer compelling evidence for cross-linguistic influence theories and demonstrate the significant role of L1 typology in L2 acquisition. The consistent occurrence of certain features across learners, combined with individual variation in others, suggests a complex interplay between universal acquisition patterns and language-specific influences. Such findings underscore the need for more sophisticated research methodologies, particularly longitudinal studies that can track developmental trajectories in the acquisition of challenging features such as articles and phonological contrasts. Furthermore, the complex interaction between different linguistic domains such as phonological, morphological, syntactic and pragmatic suggests the need for integrated research approaches. Future investigations should particularly examine how individual differences and various external factors influence the degree and persistence of L1 transfer. Such research could significantly enhance our understanding of both general second language acquisition processes and the specific challenges faced by L1 Korean-L2 English learners.

Conclusion

This chapter introduced common sources of non-target-like forms that L1 Korean-L2 English learners make due to the influence of their native language. It has mainly focused on phonetic and grammatical aspects to illustrate the basic and most prominent characteristics of the interlanguage of L1 Korean-L2 English learners, which can impede effective communication. However, there are many more sources of L1-transfer from Korean to English that could not be introduced in this chapter, such as lexical and semantic discrepancies, pragmatic differences that can lead to errors at the discourse level, as well as sociocultural factors, including cultural differences. Such discrepancies between Korean and English can result in miscommunication. For instance, the English word *wear* translates into more than 10 different words in Korean, depending on where it is worn or what is being worn. This difference in semantic concepts between Korean and English can make it difficult for L1 Korean-L2 English learners to choose the appropriate word when speaking English. Additionally, in Korean, it is common to use indirect language when refusing an invitation or offer to avoid confrontation or embarrassment. For example, L1 Korean-L2 English learners might say *Maybe I can come*, instead of directly saying *No, I can't come*, resulting in English refusals that are too vague or indirect, leading to confusion.

When discussing these characteristics, it's crucial to clearly differentiate them from pathological symptoms by properly identifying the sources of errors. As mentioned earlier, in the field of SLA, it is well-known that L1-transfer plays an important role in forming L2 learners' interlanguage, and in many cases, they are persistent, forming a language group that shows similar patterned non-target-like forms. For example, pronunciation errors should be understood as resulting from phonological system differences rather than being misinterpreted as language disorders. This approach helps language practitioners better understand the typical characteristics of Korean native speakers learning English.

However, as mentioned earlier, we should avoid overgeneralizing these characteristics since individual learners' L2 performance is also influenced by factors such as proficiency level, language background and individual differences. While L1-transfer is known to play an important role in second language acquisition, and many immigrants are affected by fossilization, recent studies (e.g. Tanner, 2013; Tanner & Van Hell, 2014) are increasingly finding that factors other than L1-transfer, such as individual differences, also play a significant role.

Notes

(1) It is still controversial since there is a 10-vowel view as well. It includes the front high rounded vowel [y] and the front mid rounded vowel [ø]. (See Lee *et al.*, 2015 for more information.)

(2) Definiteness can be defined in two different ways: 'anaphoric definites' and 'bridging definites'. With anaphoric definites, the uniqueness in the discourse is established by prior mention, while with bridging definites, uniqueness in the discourse is established by relationship to another entity in the context. (See Ionin *et al.*, 2022 for more information.)

(3) Specificity is about whether the speaker has a particular referent in mind, while definiteness is about whether the referent is known to the listener, and uniqueness is about whether there is only one possible referent in the given context. (For more information, see Ionin *et al.*, 2004, 2012; Ko *et al.*, 2010)

(4) The universal concept of boundedness refers to whether or not the property holds for all subparts (e.g. *table* has a boundary while *water* does not have a boundary). While the extension of a count noun such as *table* has minimal parts (atomic/individual tables), the extension of a mass noun such as *water* does not. That is, there is no set of atoms representing the smallest entities which have the property of being water. (For more information, see Bale & Barner, 2009; Bunt, 1985; Chierchia, 1998a, 1998b, 2010; Landman, 1989a, 1989b.)

References

Abbott, B. (2003) Definiteness and indefiniteness. In L.R. Horn and G. Ward (eds) *The Handbook of Pragmatics* (pp. 122–149). Blackwell.

Bale, A. and Barner, D. (2009) The interpretation of functional heads: Using comparatives to explore the mass/count distinction. *Journal of Semantics* 26, 217–252.

Bunt, H. (1985) *Mass Terms and Model Theoretic Semantics*. Cambridge University Press.

Chierchia, G. (1998a) Plurality of mass nouns and the notion of "semantic parameter." In S. Rothstein (ed.) *Events and Grammar* (pp. 53–103). Kluwer.

Chierchia, G. (1998b) Reference to kinds across languages. *Natural Language Semantics* 6, 339–405.

Chierchia, G. (2010) Mass nouns, vagueness and semantic variation. *Synthese* 174, 99–149.

Cho, Y.Y., Lee, H.S., Schulz, C., Sohn, H. and Sohn, S.O. (2019) *Integrated Korean: Beginning 1* (3rd edn). University of Hawai'i Press.

Choi, S.H. and Ionin, T. (2021) Plural marking in the second language: Atomicity, definiteness, and transfer. *Applied Psycholinguistics* 42 (3), 549–578.

Choi, S.H., Ionin, T. and Zhu, Y. (2018) L1 Korean and L1 Mandarin L2 English learners' acquisition of the count/mass distinction in English. *Second Language Research* 34 (2), 147–177.

Flege, J.E. (1995) Second language speech learning: Theory, findings, and problems. In W. Strange (ed.) *Speech Perception and Linguistic Experience: Issues in Cross-Language Research* (pp. 233–277). York Press.

Gass, S.M. and Selinker, L. (2008) *Second Language Acquisition: An Introductory Course* (3rd edn). Routledge.

Ha, S., Johnson, C.J. and Kuehn, D.P. (2009) Characteristics of Korean phonology: Review, tutorial, and case studies of Korean children speaking English. *Journal of Communication Disorders* 42 (3), 163–179.

Han, Z.-H. (2004) *Fossilization in Adult Second Language Acquisition*. Multilingual Matters.

Henton, C.G. (1987) The IPA consonant chart: Mugwumps, holes and therapeutic suggestions. *Journal of the International Phonetic Association* 17 (1), 15–25.

Ionin, T., Ko, H. and Wexler, K. (2004) Article semantics in L2 acquisition: The role of specificity. *Language Acquisition* 12 (1), 3–69.

Ionin, T., Choi, S.H. and Liu, Q. (2022) What transfers (or doesn't) in the second language acquisition of English articles by learners from article-less native languages? *Linguistic Approaches to Bilingualism* 12 (2), 133–162.

Ionin, T., Baek, S., Kim, E., Ko, H. and Wexler, K. (2012) That's not so different from the: Definite and demonstrative descriptions in second language acquisition. *Second Language Research* 28 (1), 69–101.

Jun, S.-A. (2005) Korean intonational phonology and prosodic transcription. In S.-A. Jun (ed.) *Prosodic Typology: The Phonology of Intonation and Phrasing* (pp. 201–229). Oxford University Press.

Kim, H. and Tremblay, A. (2021) Korean listeners' processing of suprasegmental lexical contrasts in Korean and English: A cue-based transfer approach. *Journal of Phonetics* 87, 101059.

Kim, K. and Kim, H. (2013) L1 Korean transfer in processing L2 English passive sentences. In E. Voss, S.-J.D. Tai and Z. Li (eds) *Selected Proceedings of the 2011 Second Language Research Forum: Converging Theory and Practice* (pp. 118–128). Cascadilla Proceedings Project.

Kim, M.-R. and Duanmu, S. (2004) "Tense" and "lax" stops in Korean. *Journal of East Asian Linguistics* 13 (1), 59–104.

Ko, H., Ionin, T. and Wexler, K. (2010) The role of presuppositionality in the second language acquisition of English articles. *Linguistic Inquiry* 41 (2), 213–254.

Landman, F. (1989a) Groups, i. *Linguistics and Philosophy* 12, 559–605.

Landman, F. (1989b) Groups, ii. *Linguistics and Philosophy* 12, 723–744.

Lee, E., Madigan, S. and Park, M.J. (2015) *An Introduction to Korean Linguistics*. Routledge.

Lee, S. and Cho, M.H. (2018) Predicting L2 vowel identification accuracy from cross-language mappings between L2 English and L1 Korean. *Language Sciences* 66, 183–198.

Lightbown, P.M. and Spada, N. (2013) *How Languages are Learned* (4th edn). Oxford University Press.

Long, M.H. (2003) Stabilization and fossilization in interlanguage development. In C.J. Doughty and M.H. Long (eds) *The Handbook of Second Language Acquisition* (pp. 487–535). Blackwell.

Odlin, T. (1989) *Language Transfer: Cross-Linguistic Influence in Language Learning*. Cambridge University Press.

Ortega, L. (2014) *Understanding Second Language Acquisition*. Routledge.

Schachter, J. (1974) An error in error analysis. *Language Learning* 24 (2), 205–214.

Schwartz, B.D. and Sprouse, R. (1996) L2 cognitive states and the Full Transfer/Full Access model. *Second Language Research* 12 (1), 40–72.

Selinker, L. (1972) Interlanguage. *International Review of Applied Linguistics in Language Teaching* 10, 209–231.

Seo, M. (2021) Korean learners' production of English consonant clusters with an onset liquid. *Journal of Pan-Pacific Association of Applied Linguistics* 25 (2), 1–19.

Sohn, H.-M. (1999) *The Korean Language*. Cambridge University Press.

Statistics Canada (2022) *Knowledge of languages by age and gender: Canada, provinces and territories, census divisions and census subdivisions* (Table 98-10-0216-01). https://doi.org/10.25318/9810021601-eng

Tanner, D. (2013) Individual differences and streams of processing. *Linguistic Approaches to Bilingualism* 3 (3), 350–356.

Tanner, D. and Van Hell, J.G. (2014) ERPs reveal individual differences in morphosyntactic processing. *Neuropsychologia* 56, 289–301.

U.S. Department of State, Foreign Service Institute. (n.d.) *Languages*. https://2009-2017.state.gov/m/fsi/sls/orgoverview/languages.htm

19 Speech and Language of Vietnamese-English-Speaking Children and Their Families

Kate Margetson, Van H. Tran, Helen L. Blake, Sarah Verdon, Ben Phạm and Sharynne McLeod

Introduction

Context and culture

Vietnamese people live in the Southeast Asian country of Vietnam (Việt Nam) and have a long history of learning and culture. For example, Vietnam's first national university is over 1,000 years old and was located in the Temple of Literature (Văn Miếu) from 1076 to 1779. The first wave of Vietnamese immigrants to America began in 1975, following the end of the Vietnam-American War and the withdrawal of American forces. This wave brought approximately 130,000 refugees, the majority of whom settled in Orange County, California. Prior to this, about 15,000 Vietnamese people migrated to the United States between 1960 and 1975, largely as a result of immigration laws and American involvement in Vietnam (Ciment, 2010). The second wave of immigration occurred in the early to mid-1980s, following Vietnam's border war with China. This influx increased the Vietnamese population in the United States to over 245,000, with many residing in Southern California and coastal Texas. The third wave took place in the 1990s, under the family reunification policy, bringing the Vietnamese population in the country to 1,110,207 by 2000. Since the first wave, Vietnamese communities have spread across several states, including Louisiana, Pennsylvania, Massachusetts, Minnesota, Illinois and Washington (Ciment, 2010). As of the most recent data, there are approximately 2 million people with Vietnamese heritage living throughout America; among those, 1.3 million people are immigrants (Batalova, 2023; US Census Bureau, 2022). In Canada, similar waves of immigration were observed, though in smaller numbers. Between 1975 and 1978, 7,700 Vietnamese immigrants arrived in Canada (Hou, 2020). This number rose to 150,000 in 2000 and nearly 300,000 people in 2023 (Statistics Canada, 2001, 2024).

The use of English and Vietnamese among Vietnamese immigrants in North America or in other English-speaking countries varies depending on their wave and generation of immigration. First wave and first-generation immigrants primarily use Vietnamese at home and in community settings, while the use of Vietnamese decreased in later waves and generations (Tran, 2021; Tran *et al.*, 2024). Since almost a quarter of the first-wave Vietnamese immigrants to North America could not speak English, the use of Vietnamese was popular at home and within the community, contributing to home language maintenance among the second generation (Christian, 1983; Hou, 2020). The maintenance of Vietnamese and bilingualism among the Vietnamese diaspora was affected by the community's attitudes towards preserving Vietnamese culture while living in another country (Tran, Verdon & McLeod, 2022). First wave and first-generation immigrants are generally more successful in maintaining home language thanks to a strong connection with Vietnamese culture that emphasizes family relationships, which results in children living with grandparents, which in turn provides more opportunities for more home language use (Christian, 1983; Tran, Verdon & McLeod, 2022).

These variations in language use across different waves of immigration led to differences in language use and proficiency among the second generation of Vietnamese immigrants. Children of first-wave immigrants maintained their Vietnamese language skills better than those of second- and third-wave immigrants, as their parents consistently spoke Vietnamese at home. The former therefore have more balanced bilingualism and a stronger bilingual identity (Tran, 2021). This is consistent with studies of children's home language maintenance and loss across the world (e.g. Verdon *et al.*, 2014).

Grammar of the Language

The Vietnamese and English languages vary, specifically in relation to phonology, morphology, syntax and prosody. Therefore, bilingual speakers have many non-shared features to acquire in each language (Phạm & Kohnert, 2014). For example, English contains many multisyllabic words, while Vietnamese largely consists of words with only one syllable. Vietnamese may be considered a monosyllabic language as each syllable is written and spoken separately; however, some words contain two or more separate syllables e.g. mũ bảo hiểm /mu^3 bɯw^4 hiem^4/ 'helmet' (Phạm *et al.*, in press). In English, grammatical features such as tense are typically marked using inflectional suffixes, while in Vietnamese, these features are marked using additional words rather than bound morphemes (Tang, 2007). For example, in English an animal is named with one word (e.g. *elephant*), whereas in Vietnamese the morpheme for animal precedes the name of the animal (e.g. *con voi* 'elephant'). Further, English is a stress-timed language, while Vietnamese is syllable-timed and uses tones to indicate meaning (Blake, 2020). The aetiologies of these languages do not overlap; therefore, the languages do not share cognates of similar form and meaning, apart from borrowed words that have been acquired more recently, such as *email* and *iPhone*. Pragmatically, English is a low-context language, where speaking directly is considered socially appropriate; whereas Vietnamese is a high-context language that relies on non-verbal features and implicit understandings of social hierarchies to convey much of its meaning (Comrie, 2011; McKinney, 2000). The differing features between English and Vietnamese may result in cross-linguistic transfer among Vietnamese and English where the phonology, morphology, syntax or pragmatics of one language is present in the other.

Developmental progression

Bilingual Vietnamese-English-speaking children's speech and language development has recently been explored through VietSpeech, a large-scale study of Vietnamese-English-speaking children aged 2;0–8;10 years old (n = 69) and adults (n = 85) in Australia (McLeod *et al.*, 2023). In the VietSpeech study, both children's speech acquisition and adults' pronunciation were influenced by cross-linguistic factors (McLeod *et al.*, 2023). Children's speech acquisition was influenced by additional factors including maturity, environment (ambient phonology) and language experience. Children's percentage of consonants correct – standard (PCC-S) was high for English (M = 82.51%) and Vietnamese (M = 70.34%). However, PCC varied according to children's language proficiency and was significantly higher when Vietnamese dialectal variants were included as correct (percentage of consonants correct – dialect, PCC-D: M = 87.76%). Vowels (in English and Vietnamese) and tones (in Vietnamese) were acquired earlier than consonants. In Vietnamese, children's plosives /b, t̪ʰ, d, c/, nasals /m, n, ɲ/, fricatives /f, s, h/, lateral approximant /l/ and semivowels /w, j/ were more accurate (>80% accurate); and voiceless plosives /p, t, k, t̪/, nasal /ŋ/ and fricatives /v, z, ʂ, ʐ, x, ɣ/ were less accurate (<80% accurate). In English, children's plosives /b, k, d, ɡ, p, t/, nasals /m, n, ŋ/, fricatives /h, f, ʃ, v/, affricate /ʧ/ and glides /w, j/ and liquid /l/ were more accurate (>80% accurate); and fricatives /s, z, ʒ, θ, ð/, affricate /ʤ/ and approximant /ɹ/ were less accurate (<80% accurate). The following phonological patterns were evident:

- *Phonological patterns in both Vietnamese and English*: velar and palatal fronting; stopping of fricatives.
- *Vietnamese-only phonological patterns*: gliding of fricatives and nasals, denasalization, nasalization, aspiration, deaspiration, glottal replacement, initial consonant deletion, final consonant deletion and semivowel deletion.

- *English-only phonological patterns*: stopping of affricates, deaffrication, gliding of liquids, prevocalic voicing, postvocalic devoicing, fricative simplification, liquid simplification, backing, consonant cluster simplification, cluster reduction and epenthesis.

Cross-linguistic transfer of phonological patterns has been found to occur in Vietnamese-English-speaking children's speech, e.g. gliding of fricatives in English (Margetson *et al.*, 2023). Compared with other family members, VietSpeech children's speech most often matched their mother's speech (McLeod *et al.*, 2023).

Children in the VietSpeech research also completed language screening tests in English and Vietnamese, and these language samples demonstrate the way that cross-linguistic transfer can present in typically developing bilingual Vietnamese-English speakers (Faulks, 2023). For example:

'he caught the two mouses' (C004, aged 6;11)

In Vietnamese, plurals are typically marked by using a quantifying word before the noun e.g. *nhiều* 'many' or *mấy* 'several,' whereas in English plurals are marked either by adding a plural -s or using the more complex irregular verb form, such as in the case of the word *mice*. In this example, the child has marked the plural in both the English and Vietnamese style, using the quantifying word *two* but has also pluralized the word mouse. In this example, the child has overgeneralized the use of plural -s instead of using the irregular verb form, which may be an indication of their young age and a typical developmental trajectory in English.

'she hurt his eye with the dog' (C007, aged 4;8)

This example demonstrates cross-linguistic influence in relation to pronouns. The child is attempting to use pronouns in English but uses pronouns of different genders to refer to the same person, indicating some confusion. This is likely because in Vietnamese, gender is not marked directly within pronouns, but instead, is indicated by using specific terms like *anh* 'he,' *chị* 'she,' which are considered classifiers and are used alongside a gender-neutral pronoun like *ấy;* for example, *anh* ấy means 'he' and *chị ấy* means 'she' (Faulks, 2023).

Language development of bilingual Vietnamese-English-speaking children and monolingual Vietnamese-speaking children has also been studied in the United States and Vietnam (Phạm, 2024). This research included exploration of bilingual Vietnamese-English-speaking children's grammatical development (Dam *et al.*, 2020); monolingual Vietnamese-speaking children's vocabulary, phonological awareness and reading development (Phạm & Snow, 2020); features and identification of developmental language disorder (DLD) in monolingual Vietnamese-speaking children (Phạm *et al.*, 2019, 2023); and vocabulary intervention for bilingual Vietnamese-English-speaking children (Phạm *et al.*, 2018).

As the speech-language pathology profession in Vietnam continues to grow, tools such as the Vietnamese Language Assessment (VLA; Ivey *et al.*, 2019) have been developed to measure typical language development and identify the presence of DLD in Vietnamese-speaking children. The VLA is similar to the Renfrew Action Picture Test in that it shows children a series of pictures designed to elicit a range of vocabulary and grammar items in order to assess their language skills. Additionally, the VLA also considers receptive language by investigating children's comprehension skills (Verdon *et al.*, 2025).

Adult forms

English language ability is a major factor impacting the communication of Vietnamese Americans, along with occupation and external factors such as government policy and societal receptivity (Kula *et al.*, 2021). Factors that may influence the English proficiency of Vietnamese-English-speaking adults include age of English acquisition, formal instruction, amount of English versus Vietnamese language use, language learning aptitude, quantity and quality of interactions with native English speakers, as well as cross-linguistic factors (Blake & McLeod, 2019b).

Vietnamese American adults' language proficiency may influence their English speech accuracy. In the VietSpeech study, adults' overall English PCC-S was high (M = 85.73%), but consonant accuracy differed according to their language proficiency. Adults who were more proficient in English than Vietnamese had the highest English PCC-S (M = 95.71%), compared with those with similar proficiency in both languages (M = 90.68%) or those who were more proficient in Vietnamese (M = 77.90%). Adults most accurately produced the English consonants that are shared between Vietnamese and English /m, n, f, h, l, j, w/ (over 90% accuracy). The next most accurate consonants were /p, b, t, d, k, ŋ, s, ɹ/ (between 80–90% accuracy), followed by /v, z, ʃ, ʧ/ (between 70–80% accuracy). The least accurately produced consonants were /ɡ, θ, ð, ʒ, ʤ/ which do not occur in Vietnamese (less than 70% accuracy). Similar to the children in VietSpeech, the adults' mean Vietnamese PCC was significantly higher when dialectal variants were accepted (PCC-S M = 80.47%; PCC-D M = 98.04%) (McLeod *et al.*, 2023).

Many of the first wave of Vietnamese immigrants to the United States were from more developed cities, were educated and had some proficiency in English, while those in the second and third waves arrived with limited English language and professional skills and less education. Consequently, parents from the later waves may have difficulty supporting their children's educational and language development

(Kula *et al.*, 2021). Culturally responsive bilingual support services and English language learning can assist Vietnamese-speaking adults to bridge the gap between home and school, as well as allow them to participate in the society of their adopted country.

Speech accuracy in intergenerational families

Speech accuracy in Vietnamese-English-speaking families has been studied across generations. A study of a three-generation bilingual family in the United States revealed differences in Vietnamese and English speech production between the two grandparents (first generation), two parents (second generation) and two children aged 9 years old and 16 years old (third generation) (Hogan *et al.*, 2024). Vietnamese speech accuracy (PCC-R) was high across generations. Consistent with VietSpeech (McLeod *et al.*, 2023), Vietnamese voiced plosives were more accurate than voiceless plosives in the second and third generation (Hogan *et al.*, 2024). The difference in voicing accuracy may have been due to cross-linguistic transfer, that is, the influence of English on Vietnamese, because voiceless plosives in Vietnamese and English have different phonetic realisation (Hwa-Froelich *et al.*, 2002). English speech accuracy increased across generations, generally aligning with increased daily usage of English (PCC-R first generation = 56.47%; second generation = 68.35%; third generation = 99.64%). Voiceless English consonants were easier for the adults to produce than voiced; plosives and nasals were easier than fricatives, affricates and approximants; and glottals, labiovelars and bilabials were the easiest places of articulation. Consonant cluster accuracy also increased from first to third generations, consistent with previous literature indicating Vietnamese speakers who are acquiring English may have difficulty producing consonant clusters (Hwa-Froelich *et al.*, 2002; Osburne, 1996; Sato, 1984; Tang, 2007). Word-final English consonants were most difficult for the first and second generations to produce, aligning with a study that found adult Vietnamese-English speakers may omit word-final English consonants (Benson, 1988). Some of the mothers' Vietnamese speech productions matched the children's productions, consistent with VietSpeech findings that mothers' speech may influence children's speech (Hogan *et al.*, 2024; McLeod *et al.*, 2023).

A similar three-generation study was conducted in Australia with a bilingual Vietnamese-English-speaking family (McLeod *et al.*, 2022a). The authors suggest that some of the children's speech productions that did not match the target words could be attributed to typical influences on multilingual speech, rather than speech sound disorder. Differences in children's productions could be attributed to development (i.e. phonological processes), cross-linguistic transfer (e.g. using an English consonant while speaking Vietnamese) or dialect (e.g. a consonant from one Vietnamese dialect is used while speaking another dialect) (McLeod *et al.*, 2022a). Further case studies with Vietnamese-English-speaking children (see Margetson *et al.*, 2023, 2024) also highlight the implications of similar speech differences in the differential diagnosis of speech sound disorders in multilingual children.

Clinical Implications for Researchers

Since Vietnamese is in the top 20 languages spoken in the world (Eberhard *et al.*, 2024), there are many Vietnamese speech and language resources for researchers. There is literature written in English; however, there is also extensive literature published in Vietnamese (e.g. Vietnamese linguistics journals published in Vietnam), French, Russian and other languages (Phạm & McLeod, 2016). For example, publications in Vietnamese provide details of Vietnamese phonology, language and dialects (Hữu & Vương, 1980; Huỳnh, 1996; Phạm, 1988), report on studies of children with speech sound disorders (Hoang *et al.*, 2019; Nguyen & Phạm, 2014) and identify assessments available for Vietnamese-speaking children (Ngo, 2019; Trần *et al.*, n.d.).

The VietSLP team at San Diego State University has undertaken the most comprehensive research regarding bilingual Vietnamese-English-speaking children's *language* (https://vietslp.sdsu.edu/) and the VietSpeech team at Charles Sturt University in Australia has undertaken the most comprehensive research regarding bilingual Vietnamese-English-speaking children's *speech* (https://www.csu.edu.au/research/vietspeech/info). Additionally, the Multilingual Children's Speech website contains information about children's speech acquisition, assessments and interventions in over 100 languages, including Vietnamese (https://www.csu.edu.au/research/multilingual-speech/home).

Researchers working with bilingual Vietnamese-English-speaking children, adults and professionals need to be mindful of their own cultural responsiveness (Verdon, 2025). Reflecting on who you are as a person, professional and researcher in this context (as in any other context) is an important first step. Next, learning about the history of Vietnam, Vietnamese culture, traditions, food and migration patterns provides foundational knowledge. The first wave of migration to many English-speaking countries came from Saigon in Southern Vietnam during the Vietnam-American War in the 1970s. Most of these migrants spoke the Southern Vietnamese dialect (which has different consonants, vowels and tones from Standard and Northern Vietnamese) (Pham & McLeod, 2016). Many fled with limited resources. At the end of the war, Saigon was renamed Ho Chi Minh City, and some of the first wave of migrants associate the current Vietnamese flag with the war. The second wave of migrants to many English-speaking countries is often called economic migrants, who migrated for work or education. These migrants often came from Northern Vietnam and required financial resources to facilitate migration. Researchers who fail to consider the migration backgrounds of Vietnamese people may impact relationships, trust and data interpretation. In order to undertake culturally responsive research, it is essential to include Vietnamese people within the research team, either as paid team members or consultants. For example, the VietSpeech research team includes bilingual Vietnamese-English speaking team members, including those living in Vietnam and Australia and those with Northern and Southern Vietnamese heritage (McLeod *et al.*, 2023).

Clinical Implications for Practitioners

Implications when working with children

Speech-language pathologists (SLPs) can assess bilingual Vietnamese-English-speaking children's language through collecting and analyzing language samples in both languages, with the support of an interpreter, if needed (Dam *et al.*, 2020). Due to differences in features such as consonants, vowels, semivowels, tones and vocabulary across Vietnamese dialects, some Vietnamese authors suggest dialect should also be considered in speech and language assessments (Nguyễn, 2011; The Vietnamese Ministry of Education and Training, 2006). This could include case history information about the dialect spoken at home (including prestige and perceptions of dialect), as well as the use of dialect appropriate assessment tools (Phạm & McLeod, 2016). When diagnosing developmental language disorder, it is important to consider linguistic strengths and areas of difficulty that are common to both languages and language-specific, in the context of the differences between Vietnamese and English grammar and morphology, and the individual child's language proficiency. SLPs who work with bilingual Vietnamese-English-speaking children can expect to see high levels of speech accuracy in both languages (McLeod *et al.*, 2023). However, individual children's language proficiency must always be considered when analyzing bilingual children's speech as proficiency can impact accuracy. If children's speech productions do not match adult targets, then potential reasons for mismatches other than speech sound disorder can be considered. For example, cross-linguistic transfer, dialect or the influence of adult family members' speech productions (McLeod *et al.*, 2022a). For a diagnosis of speech sound disorder, evidence of the disorder should be present in both Vietnamese and English (Margetson *et al.*, 2024; Pert, 2023). Learning modules and resources for working with bilingual Vietnamese-English-speaking children are available through VietSLP https://vietslp.sdsu.edu/ and VietSpeech https://www.csu.edu.au/research/vietspeech/info.

Additionally, power differential plays an important role in communication, as Vietnamese speakers are culturally less likely to challenge or disagree with those in a position of higher authority. This has important implications for adult-child relationships in education and intervention settings where children may experience conflict between the social expectations of their home language and the dominant English language (McKinney, 2000).

It also has implications for assessment, where children may be unwilling to 'guess' or attempt an answer during assessment if they are not sure that they know the answer or understand what is expected of them.

Implications when working with adults

Given the differences between Vietnamese and English phonology noted above, bilingual Vietnamese-English–speaking adults may seek support from SLPs, voice coaches or language teachers if they believe their intelligibility in English is negatively impacting their participation in major life areas (Blake & McLeod, 2019a). Spoken English proficiency has been proven to impact bilingual speakers' ability to participate in education, employment and community life in English-dominant countries (Blake *et al.*, 2017, 2018; Chin *et al.*, 2006). SLPs intending to provide these services are encouraged to incorporate a holistic approach by following protocols such as those recommended within the Intelligibility Enhancement Assessment and Intervention Protocols (Blake, 2019a, 2019b). Blake *et al.* (2020) have described implementing these protocols with Giang (pseudonym), a 37-year-old bilingual Vietnamese-English–speaking female undertaking a PhD in Management.

Before undertaking any clinical assessment, the individual's home language should be investigated in order to formulate predictions about the speakers' potential difficulties in English. For example, as stated above, a bilingual Vietnamese-English speaker may have difficulty with features of English such as consonants that do not occur in Vietnamese (/ɡ, θ, ð, ʒ, ʤ/), final consonants, consonant clusters, polysyllabic words and stress in English. At initial assessment, Giang's English speech contained systematic variations in pronunciation consistent with these expectations. She substituted and deleted English sounds not in Vietnamese (e.g. *threw* /θɹu/ was produced as [tɹu] and *catch* /kæʧ/ as [kæt]), deleted final consonants (e.g. *nine* /naɪn/ was produced as [naɪ]), reduced consonant clusters in all word positions (e.g. *price* /pɹaɪs/ was produced as [ɹaɪs]) and had difficulty with stress in polysyllable words (e.g. *'delicate* as *deli'cate*). A holistic and structured assessment should contain typical elements of a speech-language pathology assessment (e.g. case history that includes any difficulties acquiring home language, single word and connected speech sample) as well as an investigation of the individual's perceptions of their own oral communication skills in English in order to provide insight into the impact of intelligibility on their functioning and participation. Giang reported that although she had been studying English since she was 12 years old, her pronunciation did not meet her own professional expectations as an academic and researcher and impacted her confidence communicating and presenting her research.

Post intervention, Giang's percentage of consonants correct increased from 62.5% to 85.0%, her word stress accuracy increased and she perceived she had less difficulty communicating in English. Giang reported that before intervention she was unaware that substituting or deleting one English sound could make a different word: 'I think ...people can understand for example, ... [if] I say "play," it means "place".' Intervention should provide multilingual speakers with awareness of those features of their English speech most influencing their intelligibility, include perception and production training, and incorporate specific training in conversation breakdown and repair strategies that can promote confidence communicating, as well as make it easier for conversation partners to understand what is being said. SLPs can also facilitate conversation opportunities and, where possible, provide conversation partner training in accent listening and interactional competence.

Conclusion

Vietnamese is in the top 20 languages of the world, and there has been extensive migration of Vietnamese people across the world, including to North America. There have been a number of research programs focused on bilingual Vietnamese-English-speaking children's speech and language that have outlined evidence-based practices for working with this population and their families.

References

Batalova, J. (2023) *Vietnamese Immigrants in the United States*. Migration Policy Institute. See https://www.migrationpolicy.org/article/vietnamese-immigrants-united-states#:~:text=More%20than%201.3%20million%20Vietnamese,all%2046.2%20million%20U.S.%20immigrants

Benson, B. (1988) Universal preference for the open syllable as an independent process in interlanguage phonology. *Language Learning* 38 (2), 221–235. https://doi.org/10.1111/j.1467-1770.1988.tb00410.x

Blake, H.L. (2019a) *Intelligibility Enhancement: Assessment Protocol*. Author.

Blake, H.L. (2019b) *Intelligibility Enhancement: Intervention Protocol*. Author.

Blake, H.L. (2020) *Vietnamese Language Summary*. Author.

Blake, H.L. and McLeod, S. (2019a) Intelligibility enhancement. In J.S. Damico and M.J. Ball (eds) *The SAGE Encyclopedia of Human Communication Sciences and Disorders* (pp. 926–928). SAGE Publications.

Blake, H.L. and McLeod, S. (2019b) Speech-language pathologists' support for multilingual speakers' English intelligibility and participation informed by the ICF. *Journal of Communication Disorders* 77, 56–70. https://doi.org/10.1016/j.jcomdis.2018.12.003

Blake, H.L., McLeod, S., Verdon, S., and Fuller, G. (2018) The relationship between spoken English proficiency and participation in higher education, employment and income from two Australian censuses. *International Journal of Speech-Language Pathology* 20 (2), 202–215. https://doi.org/10.1080/17549507.2016.1229031

Blake, H.L., Bennetts Kneebone, L. and McLeod, S. (2019) The impact of oral English proficiency on humanitarian migrants' experiences of settling in Australia. *International Journal of Bilingual Education and Bilingualism* 22 (6), 689–705. https://doi.org/10.1080/13670050.2017.1294557

Blake, H.L., McLeod, S. and Verdon, S. (2020) Intelligibility enhancement assessment and intervention: A single-case experimental design with two multilingual university students. *Clinical Linguistics and Phonetics* 34 (1–2), 1–20. https://doi.org/10.1080/02699206.2019.1608470

Chin, J.J., Kang, E., Kim, J.H., Martinez, J. and Eckholdt, H. (2006) Serving Asians and Pacific Islanders with HIV/AIDS: Challenges and lessons learned. *Journal of Health Care for the Poor and Underserved* 17 (4), 910–927. https://doi.org/10.1353/hpu.2006.0119

Christian, D. (1983) Adolescent and young adult English of Vietnamese refugees. Center for Applied Linguistics, Washington, D.C. https://files.eric.ed.gov/fulltext/ED248715.pdf

Ciment, J. (2010) The Vietnamese American experience: History and culture. In H. Ling and A.W. Austin (eds) *Asian American History and Culture: An Encyclopedia*. Taylor & Francis Group. See https://www.taylorfrancis.com/chapters/edit/10.4324/9781315706306-411/vietnamese-american-experience-history-culture-james-ciment

Comrie, B. (2011) *The World's Major Languages* (2nd edn). Routledge.

Dam, Q., Phạm, G., Potapova, I. and Pruitt-Lord, S. (2020) Grammatical characteristics of Vietnamese and English in developing bilingual children. *American Journal of Speech-Language Pathology* 29 (3), 1212–1225. https://doi.org/10.1044/2019_AJSLP-19-00146

Eberhard, D.M., Simons, G.F. and Fennig, C.D. (2024) *Ethnologue: Languages of the World* (27th edn). SIL International. See http://www.ethnologue.com

Faulks, S. (2023) Multilingual language assessment for Vietnamese-Australian children. Unpublished honours thesis, Charles Sturt University, Australia.

Hoang, Q.V., Tra, T.T., Nguyen, H.T.T., Tran, D.T.M. and Cao, A.P. (2019) Speech characteristics of children with speech sound disorders visiting Pediatrics Hospital No. 1 and Phạm Ngoc Thach University Clinic from January to June 2018 [Đặc điểm âm lời nói của trẻ bị rối loạn âm lời nói đến khám tại bệnh viện nhi đồng 1 và trường Đại học Y khoa Phạm Ngọc Thạch từ tháng 1 đến tháng 6 năm 2018]. *Medicine Journal in Ho Chi Minh City* [*Tạp chí Y Học Thành phố Hồ Chí Minh*] 23 (4), 199–202.

Hogan, A.J., Gibson, T.A. and Luong, V. (2024) Speech production in Vietnamese-English bilingual speakers living in a 3-generation home. *International Journal of Bilingual Education and Bilingualism* 27 (10), 1375–1389. https://doi.org/10.1080/13670050.2024.2355533

Hou, F. (2020) The resettlement of Vietnamese refugees across Canada over three decades. *Journal of Ethnic and Migration Studies* 47 (21), 4817–4834. https://doi.org/10.1080/1369183X.2020.1724412

Hữu, Q. and Vương, L. (1980) *Khái quát về lịch sử tiếng Việt và ngữ âm tiếng Việt hiện đại [Overview of Vietnamese Language History and Modern Vietnamese Phonology]*. Giáo dục.

Huỳnh, C.T. (1996) Tiếng Việt và vấn đề phân vùng phương ngữ [Vietnamese language and regions of dialects]. In Viện Ngôn ngữ học Việt Nam (ed.) *Ngữ học trẻ '96* (pp. 30–33). Hội ngôn ngữ học Việt Nam.

Hwa-Froelich, D., Hodson, B.W. and Edwards, H.T. (2002) Characteristics of Vietnamese phonology. *American Journal of Speech-Language Pathology* 11 (3), 264–273. https://doi.org/10.1044/1058-0360(2002/031)

Ivey, A., Verdon, S. and Pham, B. (2019) *The Vietnamese Language Assessment*. Trinh Foundation Australia.

Kula, S.M., Tran, V.Q., Garcia, I.E., Saito, L.E. and Paik, S.J. (2021) Vietnamese Americans: History, education, and societal context. *Journal of Southeast Asian American Education & Advancement* 16 (1), 1–25. https://doi.org/https://www.jstor.org/stable/10.2307/48684461

Margetson, K., McLeod, S. and Verdon, S. (2023) Cross-linguistic transfer and ambient phonology: Impact on diagnosis of speech sound disorders in a longitudinal bilingual case study. *Journal of Monolingual and Bilingual Speech* 4 (3), 311–339. https://doi.org/10.1558/jmbs.23672

Margetson, K., McLeod, S. and Verdon, S. (2024) Diagnosing speech sound disorder in bilingual Vietnamese-English–speaking children: Are English-only assessments sufficient? In E. Babatsouli (ed.) *Multilingual Acquisition and Learning: An Ecosystemic View to Diversity* (pp. 217–245). John Benjamins Publishing.

McKinney, B.C. (2000) Intercultural communication differences between the United States and Vietnam with implication for future relations. *Peace Research* 32 (3), 23–33.

McLeod, S., Margetson, K., Wang, C., Tran, V.H., Verdon, S., White, K. and Phạm, B. (2022a) Speech acquisition within a 3-generation Vietnamese-English family: The influence of maturation and ambient phonology. *Clinical Linguistics and Phonetics* 36 (4–5), 470–493. https://doi.org/10.1080/02699206.2020.1862915

McLeod, S., Verdon, S., Tran, V.H., Margetson, K. and Wang, C. (2022b) SuperSpeech: Multilingual speech and language maintenance intervention for Vietnamese-Australian children and families via telepractice. *Language, Speech, and Hearing Services in Schools* 53 (3), 675–697. https://doi.org/10.1044/2021_LSHSS-21-00146

McLeod, S., Verdon, S., Margetson, K., Tran, V.H., Wang, C., Phạm, B., To, L. and Huynh, K. (2023) Multilingual speech acquisition by Vietnamese-English–speaking children and adult family members. *Journal of Speech, Language, and Hearing Research* 66 (7), 2184–2229. https://doi.org/10.1044/2023_JSLHR-21-00669

Ngo, T.P.T. (2019) Tools to identify students with speech dificulties [Một số công cụ nhận diện học sinh khó khăn về nói]. *Tạp chí Khoa học Giáo dục Việt Nam* 19, 92–97. http://lib.yhn.edu.vn/bitstream/YHN/5368/1/N599.pdf

Nguyen, K.T.L. and Phạm, L.H. (2014) Common errors in 2-4-year-old children (in Ho Chi Minh City) [Lỗi phát âm âm tiết thường gặp ở trẻ 2-4 tuổi (tại thành phố Hồ Chí Minh)]. *Science Journal of Ho Chi Minh City University of Pedagogy [Tạp chí Khoa học trường Đại học Sư phạm thành phố Hồ Chí Minh]* 57 (91), 9–21.

Nguyễn, T.L.K. (2011) Nội dung đánh giá khả năng phát âm âm tiết tiếng Việt của trẻ mẫu giáo [The assessment content of pronunciation ability of Vietnamese syllable of preschoolers]. *Ngôn ngữ* 9, 6–17.

Osburne, A.G. (1996) Final cluster reduction in English L2 speech: A case study of a Vietnamese speaker. *Applied Linguistics* 17 (2), 164–181. https://doi.org/10.1093/applin/17.2.164

Pert, S. (2023) *Working with Children Experiencing Speech and Language Disorders in a Bilingual Context: A Home Language Approach*. Routledge. https://doi.org/10.4324/9781003125563

Phạm, B., Margetson, K., McLeod, S., Verdon, S. and Tran, V.H. (2026, in press) Vietnamese speech development. In S. McLeod (ed.) *The Oxford Handbook of Speech Development in Languages of the World*. Oxford University Press.

Phạm, B. and McLeod, S. (2016) Consonants, vowels and tones across Vietnamese dialects. *International Journal of Speech-Language Pathology* 18 (2), 122–134. https://doi.org/10.3109/17549507.2015.1101162

Phạm, B. and McLeod, S. (2019) Vietnamese-speaking children's acquisition of consonants, semivowels, vowels, and tones in Northern Viet Nam. *Journal of Speech, Language, and Hearing Research* 62 (8), 2645–2670. https://doi.org/10.1044/2019_JSLHR-S-17-0405

Phạm, B., and McLeod, S. and Le, X.T.T. (2016) Development of the Vietnamese speech assessment. *Journal of Clinical Practice in Speech-Language Pathology* 18 (3), 126–130.

Phạm, B., McLeod, S. and Harrison, L.J. (2017) Validation and norming of the Intelligibility in Context Scale in Northern Viet Nam. *Clinical Linguistics & Phonetics* 31 (7–9), 665–681. https://doi.org/10.1080/02699206.2017.1306110

Phạm, G., Donovan, D., Dam, Q. and Contant, A. (2018) Learning words and definitions in two languages: What promotes cross-language transfer? *Language Learning* 68, 206–233. https://doi.org/10.1111/lang.12274

Pham, G. and Kohnert, K. (2014) A longitudinal study of lexical development in children learning Vietnamese and English. *Child Development* 85 (2), 767–782. https://doi.org/10.1111/cdev.12137

Phạm, G., Simpson, A. and Nguyen, K. (2023) Vietnamese children with and without DLD: Classifier use and grammaticality over time. *Journal of Communication Disorders* 101, 106297. https://doi.org/10.1016/j.jcomdis.2022.106297

Phạm, G. and Snow, C.E. (2020) Beginning to read in Vietnamese: Kindergarten precursors to first grade fluency and reading comprehension. *Reading and Writing: An Interdisciplinary Journal*. https://doi.org/10.1007/s11145-020-10066-w

Phạm, G.T. (2023) A narrative approach to synthesizing research on Vietnamese bilingual and monolingual children. *Journal of Speech, Language, and Hearing Research* 66 (12), 4756–4770. https://doi.org/10.1044/2023_JSLHR-23-00047

Phạm, G.T. (2024) A narrative approach to synthesizing research on Vietnamese bilingual and monolingual children. *Journal of Speech, Language, and Hearing Research.* https://doi.org/10.1044/2023_JSLHR-23-00047

Phạm, G.T., Pruitt-Lord, S., Snow, C.E., Nguyen, Y.H.T., Phạm, B., Dao, T.B.T., Tran, N.B.T., Phạm, L.T., Hoang, H.T. and Dam, Q.D. (2019) Identifying developmental language disorder in Vietnamese children. *Journal of Speech, Language, and Hearing Research* 62 (5), 1452–1467. https://doi.org/10.1044/2019_JSLHR-L-18-0305

Phạm, V.H. (1988) Về đặc trưng một số đường đồng ngữ trong các phương ngữ tiếng Việt [About typical characterisitcs of the same linguistic lines in Vietnamese dialects]. In Viện ngôn ngữ học Việt Nam (ed.) *Tiếng Việt và các ngôn ngữ Đông Nam Á [Vietnamese and South East Asian languages]*. Khoa học xã hội.

Sato, C.J. (1984) Phonological processes in second language acquisition: Another look at interlanguage syllable structure. *Language Learning* 34 (4), 43–58. https://doi.org/10.1111/j.1467-1770.1984.tb00351.x

Statistics Canada (2001) *The Vietnamese Community in Canada.* See https://www150.statcan.gc.ca/n1/pub/89-621-x/89-621-x2006002-eng.htm

Statistics Canada (2024) *A Statistical Snapshot of Asians in Canada.* See https://www.statcan.gc.ca/o1/en/plus/6178-statistical-snapshot-asians-canada

Tang, G.M. (2007) Cross-linguistic analysis of Vietnamese and English with implications for Vietnamese language acquisition and maintenance in the United States. *Journal of Southeast Asian American Education & Advancement* 2 (1), 1–33. https://www.jstor.org/stable/48684597

The Vietnamese Ministry of Education and Training (2006) *Giáo dục hòa nhập trẻ khuyết tật ở tiểu học [Inclusive Education for Primary Students with Disabilities]*. Giáo dục.

Trần, D.Q., Content, A., Nguyễn, K.T.L., Nguyễn, P.T.H., Huỳnh, T.M. and Hoàng, V.T. (n.d.) *Bộ trắc nghiệm đánh giá khả năng ngôn ngữ và khả năng tính toán của trẻ từ 6 đến 9 tuổi. [Evaluation Test of Language Ability and Capacity Calculation of Child from 6 to 9 Years]*. Libre University of Brussels, Catholic University of Louvain, Ho Chi Minh City University of Education.

Tran, V.T.H. (2021) Home language maintenance among Vietnamese-Australian families. PhD thesis, Charles Sturt University.

Tran, V.H., Verdon, S. and McLeod, S. (2022) Consistent and persistent: Successful home language maintenance among Vietnamese-Australian families. *Journal of Home Language Research* 5 (1), 1–19. https://doi.org/10.16993/jhlr.43

Tran, V.H., Wang, C., McLeod, S. and Verdon, S. (2022) Vietnamese-Australian children's language proficiency and use. *International Journal of Bilingualism* 25 (6), 1735–1763. https://doi.org/10.1177/13670069211034587

Tran, V.H., McLeod, S., Verdon, S., Margetson, K. and Phạm, B. (2024) Vietnamese-Australian families: Children's language competence and home language maintenance. In L. Mahony, S. McLeod, A. Salamon and J. Dwyer (eds) *Early Childhood Voices: Children, Families, Professionals* (pp. 135–150). Springer International Publishing. https://doi.org/10.1007/978-3-031-56484-0_10

US Census Bureau (2022) American Community Survey. Access from Steven Ruggles, Katie Genadek, Ronald Goeken, Josiah Grover, and Matthew Sobek. Integrated Public Use Microdata Series: Version 7.0 [dataset]. University of Minnesota. https://usa.ipums.org/usa/

Verdon, S., McLeod, S. and Winsler, A. (2014) Language maintenance and loss in a population study of young Australian children. *Early Childhood Research Quarterly* 29, 168–181. https://doi.org/10.1016/j.ecresq.2013.12.003

Verdon, S., Phạm, B. and Ivey, A. (2025, in submission) *Conceptualisation of the Vietnamese Language Screener.*

Verdon, S. (2025) Cultural considerations regarding children's speech development. In S. McLeod (ed.) *The Oxford Handbook of Speech Development in Languages of the World.* Oxford University Press.

20 Cantonese English in North America

An L2 Perspective for Researchers and Clinicians

Carol K.S. To and Kevin K.H. So

Introduction

Context

Cantonese is spoken by about 87 million people worldwide, including significant communities in Hong Kong, Macau, Mainland China, and diaspora populations around the world (Eberhard *et al.*, 2023). Cantonese-speaking communities in North America are most prominent in cities with large immigrant populations, such as San Francisco, Vancouver, New York and Toronto. These cities boast vibrant Chinatowns *Tong Yun Gai* 'Tang people's street', where Cantonese is widely spoken.

Cantonese speakers have long been a part of North American society, contributing to the growth and development of Chinese-American and Chinese-Canadian communities. Key historical events played a role in shaping the Cantonese communities in North America. For instance, in the United States, cities such as San Francisco have deep historical connections to Cantonese-speaking immigrants dating back to the mid-19th century during the California Gold Rush and the construction of the Transcontinental Railroad, when many Chinese laborers arrived from the Guangdong province (Chan, 1991; Yu, 2013). After the period of British political control over Hong Kong (1842–1997), many Hong Kong citizens sought opportunities abroad in countries like the United States, Canada and Australia (Li, 2005). Vancouver and Toronto have become prominent destinations for migration leading to the establishment of sizable Cantonese-speaking diaspora communities abroad (Tse, 2001). With increasing migration from Mainland China, there has been a demographic shift in some regions toward Putonghua-speaking Chinese communities (Lai, 2012). Nevertheless, Cantonese still retains its importance as a community language in these established diaspora regions and continues to hold significant cultural and symbolic value within its communities (Liang & Li, 2021). However, language use within the

Cantonese-speaking population in North America is undergoing a transition. In younger generations, especially those born in North America, Cantonese is often maintained alongside English but, in some cases, a language shift occurs where English becomes dominant, and Cantonese is used less frequently, particularly in professional and educational settings (Nagy, 2018). These dynamics create a complex sociolinguistic environment where bilingualism and language maintenance become central to identity and communication (Tse & Li, 2020).

Pragmatics and cultural values

The pragmatics of communication in Cantonese-speaking communities are intensely shaped by Confucian values, which emphasize respect for hierarchy, social harmony and appropriate conduct. These cultural values significantly influence both turn-taking and conversation management, particularly in interactions that reflect hierarchical relationships, such as between parents and children. In these settings, communication is often more directive, with parents frequently using clear, authoritative instructions rather than engaging in open-ended dialogue or negotiation. This approach not only reinforces parental authority but also cultivates an expectation of compliance in children – reflecting Confucian ideals of respecting elders and maintaining social order. For example, Cantonese-speaking parents may use indisputable commands or direct requests (e.g. *Do your homework now*) to guide their children, who are supposed to follow strictly. This contrasts with English-speaking cultures, where dialogic interactions that encourage questioning and negotiation are more common, reflecting a more egalitarian approach to parent-child communication.

Cantonese speakers may use distinct syntactic structures to perform different speech acts as a result of the transfer from Cantonese and differences in pragma-linguistic competence. For example, Cantonese speakers tend to use fewer bi-clausal indirect expressions (e.g. *I am wondering if you…*) to signal politeness in making requests (Lee, 2011). In expressing disagreement, Chinese speakers in general might use stronger forms of disagreement, such as sentences containing *no*/*not* (e.g. *You can't say that*), which are relatively rare among English speakers (Zhu & Wang, 2022).

In terms of turn-taking, Cantonese speakers generally follow a hierarchical structure in formal settings, showing deference to authority figures and waiting for clear signals before taking a turn (Kádár & Pan, 2011). However, in informal settings, such as among peers or within families, overlapping speech is often seen as a sign of engagement and active participation (Tao & Tao, 2016). In English-speaking cultures, on the other hand, overlapping speech is more likely to be viewed as interruptive, especially in formal contexts (Tannen, 2005). These differences in the pragmatic use of language might lead to misinterpretation of politeness or even pragmatic failure.

Eye contact and gestures also play critical roles in signaling respect and social hierarchy. Direct and prolonged eye contact with elders or superiors may be seen as disrespectful or confrontational in Chinese culture, reflecting deference or humility (Scollon & Scollon, 2001). Gestures, too, are typically more restrained compared to the more expressive use of body language in English-speaking cultures, where eye contact and gestures are often used to indicate engagement and openness (Matsumoto & Hwang, 2013).

Understanding these differences is essential for effective cross-cultural communication, particularly in avoiding misunderstandings that may arise from applying one culture's conversational norms to another (Spencer-Oatey & Kádár, 2016). Bilingual children learning English might benefit from explicit pragmatic instruction that highlights the salience of target pragmatic behavior and promotes more efficient gains than general exposure (Rose, 2005).

Typological Linguistic Features

The linguistic features of Cantonese and English differ significantly across various domains, presenting unique challenges and considerations for Cantonese-English bilinguals. The following sections will explore the key linguistic domains – phonology, morphosyntax and vocabulary – focusing on how Cantonese influences English language learning and usage, particular transfer patterns and the potential implications for speech and language development.

Phonology

The phonological systems of Cantonese and English differ in several key ways, influencing how Cantonese-English bilinguals produce and perceive English sounds (Chan & Li, 2000).

Syllable structure and phonotactic rules

Cantonese has a relatively simple syllable structure compared to English. The typical syllable follows a (C)V(C) pattern, where consonant clusters are not allowed in either the onset or coda (Bauer & Benedict, 1997). This simplicity contrasts sharply with English, where syllables often feature complex consonant clusters at the beginning or end of words. For example, English allows for words like *strengths* (CCCVCCCC), where clusters appear in both onset and coda positions. When Cantonese speakers learn English, the lack of consonant clusters in their L1 leads to consonant cluster reduction in L2 English (Hansen Edwards, 2006). This phenomenon is especially evident in syllable codas, where final consonants may be deleted (e.g. [1]–[2]). Similarly, when a diphthong is followed by a final nasal in English, Cantonese speakers may delete the nasal consonant entirely (e.g. [3]) (Deterding *et al.*, 2008).

[1]	*friend* /fɹɛ**nd**/ → [fre**n**] or [fe**n**]	Simplifying the final consonant cluster
[2]	*lift* /lɪ**ft**/ → [lɪf]	Omitting the final /t/
[3]	*fine* /faɪ**n**/ → [faɪ]	Omitting the final /n/

For some final consonant clusters, Cantonese speakers frequently insert a vowel to break up the consonants in English words that end in clusters. This process, known as epenthesis, involves the insertion of a vowel (usually /ə/) to simplify the cluster (Setter *et al.*, 2010) (see e.g. [4]). The vowel insertion can occur either between the singleton consonants of the cluster or at the very end of the word. This transfer pattern causes English words to sound more syllabified than usual (Chan & Li, 2000).

Segmental features

One key difference between Cantonese and English sound systems is the lack of a voicing distinction in Cantonese plosives, fricatives and affricates (Bauer & Benedict, 1997). Instead, Cantonese distinguishes between unaspirated and aspirated plosives and affricates (Zee, 1999). Cantonese speakers often produce the English voiced obstruents, like /b/, /d/, /g/, as voiceless e.g. [p], [t], [k] (Chan & Li, 2000). This type of transfer error can happen in word-final, initial and medial positions (e.g. [5]–[7]) (Hung, 2000).

[4]	*film* /fɪlm/ → [fɪləm]	Inserting a vowel between the /l/ and /m/
[5]	*bag* /ˈbæg/ → [bæ**k**]	Replacing the final /g/ by an unreleased [k]
[6]	*dog* /**d**ɔg/ → [**t**ɔk]	Replacing the initial /d/ by an unreleased [t]
[7]	*rabbit* /ˈɹæ**b**ɪt/ → [ræpɪt]	Replacing the medial /b/ by an unreleased [p̚]

Another difficulty at the segmental level lies in the production of English sounds whose place of articulation does not exist in Cantonese. For example, interdentals /θ/ and /ð/ (e.g. [8]–[9]) and the post-alveolar sounds, e.g. /ʃ/, /ʒ/ ([10]). Speakers often substitute them with a similar sound from their L1 inventory (Chan & Li, 2000), such as [f] or [t] for /θ/, [d] for /ð/ and [s] for /ʃ/ (Setter *et al.*, 2010).

[8]	*think* /θɪŋk/ → [**t**ɪŋk]	Replacing /θ/ by [t]
[9]	*this* /ðɪs/ → [**t**ɪs]	Replacing /ð/ by [t]
[10]	*she* /ʃi/ → [**s**y]	Replacing /ʃ/ by [s]

Similar transfer patterns were also noted in English rimes. The English tense-lax distinction does not exist in the same way in Cantonese (Chan & Li, 2000). English tense vowels like /iː/ are longer and more peripheral, while English lax vowels like /ɪ/ are shorter and more centralized (Ladefoged & Johnson, 2014). Without a direct equivalent contrast in Cantonese, speakers may substitute the tense vowel with a lax one or vice versa, like the pair of /ɪ, i/ (e.g. [11]–[12]) (Hung, 2000). Other vowel pairs that often confuse include /ɛ, æ/ and /ʊ, uː/ (e.g. [13]–[14]) (Deterding *et al.*, 2008). Some rimes consisting of a diphthong followed by a consonant were often substituted with the closest monophthongs (e.g. [15]–[16]) (Cheung, 2007).

[11]	*milk* /mɪlk/ → [miu]	Replacing /ɪ/ by [i]
[12]	*sheep* /ʃiːp/ or *ship* /ʃɪp/ → [ʃiːp]	Merging /ɪ/ with [iː]
[13]	*bed* /bɛd/ or *bad* /bæd/ → [bed]	Merging /æ/ with [e]
[14]	*put* /pʊt/ → [puː]	Substituting /ʊ/ with [uː]
[15]	*point* /pɔɪnt/ → [pɔn]	Substituting /ɔɪ/ with [ɔ]
[16]	*name* /neɪm/ → [nem]	Substituting /eɪ/ with [e]

Suprasegmental features: Syllable-timed rhythm

A prominent feature of Cantonese English is its prosodic characteristics. Cantonese, as a tone and syllable-timed language, ensures that each syllable takes roughly the same amount of time to produce and carries a lexical tone (Setter *et al.*, 2010). In contrast, English is stress-timed, where stressed syllables occur at regular intervals and unstressed syllables are shortened, reducing the vowels (Roach, 2009). In Cantonese English, speakers often produce syllables with equal length, regardless of stress (Chan & Li, 2000). For example, a word like *banana* is typically pronounced with stress on the second syllable in English [bəˈnænə]. A Cantonese English speaker might give each syllable equal prominence, producing [bænɑːnɑː], which affects fluency and perceived naturalness in speech (Deterding *et al.*, 2008). Moreover, the syllable-timed rhythm often influences sentence-level prosody, leading to a more staccato or segmented speech pattern (Setter, 2006).

Cantonese speakers with higher English proficiency may be aware of the presence of syllable stress in multisyllabic words. However, they may stress the wrong syllable (Zhang *et al.*, 2008). For example, for the word *mechanism* (/ˈmɛkənɪzəm/), stress often shifted away from the first syllable to the second [mɛˈkɛnɪzəm]. Another example is the word *distribution* (/ˌdɪstrɪˈbjuːʃən/) which may be produced as [ˈdɪstrɪbjuːʃən], with stress incorrectly placed on the first syllable (Hung, 2000).

In English, unstressed syllables often undergo vowel reduction, where vowels are reduced to a schwa /ə/. This reduction is an essential characteristic of English fluency and naturalness (Ladefoged & Johnson, 2014).

However, Cantonese lacks systematic vowel reduction, and vowels are typically produced with full quality, even in unstressed positions, giving an impression of over-articulation (e.g. [17]–[18]) (Setter & Jenkins, 2005).

[17]	*sentence* /ˈsɛntəns/→ [ˈsɛntɛns]	full vowel articulation
[18]	*police* (/pəˈlis/) → [p**o**ˈlis]	full vowel articulation

The following is a sample text illustrating mismatches typically produced by a Cantonese-English bilingual.

Miss Chan will have lunch at twelve.
[mɪˈsiː tsʰen wiːu həf ˈlʌnˈtʃy et tʃeˈloʊˈʃu]

But she only goes back to work at three.
[p̚at̚ˈʃy ˈʊŋˈ li ˈgoʊ p̚æk̚tu ˈwɵk̚et̚fiː]

So, she cannot help us.
[ˈsoʊ ˈʃy ˈkæn nɒt̚hel ɐs]

Another phenomenon related to the prosodic transfer domain is the reduced co-articulation in Cantonese English. Co-articulation refers to the influence of surrounding sounds on the production of a particular phoneme (Hardcastle & Hewlett, 1999). In English, co-articulation is more fluid, with sounds blending to create smoother transitions between words and syllables (Farnetani & Recasens, 2010). For example, the English phrase *pick it up* might be pronounced as [pɪkɪtʌp], with the sounds blending smoothly. Similarly, the phrase *told you* (/toʊld juː/) may undergo assimilation and coarticulation, where the /d/ in *told* and the /j/ in *you* blend together, producing something like [toʊldʒu], where the /j/ sound of *you* becomes part of an affricate /dʒ/ (Roach, 2009). Such a co-articulation phenomenon may be difficult for Cantonese English L2 learners to comprehend because the realization and the target sounds are too distinct, even though the actual meaning is simple (Chan & Li, 2000). In terms of production, the reduced co-articulation in Cantonese English can contribute to the perception of a 'choppy' or less fluid speech rhythm (Gut, 2012).

Morphosyntax

Morphosyntactic differences between Cantonese and English pose challenges for Cantonese-English bilinguals, particularly in argument structure, part of speech, pronoun use and verb morphology (Chan, 2004).

Argument structure

Argument structure refers to the way that verbs interact with the nouns or pronouns (subjects, objects, etc.) that are required to complete their meaning (Goldberg, 1995). While both languages generally follow a subject-verb-object (SVO) word order, there are important distinctions in how verbs and their arguments are structured, especially in areas like pro-drop and word order, transitivity and the use of prepositions (Matthews & Yip, 2011).

Pro-drop and word order

Compared to English, Cantonese exhibits more flexibility in sentence structure due to its use of topic-comment structures even though both share the same basic word order (Yip & Matthews, 2007). First, Cantonese is a pro-drop language, meaning subject pronouns can be omitted when they are pragmatically clear (Huang, 1984). For example, in Cantonese, it is common to omit the subject in phrases like 食飯 /sɪk6 fan6/, which can be translated as 'I'm/we/you are eating.' When learning English, Cantonese speakers may transfer this pro-drop feature, leading to sentences in which necessary subject pronouns are omitted, e.g. *he is going* is rendered as **is going* (Chan, 2004).

Second, Cantonese has a topic-comment structure that allows for greater flexibility in sentence order (Li & Thompson, 1981). For instance, a sentence like *As for this book, I already read it* could be structured with the topic first, followed by a comment about the topic. In Cantonese, this would be 呢本書，我已經睇咗 /nei1 pun2 sy1 ŋɔ6 ji5 kɪŋ1 tʰɐi2 tsɔ2/ 'This book, I already read.' Cantonese speakers may carry this structure into English, producing sentences like *This book, I already read* rather than the more pragmatically unmarked *I've already read this book* (Yip & Matthews, 2000).

Transitivity of verbs

In English, some verbs are strictly transitive (must have a direct object) or intransitive (cannot take a direct object). For example, *put* in English is a ditransitive verb and requires both a direct object and a prepositional phrase: *I put the book on the table*. In contrast, in Cantonese, verb structure and argument requirements are more flexible, and context often dictates whether an object is required, sometimes allowing verbs to be used transitively or intransitively (Matthews & Yip, 2011). As a result, Cantonese speakers may omit the direct object when using *put* in English (Chan, 2004). For example, *I put the book on the table* will become **Put book or *Put on the table*.

Prepositions play a crucial role in argument structure in English, particularly with ditransitive verbs like *give*, *put* and *tell* to specify the relationship between the action and the participants/objects involved (Huddleston & Pullum, 2002). Cantonese does not require prepositions to convey the same meaning (Yip & Matthews, 2007), leading to preposition omission or misuse in English by Cantonese speakers (Chan, 2010). For example, **I told the news, or *I told to her*.

Morphological markings

Cantonese does not mark case, animacy and gender in the same way English does in pronouns (Matthews & Yip, 2011). Spoken Cantonese uses a single third-person pronoun 佢 /kʰɵy5/ for *he*, *him*, *she*, *her* and *it*, and 我 /ngo5/ for *I* and *me* (Yip & Matthews, 2000). This lack of morphological distinction in Cantonese pronouns often leads to difficulties for Cantonese speakers when acquiring the English pronominal system (Chan, 2010). They may produce case errors (Chan, 2004) (e.g. [19]–[20]), and gender confusion in English pronoun use (e.g. [21]) (Yip & Matthews, 2007). The possessive structure in Cantonese, using the particle 嘅 /ge3/, contrasts with the English system of possessive pronouns and the *'s* genitive. This difference can lead to errors in English such as *His book* → **He's book*, *His book* → **The book of he*, or *This is his book* → **This is him book* (Chan, 2004).

[19] *He is going to school.* → **Him is going to school.*

[20] *She and I are friends.* → **Me and her are friends.*

[21] *She is my mom.* → **He is my mom.*

English articles *a*, *an* and *the* are determiners in noun phrases that provide information about whether the entity being described is definite or indefinite, singular and countable or uncountable. The definiteness marking in Cantonese is very different (Matthews & Yip, 2011), and there is no (un)countable differentiation in Cantonese (Chan, 2004, 2016). These typological differences result in frequent article issues in Cantonese English interlanguage even for speakers whose English proficiency is not low [22]–[23].

[22] *I buy an apple* → **I buy apple*

[23] *I go to school* → **I go to the school*

The plural in English is usually indicated by the suffix *-s* and *-es* or morphological changes to the noun. In Cantonese, plurality is typically conveyed through context or numerals with classifiers (Matthews & Yip, 2011). As a result, Cantonese speakers may omit plural markers in English, (e.g. *I have two apples* → **I have two apple*) or overgeneralize the plural marker (e.g. **childrens*, **peoples*) (Chan, 2004).

Cantonese does not have a formal tense system like English, where verb forms change to indicate past, present or future (Li & Thompson, 1981). Instead of using different verb forms, Cantonese expresses time using aspect markers (e.g. 咗 /tsɔ2/), context, and explicit temporal adverbials (e.g. 今日 /kɐm1jɐt6/ "today") (Matthews & Yip, 2011). These markers provide information about whether an action is completed, ongoing or habitual, but they do not specifically indicate tense in the way English does. These differences are challenging for Cantonese speakers, and errors like **I go to school yesterday*, and tenses often require explicit learning, whether through formal education or exposure to the language in context.

Parts of speech

Cantonese words often exhibit multifunctionality as syntactic constituents, meaning that the same lexical item can serve different grammatical roles (e.g. noun, verb or adjective) depending on context. Unlike English, Cantonese lacks inflectional morphology and derivational processes to mark such changes explicitly (Leung & Li, 2016). For example, the word 跑步 /pʰau2 pou6/ 'run' can serve as the subject, predicate or object without any derivational change. This difference poses challenges for Cantonese learners in using the correct parts of speech in English sentences. For example, Cantonese speakers may not use the gerund form of verbs when it is in subject or object position (e.g. [24]–[25]).

[24] *Swimming is my hobby → *Swim is my hobby*

[25] *I love singing → *I love sing*

Vocabulary Use

For bilingual children, vocabulary acquisition in English may lag behind monolingual English speakers, especially if they are still acquiring proficiency in both languages (Bialystok, 2010). This delay is not necessarily indicative of a language disorder, but just a reflection of the bilingual's division of language exposure between their two languages (Hoff, 2012). Among various lexical items, certain words can be particularly challenging for L2 learners. These include polysemy, vocabulary with idiomatic meaning and phrasal verbs (Crossley, 2010).

Polysemes have multiple but similar meanings causing difficulties. Homonyms are also a challenge, so the word *bank* in English, for example, can mean a financial institution or the side of a river. A Cantonese-English speaking bilingual child may only be able to decode the more common meaning (i.e. bank as a financial institution) (Fang, 2016). Words with figurative or idiomatic meaning require sufficient contextual exposure before they can be fully understood or used (Liontas, 2002). For example, *ice-breaking games* might be interpreted literally as a game of breaking actual ice, rather than the idiomatic meaning of starting off a conversation. Similarly, English phrasal verbs (e.g. *give up*, *take off*, *run out*) are not easy for Cantonese speakers, as their meanings are often not intuitive and cannot be derived by understanding the verb and the preposition separately (Liao & Fukuya, 2004).

Bilinguals may also experience difficulties during conversation due to lexical gaps between their native language and the target language

(Pavlenko, 2009). A lexical gap refers to the absence of a word or phrase in a language to express a particular concept or meaning that exists in another language. For example, Cantonese-English bilinguals might struggle to express certain Cantonese cultural concepts in English due to the lack of equivalent vocabulary. This may give rise to an impression of language difficulties if they are asked to share their personal experience related to their cultural activities (Altarriba, 2003).

To specifically enhance bilingual children's vocabulary, contextualized vocabulary learning is found to be a highly effective approach, which emphasizes the importance of learning new words in meaningful contexts rather than in isolation (Schmitt, 2000). When vocabulary is introduced in authentic contexts, such as through stories, conversations or thematic content, learners can more easily grasp the nuances and varied uses of a word (Nation, 2013). This approach not only enhances retention but also improves comprehension, as learners are exposed to how vocabulary is used in different grammatical and pragmatic settings. By encountering words in real-life situations or through context-rich materials, learners can develop a deeper understanding of the meanings of words (Webb, 2005). Similarly, teaching idiomatic vocabulary to bilinguals requires strategies that make idioms relatable and memorable. By providing context, using visual aids and encouraging practice in natural situations, learners can develop a stronger grasp of idiomatic expressions (Liu, 2008).

Differentiating Cultural and Linguistic Diversity from Speech, Language and Communication Disorders

Cantonese-English bilinguals often exhibit speech and language patterns that resemble the errors made by native English-speaking children with Developmental Language Disorders (DLD), particularly in areas like the use of tense marking, articles, pronoun use and sentence complexity (Eadie, 2002; Leonard, 2014; Rice, 1996). The similarities make it challenging for clinicians to distinguish between typical second language acquisition (SLA) and true developmental language impairments (Paradis, 2013), but highlights the importance of distinguishing between language difference and language disorder.

Despite the above similarities, there are important distinctions between bilingual learners and children with speech and language disorders (SLD) (e.g. Babatsouli, 2023, 2024). In terms of the nature of the errors, errors produced by bilingual learners mostly stem from transfer from L1 to L2, while in children with SLD, the errors indicate underlying language processing difficulties. The major observable differences between bilinguals are related to error patterns and error persistence over time. Children with DLD tend to make consistent grammatical errors regardless of context or proficiency, whereas bilingual children may show inconsistent errors, depending on the context or the task complexity (Paradis, 2007; Restrepo & Kruth, 2000). Moreover, the errors produced by bilingual children tend to be generative, indicating their understanding of the language's rules and their logical application (Bedore & Peña, 2008). With increased exposure to English, errors observed in bilingual children should decrease with time, especially with adequate regular formal instruction. In contrast, children with SLD may show limited progress despite sufficient exposure. It is also important to highlight that bilingual children with DLD may struggle with grammar and syntax in both languages, while typical bilingual learners may struggle primarily with their L2. Assessing the child's performance in both their L1 and L2 would be ideal to determine the presence of language difficulties. Caregivers can be very important informants if direct assessment of their L1 may not be available. In addition, information about the child's exposure to both languages should be considered during clinical decision-making.

Dynamic assessment, which evaluates a child's ability to learn new language rules, can be an effective tool for differentiating between typical bilingual development and DLD (Peña, 1996). Unlike traditional standardized tests that provide a static measure of language ability, dynamic assessment focuses on a child's learning potential and his or her ability to respond to teaching or intervention. This makes it particularly useful for bilingual children, as it accounts for their varying language experiences and exposure. A common framework is the Test-Teach-Retest model (Lidz, 1991). The child is first assessed in a task to establish a baseline (e.g. vocabulary, narrative ability or grammatical structure) during the Test phase. Then the examiner provides structured teaching or intervention during the assessment, offering strategies or feedback that can help the child improve during the Teach phase. At this stage, the assessor may rate the client's modifiability based on the child's response to the strategies or feedback. Finally, the child is assessed again to see how much they have improved or how much they have learned from the teaching phase. This process has been demonstrated to be a promising alternative to static assessment, yielding higher accuracy in identifying language disorders in culturally and linguistically diverse children (Petersen, 2024), given its advantage in differentiating between children who are simply unfamiliar with a language or concept (due to limited exposure) and those who have difficulty learning language even with instruction, which is more indicative of a language disorder.

For speech sound assessment, stimulability testing is also a type of dynamic assessment that offers valuable insights into a bilingual child's phonological abilities (Glaspey & Stoel-Gammon, 2005). Stimulability testing assesses a child's ability to produce a target sound correctly when provided with maximum cues and support, including visual, auditory and tactile prompts (Powell & Miccio, 1996). Importantly, stimulability testing should be conducted at the syllable level, as this provides a more accurate representation of a child's phonological capabilities in connected speech (Rvachew, 2005). High stimulability suggests the sound is emerging and may develop naturally with continued exposure and practice, while low stimulability might signal a true difficulty with the sound, possibly due to a speech sound disorder rather than typical bilingual development (Gierut, 1987). Recent research by To (2022) has further highlighted the predictive value of stimulability testing, along with speech intelligibility, in determining which children with speech sound disorders are likely to normalize without intervention.

Cultural differences in pragmatics and communication styles are also highly relevant when diagnosing children with social communication disorders (SCD), particularly in bilingual or bicultural contexts like Cantonese-speaking communities. SCD is often diagnosed based on challenges in personal interaction, including difficulty with eye contact, gestures, turn-taking, and responding to directives – all of which are culturally mediated behaviors. For example, in Chinese culture, direct and prolonged eye contact may be seen as disrespectful, especially between children and authority figures like parents or teachers. A clinician unfamiliar with this cultural norm might mistakenly interpret aversion to eye contact as a sign of SCD or autism, when in fact, it may be a culturally appropriate behavior.

Similarly, the use of directives in Cantonese-speaking households, where parents often issue clear, authoritative commands, might not provide children with the same opportunities for dialogic interaction that are more common in English-speaking cultures. A child's reduced verbal output in such contexts could be wrongly interpreted as a sign of impaired social communication, when it reflects the culturally appropriate expectation for the child to comply quietly with parental instructions. Likewise, the subtle use of gestures and reserved body language in Chinese culture may be seen as a lack of expressiveness, potentially leading to misinterpretations of communicative deficits.

Implications for Researchers

Understanding cultural and linguistic differences is therefore useful for Cantonese-English bilingual research. The delineated typological differences and language transfer can provide a useful lens through which developmental research on English as a second language (ESL) can be developed. Further investigation into how these differences contribute and interact with other factors (e.g. language dominance, age of exposure) can help unfold the complexity of the development of Cantonese English. Bilingual research on language disorders also requires sensitivity to these cultural and linguistic differences. Failure to account for the differences might lead to misclassification, possibly leading to invalid conclusions. Therefore, researchers should cultivate sensitivity towards the differences in designing and implementing their research.

Clinical implications for Practitioners

These cultural and linguistic norms also underscore the critical need for culturally sensitive awareness when evaluating and diagnosing speech, language and communication disorders in children from diverse backgrounds. It is essential for educators and speech-language pathologists working with Cantonese-English bilinguals to recognize how features such as different phonological patterns, morphosyntactic structures and pragmatic behaviors influence a child's language development and communication style. Failure to account for these differences can lead to misdiagnosis or over-diagnosis, potentially labeling typical language variations as disordered. A culturally informed approach not only improves diagnostic accuracy but also ensures that interventions are more tailored and effective, addressing the unique linguistic and cultural contexts of each child (To, 2016). By fostering greater awareness of these factors, professionals can support bilingual children in achieving their full communicative potential efficiently without the risks of inappropriate interventions.

Conclusion

This chapter has explored the historical and cultural landscape underlying Cantonese speakers using English as a second language in predominantly English-speaking contexts, like the one in North America. Important typological differences and language transfer were highlighted. Awareness and understanding of the cultural and language influence are important for researchers and practitioners, especially when working on the assessment and diagnosis of multilingual speakers. It is therefore of utmost importance for researchers and practitioners to cultivate this sensitivity, through which Cantonese-English bilingual children can be understood and supported in the best way possible.

References

Altarriba, J. (2003) Does cariño equal "liking"? A theoretical approach to conceptual non-equivalence between languages. *International Journal of Bilingualism* 7 (3), 305–322.

Babatsouli, E. (2023) Ecosystemic clinical assessment of linguistic diversity: Greek-dominant speech. *Perspectives of the ASHA Special Interest Groups*, 1–23. https://doi.org/10.1044/2023_PERSP-23-00088

Babatsouli, E. (2024) Phonological disorders in child bilingualism. In M. Amengual (ed.) *The Cambridge Handbook of Bilingual Phonetics and Phonology* (pp. 309–337). Cambridge University Press.

Bauer, R.S. and Benedict, P.K. (1997) *Modern Cantonese Phonology*. Walter de Gruyter.

Bedore, L.M. and Peña, E.D. (2008) Assessment of bilingual children for identification of language impairment: Current findings and implications for practice. *International Journal of Bilingual Education and Bilingualism* 11 (1), 1–29.

Bialystok, E., Luk, G., Peets, K.F. and Yang, S. (2010) Receptive vocabulary differences in monolingual and bilingual children. *Bilingualism: Language and Cognition* 13 (4), 525–531.

Chan, A.Y.W. (2004) Syntactic transfer: Evidence from the interlanguage of Hong Kong Chinese ESL learners. *The Modern Language Journal* 88 (1), 56–74.

Chan, A.Y.W. (2010) Toward a taxonomy of written errors: Investigation into the written errors of Hong Kong Cantonese ESL learners. *TESOL Quarterly* 44 (2), 295–319.

Chan, A.Y.W. (2016) How much do Cantonese ESL learners know about the English article system? *System* 56, 66–77.

Chan, A.Y. and Li, D.C. (2000) English and Cantonese phonology in contrast: Explaining Cantonese ESL learners' English pronunciation problems. *Language, Culture and Curriculum* 13 (1), 67–85.

Chan, S. (1991) *Asian Americans: An Interpretive History*. Twayne Publishers.

Cheung, Y.L. (2007) The acquisition of English vowels by Cantonese ESL learners in Hong Kong. *Hong Kong Journal of Applied Linguistics* 10 (2), 19–36.

Crossley, S.A., Salsbury, T. and McNamara, D.S. (2010) The development of polysemy and frequency use in English second language speakers. *Language Learning* 60 (3), 573–605.

Deterding, D., Wong, J. and Kirkpatrick, A. (2008) The pronunciation of Hong Kong English. *World Englishes* 27 (1), 148–175.

Eadie, P.A., Fey, M.E., Douglas, J.M. and Parsons, C.L. (2002) Profiles of grammatical morphology and sentence imitation in children with specific language impairment and down syndrome. *Journal of Speech, Language, and Hearing Research* 45 (4), 720–732. https://doi.org/10.1044/1092-4388(2002/058)

Eberhard, D.M., Simons, G.F. and Fennig, C.D. (eds) (2023) *Ethnologue: Languages of the World*. SIL International.

Fang, S.Y., Zinszer, B.D., Malt, B.C. and Li, P. (2016) Bilingual object naming: A connectionist model. *Frontiers in Psychology* 7, 644.

Farnetani, E. and Recasens, D. (2010) Coarticulation and connected speech processes. In W.J. Hardcastle, J. Laver and F.E. Gibbon (eds) *The Handbook of Phonetic Sciences* (2nd edn, pp. 316–352). Wiley-Blackwell.

Gierut, J.A., Elbert, M. and Dinnsen, D.A. (1987) A functional analysis of phonological knowledge and generalization learning in misarticulating children. *Journal of Speech and Hearing Research* 30 (4), 462–479.

Glaspey, A.M. and Stoel-Gammon, C. (2005) Dynamic assessment in phonological disorders: The scaffolding scale of stimulability. *Topics in Language Disorders* 25 (3), 220–230.

Goldberg, A.E. (1995) *Constructions: A Construction Grammar Approach to Argument Structure*. University of Chicago Press.

Gut, U. (2012) Rhythm in L2 speech. In J. Romero-Trillo (ed.) *Pragmatics and Prosody in English Language Teaching* (pp. 83–100). Springer.

Hansen Edwards, J.G. (2006) *Acquiring a Non-Native Phonology: Linguistic Constraints and Social Barriers*. Continuum.

Hardcastle, W.J. and Hewlett, N. (eds) (1999) *Coarticulation: Theory, Data and Techniques*. Cambridge University Press.

Hoff, E., Core, C., Place, S., Rumiche, R., Señor, M. and Parra, M. (2012) Dual language exposure and early bilingual development. *Journal of Child Language* 39 (1), 1–27.

Huang, C.T.J. (1984) On the distribution and reference of empty pronouns. *Linguistic Inquiry* 15 (4), 531–574.

Huddleston, R. and Pullum, G.K. (2002) *The Cambridge Grammar of the English Language*. Cambridge University Press.

Hung, T.T. (2000) Towards a phonology of Hong Kong English. *World Englishes* 19 (3), 337–356.

Kádár, D.Z. and Pan, Y. (2011) Politeness in China. In D.Z. Kádár and S. Mills (eds) *Politeness in East Asia* (pp. 125–146). Cambridge University Press.

Ladefoged, P. and Johnson, K. (2014) *A Course in Phonetics* (7th edn). Cengage Learning.

Lai, M.L. (2012) Tracking language attitudes in postcolonial Hong Kong: An interplay of localization, mainlandization, and internationalization. *Multilingua* 31 (1), 83–111.
Lee, C. (2011) Strategy and linguistic preference of requests by Cantonese learners of English: An interlanguage and crosscultural comparison. *Multilingua* 30 (1), 99–129.
Leonard, L.B. (2014) *Children with Specific Language Impairment*. MIT Press.
Leung, M.T. and Li, H.L. (2016) Cantonese LARSP: A procedure for assessment and remediation for Cantonese-speaking children. In P. Fletcher, M.J. Ball and D. Crystal (eds) *Profiling Grammar: More Languages of LARSP* (pp. 172–197). Multilingual Matters.
Li, C.N. and Thompson, S.A. (1981) *Mandarin Chinese: A Functional Reference Grammar*. University of California Press.
Li, W. (2005) Beyond Chinatown, beyond enclave: Reconceptualizing contemporary Chinese settlements in the United States. *GeoJournal* 64 (1), 31–40.
Liang, S. and Li, Y. (2021) Transnational mobility and cross-border linguistic repertoires: A case study of Cantonese and Mandarin in Vancouver. *Journal of Multilingual and Multicultural Development* 42 (3), 245–259.
Liao, Y. and Fukuya, Y.J. (2004) Avoidance of phrasal verbs: The case of Chinese learners of English. *Language Learning* 54 (2), 193–226.
Lidz, C.S. (1991) *Practitioner's Guide to Dynamic Assessment*. Guilford Press.
Liontas, J.I. (2002) Context and idiom understanding in second languages. *EUROSLA Yearbook* 2 (1), 155–185.
Liu, D. (2008) *Idioms: Description, Comprehension, Acquisition, and Pedagogy*. Routledge.
Matthews, S. and Yip, V. (2011) *Cantonese: A Comprehensive Grammar* (2nd edn). Routledge.
Matsumoto, D. and Hwang, H.C. (2013) Cultural similarities and differences in emblematic gestures. *Journal of Nonverbal Behavior* 37 (1), 1–27.
Nagy, N. (2018) Linguistic diversity and language rights in urban Canada. *Journal of Multilingual and Multicultural Development* 39 (7), 638–656.
Nation, I.S.P. (2013) *Learning Vocabulary in Another Language* (2nd edn). Cambridge University Press.
Paradis, J. (2007) Bilingual children with specific language impairment: Theoretical and applied issues. *Applied Psycholinguistics* 28 (3), 551–564.
Paradis, J., Schneider, P. and Duncan, T.S. (2013) Discriminating children with language impairment among English-language learners from diverse first-language backgrounds. *Journal of Speech, Language, and Hearing Research* 56 (3), 971–981.
Pavlenko, A. (ed.) (2009) *The Bilingual Mental Lexicon: Interdisciplinary Approaches*. Multilingual Matters.
Peña, E.D. (1996) Dynamic assessment: The model and its language applications. *Assessment of Communication and Language* 6, 281–307.
Petersen, D.B., Konishi-Therkildsen, A., Clark, K.D., DeRobles, A.K., Frahm, A.E., Jones, K., Lettich, C. and Spencer, T.D. (2024) Accurately identifying language disorder in school-age children using dynamic assessment of narrative language. *Journal of Speech, Language, and Hearing Research*, 1–18. https://doi.org/10.1044/2024_JSLHR-23-00594
Powell, T.W. and Miccio, A.W. (1996) Stimulability: A useful clinical tool. *Journal of Communication Disorders* 29 (4), 237–253.
Restrepo, M.A. and Kruth, K. (2000) Grammatical characteristics of a Spanish-English bilingual child with Specific Language Impairment. *Communication Disorders Quarterly* 21 (2), 66–76. https://doi.org/10.1177/152574010002100201
Rice, M.L. and Wexler, K. (1996) Toward tense as a clinical marker of specific language impairment in English-speaking children. *Journal of Speech and Hearing Research* 39 (6), 1239–1257. https://doi.org/10.1044/jshr.3906.1239
Roach, P. (2009) *English Phonetics and Phonology Fourth Edition: A Practical Course*. Cambridge University Press.

Rose, K.R. (2005) On the effects of instruction in second language pragmatics. *System (Linköping)* 33 (3), 385–399.
Rvachew, S. (2005) Stimulability and treatment success. *Topics in Language Disorders* 25 (3), 207–219.
Schmitt, N. (2000) *Vocabulary in Language Teaching*. Cambridge University Press.
Scollon, R. and Scollon, S.W. (2001) *Intercultural Communication: A Discourse Approach* (2nd edn). Blackwell.
Setter, J. (2006) Speech rhythm in world Englishes: The case of Hong Kong. *TESOL Quarterly* 40 (4), 763–782.
Setter, J. and Jenkins, J. (2005) State-of-the-art review article: Pronunciation. *Language Teaching* 38 (1), 1–17.
Setter, J., Wong, C.S.P. and Chan, B.H.S. (2010) *Hong Kong English*. Edinburgh University Press.
Spencer-Oatey, H. and Kádár, D.Z. (2016) The bases of (im)politeness evaluations: Culture, the moral order and the East–West debate. *East Asian Pragmatics* 1 (1), 73–106.
Tannen, D. (2005) *Conversational Style: Analyzing Talk among Friends*. Oxford University Press.
Tao, H. and Tao, Y. (2016) Conversation analysis and language socialization. In P.A. Duff and S. May (eds) *Language Socialization* (pp. 1–17). Springer.
To, C.K.S., McLeod, S., Law, T. and Sam, K.L. (2022) Predicting which children will normalize without intervention for speech sound disorders. *Journal of Speech, Language, and Hearing Research* 65 (5), 1724–1741.
To, C.K.S. (2016) Language disorders in Cantonese-speaking children. In J.L. Patterson and B.L. Rodríguez (eds) *Multilingual Perspectives on Child Language Disorders* (pp. 123–148). Multilingual Matters. https://doi.org/10.21832/9781783094738-008
Tse, H. and Li, D.C.S. (2020) Bi-/multilingualism and identity: A study of self-reports from youths in post-colonial Hong Kong. *International Journal of Bilingualism* 24 (4), 647–661.
Tse, L. (2001) Heritage language literacy: A study of US biliterates. *Language, Culture and Curriculum* 14 (3), 256–268.
Webb, S. (2005) Receptive and productive vocabulary learning: The effects of reading and writing on word knowledge. *Studies in Second Language Acquisition* 27 (1), 33–52.
Yip, V. and Matthews, S. (2000) Syntactic transfer in a Cantonese–English bilingual child. *Bilingualism: Language and Cognition* 3 (3), 193–208.
Yip, V. and Matthews, S. (2007) *The Bilingual Child: Early Development and Language Contact*. Cambridge University Press.
Yu, H. (2013) Mountains of gold: Canada, North America, and the Cantonese Pacific. In C.B. Tan (ed.) *Routledge Handbook of the Chinese Diaspora* (1st edn, pp. 108–121). Routledge.
Zee, E. (1999). Chinese (Hong Kong Cantonese). In International Phonetic Association (Ed.), *Handbook of the International Phonetic Association: A Guide to the Use of the International Phonetic Alphabet* (pp. 58–60). Cambridge University Press.
Zhang, Y., Nissen, S.L. and Francis, A.L. (2008) Acoustic characteristics of English lexical stress produced by native Mandarin speakers. *The Journal of the Acoustical Society of America* 123 (6), 4498–4513.
Zhu, W. and Wang, J. (2022) Disagreement by Chinese speakers of English: Evidence of pragmatic transfer. *Language Sciences* 93, 101487.

21 Speech-Language Pathology for Mandarin-English Bilinguals in North America

Ran An and Qiang Li

Introduction

Mandarin Chinese (Standard Mandarin, Pǔtōnghuà, 普通话), hereon Mandarin, the official language of mainland China, plays a crucial role in the country's cultural, economic and strategic development. According to a 2022 report by the Ministry of Education of the People's Republic of China, 80.72% of the population now speaks Standard Mandarin, a notable increase from approximately 70% a decade earlier (Ministry of Education of the People's Republic of China, 2022). This standardized form of the Beijing dialect is the primary language for government, education and media in mainland China, while also being widely recognized in Taiwan, Hong Kong and other regions with some regional variations.

This chapter focuses specifically on the Mandarin spoken in mainland China, analyzing its phonological and grammatical structures and exploring their implications for bilingual individuals in North America. Mandarin serves as a heritage language for many Chinese communities abroad, influencing language use and bilingual development alongside English. For speech-language pathologists (SLPs), understanding these linguistic dynamics is critical for providing effective assessments and interventions.

This chapter examines Mandarin-English bilinguals' linguistic and cultural dynamics in North America, providing insights for SLPs. It begins with an overview of the demographic and historical context, detailing Chinese migration patterns, generational differences and regional distributions that shape communication. The chapter then delves into the linguistic features of Mandarin, exploring phonology (such as its lexical tones, phoneme inventory and absence of consonant clusters), grammar including morphology (such as pluralization of nouns, verb tense inflection, adjective inflection and tenses), syntax (covering word order and passive voice) and semantics (comparing the articles between English and Mandarin). The 'Implications for Practitioners' section outlines practical assessment strategies, including case history collection, dynamic assessments and the use of combined Mandarin and English monolingual tools. It also highlights intervention approaches, such as integrating cross-linguistic strategies, leveraging native language strengths and fostering bilingual identity to support effective treatment outcomes. The chapter concludes with 'Implications for Researchers,' exploring areas for future study to advance understanding and practice in working with Mandarin-English bilingual populations.

Demographic and Historical Context of Chinese Communities in North America

Chinese families in North America tell a story of how resilience and adversity have been woven into the very fabric of their history and migration to the country. The history of these families has been characterized by phases of exclusion and the process of inclusion into the local society. For SLPs working with Mandarin-English bilingual families, knowing this background will provide the necessary cultural knowledge to help navigate the opportunities and understand the set of barriers present in these communities.

Historical immigration trends

The first significant wave of Chinese migration to North America began in the mid-19th century. Economic opportunities such as the California Gold Rush (1848–1855) and the construction of the transcontinental railroad in the United States drew thousands of Chinese laborers, primarily from Guangdong Province. These laborers undertook strenuous and, at times, life-threatening jobs under extremely poor conditions (Chang, 2003; Takaki, 1998). Similarly, in Canada, Chinese workers contributed to the construction of the Canadian Pacific Railway, where they faced comparable hardships, including dangerous working environments and discriminatory practices (Li, 1998).

Despite the contributions made by Chinese immigrants, policies were in effect for many years that prevented the growth of the Chinese community while restricting their possibilities to improve their status in society. The process of change became evident in the mid-20th century. Laws pertaining to immigration such as the Immigration and Nationality Act of 1965 in the United States and the adoption of the point-based system in Canada led to the changes in the landscape for Chinese families. These changes not only enabled people to be joined by their families but also enabled the entry of workers, students, businesspeople and entrepreneurs, thus diversifying the Chinese population in North America. The effects of these reforms are still felt to this day in the composition and cultural nature of these communities.

Demographics and generational differences

The Chinese community is now among the largest populations of Asian origin in North America. In the United States, there are about 4.7 million people of Chinese origin, accounting for 19% of the Asian American population. In Canada, there are over 1.7 million people of Chinese descent, accounting for about 5% of the Canadian population (Pew Research Center, 2024; Statistics Canada, 2023). Within these communities, distinct generational patterns emerge:

- **First Generation**: These individuals, often born in regions such as mainland China, Hong Kong or Taiwan, maintain strong ties to their native language, including Mandarin and Cantonese, and adhere closely to traditional cultural values (Kondo-Brown, 2006).
- **Second Generation**: The second generation typically bridges two cultures, with greater fluency in English and varying proficiency in their heritage languages. Studies reveal that the absence of formal language education in these settings often leads to declining fluency in heritage languages (Cheung, 2019).
- **Third Generation and Beyond**: By the third generation, English becomes the dominant or exclusive language, reflecting broader patterns of cultural assimilation and language attrition in immigrant families (Kondo-Brown, 2006).

Regional distribution

Geographically, Chinese communities in North America are concentrated in urban centers with robust Asian cultural networks. In the United States, cities such as San Francisco, Los Angeles and New York have historically served as cultural hubs for Chinese immigrants. Similarly, Chicago, Houston and Seattle host vibrant Chinese populations (Pew Research Center, 2024). In Canada, Vancouver and Toronto are home to nearly half of all Chinese Canadians, with Vancouver often regarded as a gateway city due to its proximity to Asia and historical significance as an immigrant entry point (Statistics Canada, 2023).

Linguistic Features of Mandarin-English Bilinguals

There are significant differences between English and Mandarin Chinese in all aspects of language, including grammar, morphology, vocabulary, phonology, syntax, pragmatics and semantics. This chapter briefly discusses the following language levels: differences in phonology and grammar, with particular attention to morphology, syntax, and selected semantic distinctions related to article use.

Phonology

Phonology in Mandarin Chinese is characterized by its distinct segmental inventory, the absence of consonant clusters and its tonal nature. Mandarin Chinese has a relatively small inventory of consonants and vowels compared to other languages, yet it exhibits rich allophonic variations. Mandarin Chinese has five vowels as shown in Table 21.1, including [i] and [u] like the English high vowels, a front high rounded vowel [y], and [i] and [u] serving as the offglide of diphthongs (Li, 2016). Standard Mandarin Chinese has four diphthongs, including [əi], [əu], [ai] and [au]. They are made by combining the mid-vowel [ə] or low vowel [a] with the high vowel [i] or [u] (Duanmu, 2007: 40).

There are 19 consonants in Mandarin as in Table 21.2 (Duanmu, 2007: 24). All the consonants except [ŋ] can be the onset of a syllable, but the codas are limited to [n] and [ŋ] only, which are represented in 拼音 (*pīn yīn*, 'Pinyin') <-n> and <-ng> respectively, where their oral closure is often incomplete. Glides and consonant-glide combinations are two special groups of consonants. In Mandarin, high vowels that occur before another vowel function as glides and are transcribed as /j, ɥ, w/ (Duanmu, 2007: 23). For instance, tone 1 Pinyin <*yan*> 烟, 'smoke' is pronounced as [jan]; <yuan> 怨, 'grievance' is pronounced as [ɥan], and <wan> 弯, 'curve' is pronounced as [wan]. However, the glides do not contrast with the corresponding high vowels [i, u, y], and the two sets can be treated as variants.

Speech sound disorders in Mandarin often result in non-target-like articulation of these sounds. For example, distinguishing between retroflex and alveolar consonants can be challenging for children with articulation disorders due to the precise tongue and airflow control required

Table 21.1 Mandarin Chinese vowels

	Front		Back
High	i	y	u
Mid	ə		
Low	a		

Table 21.2 Mandarin Chinese consonants

	Labial	Dental	Retroflex	Velar
Stop	p, p^{h}	t, t^{h}		k, k^{h}
Affricate		ts, ts^{h}	tʂ^{h}, tʂ	
Fricative	f	s	ʂ, ʐ	x
Nasal	m	n		(ŋ)
Liquid		l		

(Liu & Chien, 2020). Mispronunciation in these areas can cause confusion between similar-sounding words, severely impacting intelligibility. For instance, mispronouncing /ʂ/ as /s/ can change <*shì*> 是 'to be' to <*sì*>, 四 'four,' leading to significant communication difficulties.

Furthermore, although vowel errors are less common than consonant errors, they also affect intelligibility, especially when diphthongs are involved. For instance, children may reduce diphthongs to monophthongs or substitute one vowel quality for another, such as producing /ai/ as /a/ or /e/ as /ɛ/ (Yang & Resendiz, 2024). The English vowel system poses challenges for Mandarin speakers learning English because it has a larger inventory. For example, English distinguishes between [ɪ] (in *bit*) and [i] (in *beat*), a contrast not present in Mandarin. Mandarin speakers may substitute these with their closest Mandarin equivalents, leading to errors, such as pronouncing *bit* as *beet*. English consonants that are not found in Mandarin also pose difficulties for Mandarin speakers, such as interdentals /θ/ and /ð/, as in *think* and *this*. Mandarin speakers might substitute these sounds with [s] or [z], resulting in **sink* for *think* and **zis* for *this*. Similarly, English [ɹ] and [l] sounds are hard to distinguish and produce for Mandarin speakers since Mandarin has only one liquid consonant that is somewhat between /ɹ/ and /l/.

When working with Mandarin-English bilingual clients, SLPs may collect speech samples in English at the phoneme level, word level and syllable level to evaluate the speech sounds. If the observed errors in producing phonemes are unique to English, they may reflect patterns of Mandarin-influenced English (Yang & Resendiz, 2024). Omission or addition of sounds and/or deviations of stress patterns may be observed in Mandarin-English bilinguals due to the lack of consonant clusters in Mandarin Chinese. In certain cases, consultation with a Mandarin-English bilingual SLP or a Mandarin-English interpreter is recommended when assessing speech sounds, particularly when dialectal differences in Chinese need to be considered.

Prosody

Chinese syllables are simple, typically following a consonant-vowel (CV) structure, but also comprise a CVC syllable with coda /n/ or /ŋ/. Other than the vowels /i, y, u, ə, a/, the syllable nucleus can also include a medial glide, such as [j], [ɥ] and [w], preceding the main vowels, as for /w/ before /ai/ in [k^{h}wai] 快 'fast.' Mandarin does not allow consonant clusters in the onset or coda of syllables, making its structure simpler compared to many other languages. As a result, Mandarin speakers encounter difficulties with English consonant clusters. In clinical practice, understanding Mandarin phonotactic rules is crucial for diagnosing and treating phonological disorders. For instance, children with phonological disorders might produce syllables with illegal consonant clusters or incorrect endings, like adding a schwa for *play* as [pəleɪ] or omitting coda obstruents, as in *cup* [ka], making their speech difficult to understand (Yang & Resendiz, 2024). These errors suggest a breakdown in the child's ability to plan phonologically, as they fail to adhere to the language's rules. In contrast, English syllables are more complex, e.g. *strengths* /strɛŋθs/ or *splints* /splɪnts/. Mandarin speakers might simplify clusters by omitting one or more consonants, leading to productions like **stren* for *strength* or **splin* for *splints*, which can reduce intelligibility (McBride-Chang *et al.*, 2008).

Tone

One of the most distinctive features of Mandarin is its tonal system, where pitch contours determine lexical meaning. Mandarin has four primary tones, including high-level (Tone 1), rising (Tone 2), falling-rising (Tone 3) and falling (Tone 4) (Duanmu, 2007). These tones are essential to the language's phonological system because they are contrastive. For example, the *ma* can mean 妈 <mā> 'mother' with Tone 1, 麻 <má> 'hemp' with Tone 2, 马 <mǎ> 'horse' with Tone 3, or 骂 <mà> 'scold' with Tone 4, showing how crucial tone is to communication in Mandarin (Xu, 1997; Chao, 1968).

Mandarin tones are primarily differentiated by their pitch contours, which can be analyzed acoustically in terms of fundamental frequency (F0) patterns. Tone 1 is characterized by a high-level F0, Tone 2 by a rising F0, Tone 3 by a dipping F0 and Tone 4 by a falling F0. These F0 contours are essential for distinguishing between otherwise identical syllables (Xu, 1997). For example, *shi* could mean 诗 *<shī>* 'poetry,' 十 *<shí>* 'ten,' 史 *<shǐ>* 'history' or 市 *<shì>* 'city,' depending on the F0 pattern. Acoustic analysis is often used in speech-language pathology to diagnose and treat tone-related speech disorders. For instance, individuals with hearing impairments may struggle to perceive these F0 patterns, leading to tone production errors. Research has shown that using pitch contour displays, which visually represent these F0 patterns, can be an effective intervention tool, helping individuals better perceive and produce accurate tonal contours (Li *et al.*, 2024). Moreover, studies have revealed that the production of Mandarin tones is influenced by factors such as speech rate and emotional state. Faster speech rates tend to compress F0 contours, making tones less distinct, which can lead to perceptual confusion (Xu, 1997).

Tonal errors can lead to severe communication breakdowns, especially in children with developmental speech disorders. These children might struggle with producing tones correctly, resulting in misunderstandings. Studies (e.g. Wong *et al.*, 2009) have shown that tone production errors in Mandarin-speaking children with phonological disorders often involve substituting one tone for another, flattening pitch contours, or completely omitting tonal distinctions. These errors are particularly challenging to address because they affect both the consonant and vowel levels (segmental) and the tone (suprasegmental) levels of speech. Research has also identified patterns in tonal production errors that are critical for diagnosis and treatment. For instance, Tone 3 is often the most difficult for children to master, possibly due to its complex falling-rising contour (Li & Thompson, 1977). Additionally, children with developmental language disorders (DLD) have been observed to make more tonal errors than their typically developing peers, indicating a need for targeted interventions that address both tonal and phonemic accuracy (Wong *et al.*, 2009).

Tone sandhi

Coarticulation is common in Mandarin. For example, Tone 3 often changes to Tone 2 when followed by another Tone 3 syllable, a process known as tone sandhi (Gao *et al.*, 2021). This tone sandhi is an essential aspect of natural speech and presents unique challenges in SLP. Understanding coarticulation effects is crucial in speech therapy, especially in the context of tone sandhi. For instance, children with speech sound disorders might struggle with correctly applying tone-sandhi rules, leading to unnatural or unintelligible speech patterns (Zhu & Dodd, 2000).

The complexity of tone sandhi requires SLPs to focus on individual tone production and the dynamic changes in connected speech. Therapeutic strategies might include exercises that gradually introduce tone sandhi contexts, allowing the child to practice these coarticulatory effects in increasingly complex linguistic environments. Additionally, tone sandhi rules can vary depending on dialect and speech context, adding another layer of complexity. For example, Beijing Mandarin and Taiwan Mandarin have slight differences in tone sandhi patterns, which can influence the therapeutic approach (Zhang, 2010). SLPs working with Mandarin speakers need to be aware of these regional variations to tailor their interventions effectively.

Intonation

Beyond individual tones, Mandarin's intonation patterns play a significant role in conveying meaning. While Mandarin is often considered a tone language in which lexical tones place constraints on intonational variation, recent studies have shown that intonation can influence tone perception, especially in longer utterances or questions. For example, in yes-no questions, the final tone in a sentence may be slightly raised, altering its standard F0 contour (Liu, 2009). Individuals with autism spectrum disorder (ASD) might have atypical intonation patterns that interfere with their tone production, leading to difficulties in social communication (Chan & To, 2016). These individuals might produce flat or exaggerated intonation contours, confusing listeners and affecting overall speech clarity. Interventions often involve working on both prosody and tone to improve communication effectiveness. For example, melodic intonation therapy, which emphasizes the musical aspects of speech, has been adapted for Mandarin speakers to help them improve their prosody and tone production (Zhang *et al.*, 2021). Furthermore, prosodic features like stress and rhythm also play a role in Mandarin speech. Although less prominent than in stress-timed languages like English, stress in Mandarin can still affect the perceived prominence of syllables, influencing tone perception (Xu, 1997).

Prosodic features such as stress, rhythm and intonation are crucial in spoken English, conveying meaning and intent. However, Mandarin speakers often struggle with these aspects due to differences in how Mandarin and English handle prosody. In English, stress can emphasize certain words within a sentence or distinguish between words with different meanings, such as the difference between *a record* (noun) and *to record* (verb). Mandarin, on the other hand, does not use stress similarly, making it difficult for Mandarin speakers to adjust to English stress patterns (Zhang *et al.*, 2008). Intonation, thus, is another area where they may face challenges. English uses intonation to signal questions, statements and emotions, with rising intonation typically indicating a question and falling intonation signaling a statement. Mandarin speakers might transfer their native tonal patterns to English, leading to speech that sounds either overly flat or overly melodic to native English listeners. For example, a Mandarin speaker might use a rising tone on a statement intended to be declarative, making it sound like a question to an English listener (Zhu & Wu, 2011).

Grammar

The following language sample illustrates common grammatical challenges encountered by Mandarin-English bilingual speakers, reflecting issues with grammar. It provides insight into the impact of linguistic transfer and the difficulty of adapting to English grammar rules.

Mandarin Chinese-English language sample reflecting bilinguals' challenges

Last week, I attend a conference in a more big city to learn about new idea in my field. The event has many sessions, and I listen to several talk on interesting topics. At first, I feel nervous because the building is large, and I cannot find the correct room. A staff member help me, and I finally arrive on time. The first presentation discuss technology in education, and it is one of the most informative session I attend.

During lunch break, I meet a professor from another university. He tell me about his research, which is more advanced than mine. We share contact information and agree to keep in touch. After lunch, I visit exhibition hall. There are many booth display books, tools and software.

I buy a book about communication because it seems the most useful resource for my work.

In the evening, I decide to explore the city. I find a restaurant that serve traditional dish. The food is delicious, but I think the food in my hometown is more cheap. After dinner, I walk through a park near hotel. The park is very quiet, and I take a few picture of the fountain and flower.

The language sample illustrates how Mandarin-English bilinguals may exhibit differences in aspects of English grammar that are not present in Mandarin, including pluralization, verb tense inflection, adjective comparison and article usage. These challenges are rooted in the structural differences between the two languages. SLPs working with bilingual speakers should consider these differences to differentiate between language transfer and true language disorders, ensuring effective intervention strategies.

Morphology

The typological differences between English and Mandarin Chinese are mainly due to the different language families to which they belong. English belongs to the Germanic branch of the Indo-European language family and has a rich morphological system, with variations for verb tense, noun singular and plural, and the comparative and superlative forms of adjectives. Such variation plays a vital role in English grammar, helping to distinguish time, quantity and degree. However, Mandarin Chinese belongs to the Sino-Tibetan language family and is an isolating language with basically no morphological variation. Grammatical relations are mainly expressed through word order and context. This typological difference makes bilingual Mandarin-English clients often find it challenging to master the complexity of morphological variation and tense marking in English, which may lead to grammatical errors when using English.

Singular and plural changes of nouns

In English, singular and plural noun forms are expressed through word form changes. Singular nouns usually do not have suffixes, while plural nouns are typically expressed by adding *-s* or *-es* to the word end. In addition, there are nouns with irregular plural forms, such as *child* becoming *children*, or *foot* becoming *feet*. In contrast, Mandarin Chinese nouns do not distinguish singular-plural forms. The plural is usually expressed through quantifiers or context, such as 一个苹果 <*yí gè píngguǒ*> 'one apple' in the singular and 两个苹果 <*liǎng gè píngguǒ*> 'two apples' in the plural. This invariance of noun morphology may lead English learners with a Mandarin background to make mistakes in English expressions, such as omitting the plural marker '-s' or misusing plural forms (Table 21.3).

Table 21.3 Comparison of singular and plural forms of nouns

Noun type	English examples	Mandarin Chinese examples
Singular	*one* ***apple***	一个苹果 <yí gè píngguǒ>
Plural	*two* ***apples***	两个苹果 <liǎng gè píngguǒ>
Irregular singular	*one* ***child***	一个孩子 <yí gè háizi>
Irregular plural	*two* ***children***	两个孩子 <liǎng gè háizi>

Table 21.4 Comparison of verb tense changes for English *go* and Chinese 去 <qù> 'go'

Tense	English examples	Mandarin Chinese examples
Present tense	I **go** to school.	我去学校 *<wǒ qù xué xiào>*。
Past tense	I **went** to school yesterday.	我昨天去学校了*<wǒ zuó tiān qù xué xiào le>*。
Future tense	I **will go** to school tomorrow.	我明天去学校 *<wǒ míng tiān qù xué xiào>*。
Present perfect	I **have gone** to school.	我已经去学校了*<wǒ yǐ jīng qù xué xiào le>*。
Past perfect	I **had gone** to school.	我之前已经去学校了*<wǒ zhī qián yǐ jīng qù xué xiào le>*。

Verb tense inflection

The English verb tense system is complex, and the verb form changes according to the tense. In contrast, Mandarin verb forms do not change with tense. Temporal relations are expressed through time adverbs, e.g. 昨天 <*zuótiān*> 'yesterday', aspect markers like 了 <le> which has no direct English equivalent. It functions as an aspect marker indicating action completion or a state change to indicate action completion or state change, and context. The adverb 已经 <yǐjīng> 'already' emphasizes that an action has occurred (Liu, 2015) (Table 21.4).

This difference in tense changes poses a challenge to learners with a Mandarin background, which can easily lead to ignoring the changes in verb forms in English and then making tense errors.

Adjective inflection

In English, the comparative and superlative degrees of adjectives are expressed through morphological changes. However, Mandarin adjectives do not undergo morphological changes, and the expression of comparative and superlative degrees depends on adding adverbs such as 更 <gèng> 'more' and 最 <zuì> 'most' before the adjective. For example, 高 <gāo> 'tall' becomes 更高 <gèng gāo> 'taller' when 更 <gèng> 'more' is added to indicate the comparative degree, and it becomes 最高 <zuì gāo> 'the tallest' when 最 <zuì> 'most' is added to express the superlative degree. Since adjectives in Mandarin are not conjugated, bilingual

Table 21.5 Comparative and superlative adjectives

Adjective type	English examples	Mandarin Chinese examples
Monosyllabic	big, bigger, the biggest	大 <dà>, 更大 <gèng dà>, 最大 <zuì dà>
Polysyllabic	beautiful, more beautiful, the most beautiful	漂亮 <piào liàng>, 更漂亮 <gèng piào liàng>, 最漂亮 <zuì piào liàng>

speakers may fail to adjust the adjectives when forming comparative and superlative degrees in English, which results in incorrect expressions or grammatical mistakes (Table 21.5).

Tense and aspect

Mandarin expresses tense and aspect differently as it does not use verb inflections like English. Instead, it relies on specific markers, time words and context to indicate tense. Key markers such as 在 *<zài>* 'indicating ongoing action,' 了 *<le>* 'indicating completed action' and 过 *<guò>* 'indicating experience or completion' play central roles in expressing time-related meanings (Comrie, 1985; Xiao & McEnery, 2004).

Present tense. Mandarin uses 在 *<zài>* 'indicating ongoing action' to denote actions in progress, for example, 我在看书 *<wǒ zài kàn shū>* 'I am reading a book.' Here, 在 *<zài>* emphasizes the continuity of the action, corresponding to the English present continuous tense.

Past tense. Past actions in Mandarin are typically indicated by time words or contextual cues, rather than verb changes. For example, 我昨天打电话给他了 <wǒ zuó tiān dǎ diàn huà gěi tā le> 'I called him yesterday.' The time word 昨天 <zuó tiān> 'yesterday' establishes the past tense, while the marker 了 <le> 'indicating completed action' signifies that the action has been concluded.

Contextual cues can also be used to indicate past actions. In the example, 你什么时候回来的？<nǐ shén me shí hòu huí lái de> 'When did you come back?', the listener and speaker are in the same place, and the speaker's presence implies that the action of 'coming back' has already been completed. Even without explicit time words like *yesterday*, the conversational context clearly signals that the action occurred in the past.

Present perfect tense. Mandarin expresses completed actions or experiences with markers like 已经 <yǐ jīng> 'already' or 过 <guò> 'indicating experience', for example, 我去过那个城市 <wǒ qù guò nà gè chéng shì> 'I have visited that city.' 过 <guò> signifies completion and conveys prior experience.

Future tense. Future tense in Mandarin is expressed through time words rather than grammatical markers. The time word 明天 <míng tiān> 'tomorrow' clearly indicates a future event in the example 我明天去学校 <wǒ míng tiān qù xué xiào> 'I will go to school tomorrow.'

The differences in tense expression can affect English learners from a Mandarin background, leading to challenges such as a tendency to use base verb forms and difficulties with mastering verb conjugations, often resulting in grammatical errors.

Word order

There are significant differences in grammatical structure between Mandarin Chinese and English, which manifest in the placement of prepositions, negative sentence structure, the order of multiple adjectives and the use of modifiers and attributive clauses.

First, the use of prepositions is significantly different in Mandarin and English. Using Mandarin prepositions is more flexible, and prepositional phrases are usually placed before verbs to express time, place and other relationships. For example, in 我在家学习<wǒ zài jiā xué xí> 'I study at home' the prepositional phrase 在家<zài jiā> 'at home' appears before the verb 学习<xué xí> 'study,' following the typical Mandarin Chinese sentence structure (Li & Thompson, 1981). In contrast, the use of English prepositions is relatively fixed, in being placed after verbs to form prepositional phrases, e.g. *I study at home* (Celce-Murcia & Larsen-Freeman, 1999).

Second, the structure of negative sentences differs in the two languages. Mandarin negation is realized by adding 没 *<méi>* 'have not, did not, be not, don't have' or 不 <bù> 'not' before the verb, such as 我没吃早餐 *<wǒ méi chī zǎo cān>* 'I didn't have breakfast' (Li & Thompson, 1989). 不 and 没 immediately precede the verb or anything that precedes and modifies the verb, including an adverb, a location phrase or any other prepositional phrase (Ross *et al.*, 2024).

There are also significant differences between Mandarin and English in the use of adjectives. When a single adjective modifies a noun, Mandarin and English use similar methods, with the adjective usually preceding the noun, such as 高楼 *<gāo lóu>* 'tall building.' However, when multiple adjectives are involved, differences in order between Mandarin and English begin to emerge. In Mandarin, the order is more flexible, usually based on context or a logical arrangement from the whole to the specific, such as – 辆红色的大卡车 <yī liàng hóng sè de dà kǎ chē> 'a red big truck.' In contrast, the order of adjectives in English is relatively fixed (Biber *et al.*, 1999).

Finally, Mandarin and English also show different ways in the use of modifiers and attributive clauses. In Mandarin, the modifiers of nouns (such as attributive clauses) are usually placed before the nouns and connected by the word 的 *<de>* 'of,' such as 我喜欢的那本红色的大书 *<wǒ xǐ huān de nà běn hóng sè de dà shū>* 'the big red book that I like' (Li & Thompson, 1981). In English, similar modifiers are usually placed after the nouns, such as *The big red book that I like.*

Passive voice

The construction of passive voice is also different in the two languages, especially in terms of usage frequency, grammatical structure, semantic function and emotional expression. English passive voice is very common and widely used in both formal and informal occasions. It can be used to emphasize the importance of the object or to blur or ignore the doer of the action, thus making the sentence more objective (Quirk *et al.*, 1985). However, the frequency of passive sentences in Mandarin Chinese is relatively low and used in specific contexts, especially when negative results or unclear agents are involved (Li & Thompson, 1981).

Regarding semantic function, passive sentences in Mandarin often carry negative or negative emotional connotations, especially when describing adverse consequences or when the recipient suffers adverse effects. This is consistent with Mandarin-speaking people paying more attention to context and implicit meaning in expression. Passive sentences are usually used to highlight the negative experiences of the recipient rather than simply describing objective facts (Ross *et al.*, 2024).

In terms of syntactic structure, the passive sentence structure in Mandarin is often introduced by the word 被 <*bèi*>. The agent is often omitted in actual use, especially when the actor is unclear or unimportant (Sun, 2006), as in 信被寄了<xìn bèi jì le> 'The letter was sent away.'

In addition, although Mandarin also uses passive sentences on formal occasions, compared to English, they tend to be more frequent in informal communication because Mandarin speakers often prioritize the subject as the figure, placing greater emphasis on the agent or actor, while the object or patient is treated as the ground. This preference aligns with Mandarin speakers' cognitive focus on the subject rather than the object, as described in the figure-ground theory (Li, 2014).

Definite and indefinite articles

Unlike in English that distinguishes the definite article *the* and the indefinite article *a*/*an*, Mandarin Chinese does not have an article system, but it conveys definiteness, indefiniteness or generic reference through modifiers and contextual cues. For example, consider the following dialogue:

A: 我今晚想看电影，你有推荐吗？

<wǒ jīnwǎn xiǎng kàn diànyǐng, nǐ yǒu tuījiàn ma?>

'I want to watch a movie tonight. Do you have any recommendations?'

B: 我们昨天看的电影特别棒。

<wǒmen zuótiān kàn de diànyǐng tèbié bang>

'The movie we watched yesterday was amazing.'

In A's sentence, 电影 *<diànyǐng>* 'movie' refers to an unspecified movie. The context indicates that the speaker is referring to a generic or unspecified movie. In B's response, the phrase 我们昨天看的 *<wǒmen zuótiān kàn de>* 'we watched yesterday' serves as a modifier that specifies the particular movie being referenced, compensating for the lack of a definite article like *the* in English. This example illustrates how Mandarin relies on contextual cues and modifiers, rather than an article system, to communicate definiteness, indefiniteness or generic reference. This phenomenon suggests that Mandarin-English speakers may ignore or misuse English articles affecting their expressions' accuracy.

Clinical Implications for Practitioners

The core purpose of SLPs when assessing and providing intervention for Mandarin-English bilinguals is to accurately identify language differences and barriers to ensure appropriate and practical support. Differences in their speech and language in English do not necessarily mean a language barrier but reflect the influence of different language features and cultural backgrounds (Roseberry-McKibbin, 2018). The therapist's task is to identify the reasons behind these manifestations and avoid misdiagnosing language differences as language disorders (Paradis, 2007).

Language differences and communication challenges

Language differences are one of the main challenges for SLPs when communicating with Chinese families. Although children from Chinese families mainly use English in school, their native language (such as Mandarin or Cantonese) may still be the primary language of communication within the family. This difference in the bilingual environment may cause SLPs to encounter language barriers when communicating with families, especially when discussing complex treatment plans or requiring parents to provide feedback, as Kohnert (2008) pointed out that language barriers may lead to inadequate information transmission and affect parents' understanding and implementation of treatment plans.

To address these challenges, SLPs should pay special attention to ensuring that information is conveyed when communicating with Chinese families, using the language familiar to the family as much as possible, and providing necessary interpretation or translation services (Lujan *et al.*, 2024). In addition, SLPs should recognize that language differences may not only be a matter of language itself but may also involve differences in cultural background and communication styles. Therefore, they need to continue to learn and adapt to cultural sensitivity to better support the needs of Chinese families (Sue & Sue, 2012).

Cultural background and communication patterns

Many Chinese families in North America may place strong emphasis on preserving and transmitting traditional Chinese culture, especially in relation to family structure and educational values. Collectivist values, defined as prioritizing the needs and goals of the group over the individual and emphasizing interdependence, familial obligations and respect for hierarchical relationships (Triandis, 1995), may be salient in many Chinese families, emphasizing respect for elders and the overall interests of the family. Parents often hold considerable authority within the family, and decision-making power may rest primarily with parents or grandparents. This family structure and cultural background can profoundly influence communication between SLPs and Chinese families.

Chinese families often place great importance on respecting authority, which affects their interactions with professionals like SLPs. This cultural tendency can lead to parents accepting professional guidance without questioning it, potentially resulting in a passive role during the treatment process (Gao, 1996; Hwang, 2006; Ting-Toomey, 1999). However, this may create a one-way communication dynamic, where parents or elders may rely heavily on professional advice without engaging in equal dialogue with SLPs. Understanding these dynamics, SLPs can create a more interactive and culturally sensitive relationship, encouraging open communication and active parental involvement to maximize treatment effectiveness. By doing so, SLPs can better align their interventions with the family's collective decision-making processes and cultural values.

In addition, the high context cultural background (a communication style where much of the meaning is derived from non-verbal cues, context and shared understanding rather than explicit verbal expression; Hall, 1976) of Chinese families may often lead them to prefer indirect communication methods to maintain harmonious relationships within and outside the family (Gao, 1996; Gudykunst & Kim, 2003). This indirectness may be misunderstood as a lack of interest or unwillingness to participate in the communication process between SLPs and families, thus affecting treatment progress. For this reason, SLPs could adopt more inclusive communication strategies when communicating with these families to ensure that treatment plans and suggestions are effectively conveyed while respecting culture. For example, during the treatment process, they can take the initiative to ask families about their views on cultural customs, traditions and values and consider these factors in the treatment plan. Such respect and understanding can make families feel recognized and respected, which will enhance their trust in the treatment leading to more active participation in the treatment process.

Assessment and intervention for Mandarin-English bilinguals

The assessment of Mandarin-English bilingual individuals requires culturally relevant, functional and holistic approaches that integrate standardized tools, dynamic assessments and qualitative measures. Currently, no standardized tests specifically cater to this population. As a result, SLPs need to combine Mandarin and English monolingual tests, complemented by qualitative data, to gain a comprehensive understanding of bilingual language abilities (American Speech-Language-Hearing Association [ASHA], n.d.; Bedore & Peña, 2008). See also the Action Plan as part of the ecosystemic approach (Babatsouli, 2023).

Assessment strategies

1. ***Case History***. Collecting a detailed language history is essential to understanding the linguistic environment and cultural context of bilingual individuals. Key aspects include:
   - Age and manner of language acquisition, frequency of use and proficiency in both languages.
   - Family language practices, academic instruction language and exposure to English as a second language (Rimikis *et al.*, 2013). Client interviews and ethnographic methods can enrich the case history and ensure cultural responsiveness (ASHA, n.d.).
2. ***Questionnaires***. Parent surveys and caregiver questionnaires, validated for cultural and linguistic relevance, provide valuable insights into language development, preferences and goals (Guiberson & Rodríguez, 2010). These tools are particularly effective for young children and adults recovering from neurological injuries.
3. ***Dynamic Assessment (DA)***. DA, such as test–teach–retest models or graduated prompting, helps identify bilingual individuals' learning potential and minimizes cultural bias (Gutiérrez-Clellen & Peña, 2001; Kapantzoglou *et al.*, 2012). Unlike standardized assessments, DA focuses on how individuals acquire and apply new skills, offering a more nuanced view of their abilities.
4. ***Speech and Language Sampling***. Speech and language sample analyses in both Mandarin and English allow for the observation of real-world communication skills. This approach provides insight into morphology, syntax, and phonological patterns across languages and tracks functional progress over time (Goldstein & Fabiano, 2007).

Assessment Tools and Accommodations

While standardized tests are not normed for Mandarin-English bilinguals, Chinese speaking SLPs have used tools like the Chinese Preschool Language Scale (CPLS; Zimmerman *et al.*, 2011, 学前儿童语言能力评

估量表), the Screening Tool for Delayed Language Development (S-S Method; Ren, 1986, 儿童语言发育迟缓检查法), the Peabody Picture Vocabulary Test (PPVT; Dunn & Dunn, 2007, 皮博迪图片词汇测验, Mandarin Chinese and English versions) and the Diagnostic Receptive and Expressive Assessment for Mandarin (DREAM-C; Bethel Hearing & Speaking Training Center, n.d., 梦想普通话听力理解和表达能力评估, designed for children aged 2;6–7;11), as well as its infant-toddler version, the Diagnostic Receptive and Expressive Assessment for Mandarin – Infant Toddler (DREAM-IT; Liu *et al.*, 2023). These tools can provide valuable descriptive data for assessing language abilities. Additionally, the Chinese Expressive Vocabulary Test (Zhang *et al.*, 2013, 中康 50 词) can offer supplementary insights into early vocabulary development.

The Mandarin Expressive Narrative Test (MENT; Hao *et al.*, 2018, 普通话叙事能力评估) is designed to evaluate macrostructure (e.g. character settings, initiating events) and microstructure (e.g. productivity, lexical diversity) in storytelling. The Strengths and Difficulties Questionnaire (SDQ; Goodman, 1997, adapted for Chinese populations) is a helpful socioemotional behavior assessment tool. Lastly, the Systematic Analysis of Language Transcripts (SALT; Miller & Chapman, 2002) and Computerized Language Analysis (CLAN; MacWhinney, 2000) offer robust methods for analyzing linguistic complexity and narrative structure, especially when examining bilingual or Mandarin-speaking children.

However, SLPs should be cautious about the validity, reliability, specificity and sensitivity of assessment tools (Friberg, 2010). Providing adjustments and collaborating with interpreters may be necessary to address cultural and linguistic differences. SLPs can document any modifications and interpret results cautiously to avoid misdiagnosis (ASHA, n.d.).

Intervention approaches

For Mandarin-English bilinguals, intervention can begin by utilizing Mandarin strengths as a foundation for acquiring English if they have a solid Mandarin foundation. For example, familiar grammatical structures in Mandarin can scaffold learning English syntax. The bilingual approach focuses on shared linguistic constructs to enhance skills applicable to both languages (Yavas & Goldstein, 1998). The cross-linguistic approach addresses language-specific needs, such as remediating Mandarin tone production or English final-consonant errors (Goldstein & Fabiano, 2007). Encouraging the use of Mandarin at home and in community settings helps preserve the individual's bilingual identity, supports dual-language proficiency and fosters emotional well-being (Genesee *et al.*, 2004). SLPs working with Mandarin-English bilinguals can adopt comprehensive, culturally sensitive assessment and intervention methods.

Combining monolingual tools, dynamic assessments and qualitative data allows clinicians to holistically address the linguistic and cultural complexities of this population. By recognizing the interplay between language and culture, SLPs can provide tailored, effective support that respects the client's bilingual identity.

Implications for Researchers

Mandarin-English bilingualism presents unique linguistic and cultural complexities, offering valuable opportunities for advancing research in speech-language pathology. Several critical areas warrant focused investigations:

Development of standardized assessment tools

The lack of standardized instruments appropriate for the Mandarin-English bilingual population hampers the proper measurement of language skills. Researchers need to develop new tests that are culturally and linguistically appropriate and must include both norm-referenced tests and dynamic assessments to assess bilingual language development.

Cultural dimensions of communication

The influence of cultural values, such as collectivism, high-context communication and deference to authority, on bilingual interactions with SLPs remains underexamined. Research into how these factors affect therapy outcomes could guide culturally responsive practices and improve client-clinician interactions.

Effectiveness of the intervention for the bilingual clients

There is limited research evidence on the effectiveness of the intervention approaches designed for Mandarin-English bilinguals. Research should focus on how strategies such as utilizing native language strengths, addressing language-specific needs and supporting bilingual identity affect intervention outcomes.

Technology in assessment and intervention of bilinguals

Current technologies like speech recognition software and machine learning have great potential in the assessment and intervention of bilingual languages. It would be useful for researchers to determine how these tools can improve the accuracy of diagnosis and help in the creation of effective, targeted and time-efficient treatment plans for such clients. This chapter also discusses dynamic assessment as an important approach to assessing language disorders in culturally and linguistically diverse populations such as the Mandarin-English bilinguals. Further research should ascertain whether it can identify language impairments as opposed to language differences in this type of speaker and determine the effectiveness of the approach in different settings and at different ages.

Conclusion

Mandarin-English bilingualism presents unique linguistic and cultural complexities that profoundly influence speech-language pathology practices. This chapter provides a foundation for understanding these differences and highlights the need for continuing advancements in assessment, intervention and research to better support this population. By addressing linguistic challenges and fostering cultural sensitivity, practitioners and researchers can significantly improve outcomes for bilingual individuals in diverse clinical settings.

References

American Speech-Language-Hearing Association (n.d.) Multilingual service delivery in audiology and speech-language pathology. *ASHA Practice Portal*. See https://www.asha.org/practice-portal/professional-issues/multilingual-service-delivery/ (accessed 1 December 2024).

Babatsouli, E. (2023) Ecosystemic cinical assessment of linguistic diversity: Greek-dominant speech. *Perspectives of the ASHA Special Interest Groups*, 9(3), 692–714. https://doi.org/10.1044/2023_PERSP-23-00088

Bedore, L.M. and Peña, E.D. (2008) Assessment of bilingual children for identification of language impairment: Current findings and implications for practice. *International Journal of Bilingual Education and Bilingualism* 11 (1), 1–29. https://doi.org/10.2167/beb392.0

Bethel Hearing & Speaking Training Center (n.d.) *Diagnostic Receptive and Expressive Assessment for Mandarin (DREAM-C; 梦想普通话听力理解和表达能力评估)*. See https://www.ourbethel.cn (accessed 1 December).

Biber, D., Johansson, S., Leech, G., Conrad, S. and Finegan, E. (1999) *Longman Grammar of Spoken and Written English*. Pearson Education.

Celce-Murcia, M. and Larsen-Freeman, D. (1999) *The Grammar Book: An ESL/EFL Teacher's Course* (2nd edn). Heinle & Heinle.

Chan, K.K.L. and To, C.K.S. (2016) Do individuals with high-functioning autism who speak a tone language show intonation deficits? *Journal of Autism and Developmental Disorders* 46 (5), 1784–1792. https://doi.org/10.1007/s10803-016-2709-5

Chang, I. (2003) *The Chinese in America: A Narrative History*. Viking.

Cheung, J. (2019) *Mind the Generation Gap: Heritage Language Often Lost by Third Generation*. University of Alberta.

Comrie, B. (1985) *Tense*. Cambridge University Press.

Duanmu, S. (2007) *The Phonology of Standard Chinese*. Oxford University Press.

Dunn, L.M. and Dunn, D.M. (2007) *Peabody Picture Vocabulary Test, Fourth Edition (PPVT; 皮博迪图片词汇测验, Mandarin Chinese and English Versions)*. Pearson Assessments.

Friberg, J.C. (2010) Considerations for test selection: How do validity and reliability impact diagnostic decisions? *Child Language Teaching and Therapy* 26 (1), 77–92. https://doi.org/10.1177/0265659009349972

Gao, F., Lyu, S. and Lin, C.C. (2021) Processing Mandarin tone 3 sandhi at the morphosyntactic interface: Reduplication and lexical compounds. *Frontiers in Psychology* 12, 713665. https://doi.org/10.3389/fpsyg.2021.713665

Gao, G. (1996) Self and other: A Chinese perspective on interpersonal relationships. In W.B. Gudykunst, S. Ting-Toomey and T. Nishida (eds) *Communication in Personal Relationships across Cultures* (pp. 81–101). Sage.

Genesee, F., Paradis, J. and Crago, M. (2004) *Dual Language Development and Disorders: A Handbook on Bilingualism and Second Language Learning*. Paul H. Brookes Publishing Co.

Goldstein, B.A. and Fabiano, L. (2007) Assessment and intervention for bilingual children with phonological disorders. *The ASHA Leader* 12 (2), 6–31. https://doi.org/10.1044/leader.FTR2.12022007

Goodman, R. (1997) The strengths and difficulties questionnaire: A research note. *Journal of Child Psychology and Psychiatry* 38 (5), 581–586. https://doi.org/10.1111/j.1469-7610.1997.tb01545.x

Gudykunst, W.B. and Kim, Y.Y. (2003) *Communicating with Strangers: An Approach to Intercultural Communication* (4th edn). McGraw-Hill.

Guiberson, M. and Rodríguez, B.L. (2010) Measurement properties and classification accuracy of two spanish parent surveys of language development for preschool-age children. *American Journal of Speech-Language Pathology* 19 (3), 225–237. https://doi.org/10.1044/1058-0360(2010/09-0058)

Gutiérrez-Clellen, V.F. and Peña, E.D. (2001) Dynamic assessment of diverse children: A tutorial. *Language, Speech, and Hearing Services in Schools* 32 (4), 212–224. https://doi.org/10.1044/0161-1461(2001/019)

Hall, E.T. (1976) *Beyond Culture*. Anchor Press.

Hao, Y., Sheng, L., Zhang, Y. and de Villiers, J. (2018) A narrative evaluation of Mandarin-speaking children with language impairment. *Journal of Speech, Language, and Hearing Research* 61 (5), 1121–1136. https://doi.org/10.1044/2017_JSLHR-L-16-0367

Hwang, W.C. (2006) Acculturative family distancing: Theory, research, and clinical practice. *Psychotherapy: Theory, Research, Practice, Training* 43 (4), 397–409. https://doi.org/10.1037/0033-3204.43.4.397

Kapantzoglou, M., Restrepo, M.A. and Thompson, M.S. (2012) Dynamic assessment of word learning skills: Identifying language impairment in bilingual children. *Language, Speech, and Hearing Services in Schools* 43 (1), 81–96. https://doi.org/10.1044/0161-1461(2011/10-0095)

Kohnert, K. (2008) *Language Disorders in Bilingual Children and Adults*. Plural Publishing.

Kondo-Brown, K. (2006) *Heritage Language Development: Focus on East Asian Immigrants*. John Benjamins Publishing.

Li, B. (2014) A comparative study of English and Chinese passives from the perspective of figure-ground theory. *Theory and Practice in Language Studies* 4 (7), 1370–1375. https://doi.org/10.4304/tpls.4.7.1370-1375

Li, C.N. and Thompson, S.A. (1977) The acquisition of tone in Mandarin-speaking children. *Journal of Child Language* 4 (2), 185–199. https://doi.org/10.1017/S0305000900001598

Li, C.N. and Thompson, S.A. (1989) *Mandarin Chinese: A Functional Reference Grammar*. University of California Press.

Li, P.S. (1998) *The Chinese in Canada*. Oxford University Press.

Li, Q. (2016) An investigation of sonority theory in Mandarin Chinese. In M.J. Ball and N. Müller (eds) *Challenging Sonority: Cross-Linguistic Evidence* (pp. 97–109). Equinox Publishing. https://doi.org/10.1558/equinox.25671

Li, S., Wang, Y., Yu, Q., Feng, Y. and Tang, P. (2024) The effect of visual articulatory cues on the identification of Mandarin tones by children with cochlear implants. *Journal of Speech, Language, and Hearing Research* 67 (7), 2106–2114. https://doi.org/10.1044/2024_JSLHR-23-00559

Liu, F. (2009) Intonation systems of Mandarin and English: A functional approach (Publication No. 3350885). Doctoral dissertation, University of Chicago. ProQuest Dissertations & Theses Global.

Liu, H.M. and Chien, H.Y. (2020) Speech sound errors of Mandarin-speaking preschool children with co-occurring speech sound disorder and developmental language disorder. *Clinical Linguistics & Phonetics* 34 (12), 1130–1148. https://doi.org/10.1080/02699206.2020.1724334

Liu, M. (2015) Tense and aspect in Mandarin Chinese. In W.S.-Y. Wang and C. Sun (eds) *The Oxford Handbook of Chinese Linguistics* (pp. 274–289). Oxford University Press.

Liu, X.L., Lee, W., Rolfhus, E., Hutchings, T., Yao, L., Xie, J., Xu, Y., Peng, Y. and de Villiers, J. (2023) The development of a parent report instrument of early communication and language skills of infants and toddlers in mainland China. *International Journal of Language & Communication Disorders* 58 (1), 1–16. https://doi.org/10.1111/1460-6984.12874

Lujan, K., Geerdes, K., Morelock, M. and An, R. (2024) Nationwide survey: Disparities in speech-language pathology service knowledge between Hispanic communities and the general public through explanatory mixed methods. *SACAD: John Heinrichs Scholarly and Creative Activity Days* 2024 (62). https://scholars.fhsu.edu/sacad/vol2024/iss2024/62

McBride-Chang, C., Tong, X., Shu, H., Wong, A.M.Y., Leung, K.-W. and Tardif, T. (2008) Syllable, phoneme, and tone: Psycholinguistic units in early Chinese and English word recognition. *Scientific Studies of Reading* 12 (2), 171–194. https://doi.org/10.1080/10888430801917290

MacWhinney, B. (2000) *The CHILDES Project: Tools for Analyzing Talk* (3rd edn). Lawrence Erlbaum Associates.

Miller, J. and Chapman, R. (2002) *Systematic Analysis of Language Transcripts (SALT)* (Version 9). University of Wisconsin.

Ministry of Education of the People's Republic of China (2022, 21 October) *A Review of Achievements in the Development of Chinese Language (2012–2021).* See https://en.moe.gov.cn/documents/reports/202210/t20221022_671530.html

Paradis, J. (2007) Bilingual children with specific language impairment: Theoretical and applied issues. *Applied Psycholinguistics* 28 (4), 551–576. https://doi.org/10.1017/S0142716407070300

Pew Research Center (2024) *Chinese Americans: A Survey Data Snapshot*. Pew Research Center. https://www.pewresearch.org/2024/08/06/chinese-americans-a-survey-data-snapshot

Quirk, R., Greenbaum, S., Leech, G. and Svartvik, J. (1985) *A Comprehensive Grammar of the English Language*. Longman.

Ren, Z. (1986) *儿童语言发育迟缓检查法 (S-S 法) [Screening Tool for Delayed Language Development (S-S Method)]*. Beijing Language and Culture University Press.

Rimikis, J.J., Pindzola, R.H. and Larsen, D.E. (2013) *Language Disorders across the Lifespan*. Delmar Cengage Learning.

Roseberry-McKibbin, C. (2018) *Multicultural Students with Special Language Needs: Practical Strategies for Assessment and Intervention* (5th edn). Academic Communication Associates.

Ross, C., Ma, J.-H.S., Chen, P.-C., He, B. and Yeh, M. (2024) *Modern Mandarin Chinese Grammar: A Practical Guide* (3rd edn). Routledge. https://doi.org/10.4324/9781003335078

Statistics Canada (2023) *Chinese New Year and Quality of Life among Chinese in Canada*. Statistics Canada. https://www.statcan.gc.ca/o1/en/plus/2816-chinese-new-year-and-quality-life-among-chinese-canada

Sue, D.W. and Sue, D. (2012) *Counseling the Culturally Diverse: Theory and Practice* (6th edn). Wiley.
Sun, C. (2006) *Chinese: A Linguistic Introduction*. Cambridge University Press.
Takaki, R. (1998) *Strangers from a Different Shore: A History of Asian Americans*. Little, Brown.
Ting-Toomey, S. (1999) *Communicating across Cultures*. Guilford Press.
Triandis, H.C. (1995) *Individualism and Collectivism*. Westview Press.
Wong, A.M.-Y., Ciocca, V. and Yung, S. (2009) The perception of lexical tone contrasts in Cantonese children with and without specific language impairment (SLI). *Journal of Speech, Language, and Hearing Research* 52 (6), 1493–1509. https://doi.org/10.1044/1092-4388(2009/08-0170)
Xiao, R. and McEnery, T. (2004) *Aspect in Mandarin Chinese: A Corpus-Based Study*. John Benjamins Publishing. https://doi.org/10.1075/slcs.67
Xu, Y. (1997) Contextual tonal variations in Mandarin. *Journal of Phonetics* 25 (1), 61–83.
Yang, J. and Resendiz, M. (2024) Assessing speech production in Mandarin-English bilingual children: Comparison of Mandarin and English sound systems and special considerations. *Perspectives of the ASHA Special Interest Groups* 9 (3), 715–737. https://doi.org/10.1044/2023_PERSP-23-00101
Yavas, M. and Goldstein, B.A. (1998) Phonological assessment and treatment of bilingual speakers. *American Journal of Speech-Language Pathology* 7 (2), 49–60.
Zhu, C. and Wu, X. (2011) A study of yes/no questions in English and Chinese: With special reference to Chinese EFL learners' understanding of their forms and functions. *Journal of Pragmatics* 43 (2), 632–647. https://doi.org/10.1016/j.pragma.2010.09.009
Zhu, H. and Dodd, B. (2000) The phonological acquisition of Putonghua (Modern Standard Chinese). *Journal of Child Language* 27 (1), 3–42.
Zhang, H., Wu, Y. and Li, X. (2013) *Chinese Expressive Vocabulary Test (中康 50 词)*. Beijing Normal University Press.
Zhang, J. (2010) Issues in the analysis of Chinese tone. *Language and Linguistics Compass* 4 (12), 1137–1153. https://doi.org/10.1111/j.1749-818X.2010.00259.x
Zhang, X.-Y., Yu, W.-Y., Teng, W.-J., Lu, M.-Y., Wu, X.-L., Yang, Y.-Q., Chen, C., Liu, L.-X., Liu, S.-H. and Li, J.-J. (2021) Effectiveness of melodic intonation therapy in Chinese Mandarin on non-fluent aphasia in patients after stroke: A randomized control trial. *Frontiers in Neuroscience* 15. https://doi.org/10.3389/fnins.2021.648724
Zhang, Y., Nissen, S.L. and Francis, A.L. (2008) Acoustic characteristics of English lexical stress produced by native Mandarin speakers. *Journal of the Acoustical Society of America* 123 (6), 4498–4513. https://doi.org/10.1121/1.2902165
Zimmerman, I.L., Steiner, V.G. and Pond, R.E. (2011) *Preschool Language Scales, Fifth Edition (CPLS; 学前儿童语言能力评估量表)*. Pearson Assessments.

22 Acquisition of Catalan by Multilingual Adults with L1 Mandarin

Influence from Previous Language Knowledge and Social Context

Ruochen Ning

Introduction

Context and culture

Catalan: Geographical distribution and current status

Catalan is a Romance language spoken by approximately 10 million people across Spain, France, Italy and Andorra (Prieto *et al.*, 2015). Within the Spanish territory, Catalan is present in Catalonia, Valencia, the Balearic Islands and parts of Aragon and Murcia (Vernet & Pons, 2011). It is also spoken in southern France's Roussillon region, the city of l'Alguer in Sardinia, Italy, and is the official language of Andorra (Wheeler *et al.*, 1999). Notably, most Catalan speakers are bilingual, also speaking other official or majority language(s) depending on their location. Apart from being the sole official language of Andorra, Catalan holds co-official status in Spain's regions of Catalonia, Valencia and the Balearic Islands, alongside Spanish. In Italy, Catalan is recognized as a minority language under Article 2 of Law 482/1999, which acknowledges Catalan as the traditional language of the municipality of l'Alguer in Sardinia. Regionally, the Sardinian Law 26/1997 granted Catalan minority status within a framework primarily aimed at protecting the Sardinian language (Caria, 2014). In France, Catalan is designated as a 'regional language', a term that lacks a precise legal definition and does not ensure its use in public administration within the historical territory of Northern Catalonia (Apaolaza, 2015; Peytaví Deixona, 2021). This area, encompassed by the region of France known as the 'Oriental Pyrenees Department', includes the traditionally Catalan-speaking districts of Roussillon, Vallespir, Conflent, Cerdagne and Capcir (Pons, 2020).

The majority of Catalan speakers are found in Spain, in the region of Catalonia and Valencia, with smaller populations in the Balearic Islands and other territories (Prieto *et al.*, 2015). In this chapter, we will examine the acquisition of Catalan by Chinese multilingual adults in Catalonia. Our focus on Catalonia, as opposed to other Catalan-speaking regions, is justified by its substantial number of speakers, unique sociolinguistic context and robust efforts to promote the use of Catalan and sustain bilingualism. The choice to study Chinese multilingual adults stems from the considerable population of Chinese immigrants in Catalonia, more than 60,000 until 2023,[1] which provides a relevant demographic for this study. Additionally, the significant linguistic distance between their first language (L1) and Catalan, as well as the cultural differences between their native country and the host society, highlight the obstacles they may encounter. In the context of globalization, some Chinese immigrants in Catalonia, especially the young generation, choose to move to North America for various reasons, including career development and education for their descendants. They may encounter new language issues, such as mastering English, in the new host society. Unlike children, these adults usually do not benefit from formal education at school with the target language as the instruction medium, thereby facing greater challenges in language acquisition.

In the following sections of this chapter, I will first introduce the sociolinguistic context in Catalonia and its language policies. I will then briefly describe the current situation of Chinese immigrants in Catalonia. To give a clear idea of the differences between Mandarin and Catalan, I compare the two languages from both phonological and grammatical aspects. After the comparison, I provide a small story in Catalan as a language sample to analyze possible influences from learners' L1 Mandarin and L2 Spanish. At the end of this chapter, I give relevant suggestions to researchers and speech-language practitioners about adults with such a linguistic background in North America based on findings from the current study.

Catalonia: Sociolinguistic Situation and Political Landscape

Language is a crucial symbolic resource, and nations have always invested other resources such as laws, services and educational systems to control the languages spoken within their boundaries (Andresen, 2016). From a political perspective, language and the nation-state are closely related. Thus, the word for a language often means people of that nation as well, like French, German and Italian. That's why *language* and *dialect* are in fact political concepts in that language is the official and the symbolic, while dialects are marginalized.

This One Nation One Language ideology could be seen in Catalonia in the linguistic repression during Franco's regime. During Francisco Franco's dictatorship (1939–1975), the Catalan language faced systematic repression as part of a broader strategy to enforce Spanish national unity and eliminate regional identities. The regime implemented a series of legal, political and cultural measures to eradicate Catalan from public life, education and administration. Catalan was banned in schools, courts and government institutions, and public officials were prohibited from using it in official capacities. Publishing in Catalan was censored, traditional cultural expressions were suppressed and even street signs were forcibly changed to Spanish (Palau, 2011). This linguistic repression was not merely an attempt at assimilation but rather a deliberate act of cultural and political subjugation, reinforcing the hegemony of Spanish as the only legitimate national language. In response, the Catalan people resisted through clandestine cultural initiatives, underground publishing and linguistic activism, viewing the preservation of their language as an act of political defiance and cultural survival. The fight to reclaim Catalan was not only about linguistic rights but also about preserving historical identity, regional autonomy and democratic freedoms.

After Franco's death, to promote and revitalize Catalan, public authorities have implemented numerous language policies that aimed at encouraging its use among the population, as part of the broader linguistic normalization process (Pons, 2020).

Language law and language policies

La Normalització Lingüística (Linguistic Normalization), implemented in 1983 by the Generalitat de Catalunya, aimed to reverse the language shift from Catalan to Spanish and promote Catalan in the aftermath of dictatorship and linguistic repression (Newman & Trenchs-Parera, 2015). Key aspects of this policy included providing a supportive framework for the Catalan language while avoiding antagonizing the Spanish-speaking population (Newman & Trenchs-Parera, 2015). For instance, the policy mandated the use of Catalan in public administration and education, ensuring that Catalan became the primary language of instruction in schools and universities (Roller, 2002). The media also played a significant role in this normalization process. Catalan-language television and radio stations, such as TV3 and Catalunya Ràdio (Catalonia Radio), were established to provide content in Catalan, helping to increase its presence in everyday life (Camps-Durban, 2022). Additionally, the publication of books, newspapers and magazines in Catalan was encouraged and supported by the government (Crameri, 2008).

One of the notable successes of *Normalització Lingüística* is the widespread use of Catalan in education. Today, Catalan is the main language of instruction in most schools and universities in Catalonia, with students achieving high levels of proficiency (Garvía & Santana, 2020; Muñoz, 2005). This has helped to ensure that younger generations are fluent in Catalan, securing its future as a living language.

Then, in 2004, the *Pla per la Llengua i la Cohesió Social* (Plan for Language and Social Cohesion) was inaugurated, addressing the demographic stability of the Catalan language amidst potential threats from globalization and international immigration, while also aiming to preserve social cohesion in a linguistically diverse society (Besalú & Besalú Costa, 2006). This policy builds on the infrastructure established by the earlier *Normalització Lingüística*, which successfully promoted the use of Catalan in public life (Newman & Trenchs-Parera, 2015). Recognizing the evolving challenges of the 21st century, the Plan for Language and Social Cohesion seeks to ensure that Catalan remains a vibrant and widely spoken language in Catalonia.

This policy highlights the promotion of societal multilingualism, which acknowledges the linguistic diversity brought about by immigration. It encourages the learning of Catalan among immigrants through language courses and integration programs, thereby fostering a sense of belonging and participation in Catalan society. For example, the *Consorci per a la Normalització Lingüística* (Consortium for Linguistic Normalization) offers free Catalan courses at A1 and A2 level,[2] helping newcomers to gain basic knowledge of the Catalan language and thus integrate more effectively into the host society (Branchadell, 2015; Conesa & Ibarz, 2015).

Linguistic parochialism vs linguistic cosmopolitanism

In Catalonia, the use and choice of language remain subjects of ongoing debate, reflecting the region's complex sociolinguistic landscape. Catalan residents exhibit diverse attitudes and language ideologies, which can be broadly categorized into two prevailing perspectives: linguistic parochialism and linguistic cosmopolitanism (Newman *et al.*, 2008; Trenchs-Parera & Newman, 2009).

Linguistic parochialism in Catalonia refers to attitudes that strongly favor one language over the other, often rejecting compromise or accommodation. This phenomenon manifests in two primary forms: pro-Catalan parochialism and pro-Spanish parochialism (Trenchs-Parera & Newman, 2009). Pro-Catalan parochialism supports the use of the Catalan language and rejects compromise with Spanish or the Spanish state. This attitude is closely associated with a strong Catalan national identity and support for Catalan linguistic and national aspirations. Proponents of this view often advocate for policies that prioritize Catalan in public life, seeing the language as a crucial element of Catalonia's cultural heritage and autonomy. For example, they may support the enforcement of Catalan as the primary language of instruction in schools and the exclusive use of Catalan in official government communications (Oller *et al.*, 2021). On the other hand, pro-Spanish parochialism favors the Spanish language and dismisses Catalan linguistic and national aspirations.

This view is more common among individuals whose first language is Spanish or who identify more strongly with a Spanish national identity. Proponents of this perspective may argue that Spanish, being the official language of Spain, should take precedence in public and official domains (Trenchs-Parera & Newman, 2009). They might oppose policies that they perceive as marginalizing Spanish speakers or undermining the unity of Spain. For instance, they may criticize the mandatory use of Catalan in education and public administration, advocating instead for a bilingual approach that gives equal status to both languages. This stance can be seen as a reaction to the perceived overemphasis on Catalan and the fear that such policies could lead to social division or discrimination against Spanish speakers (Kozhanovsky, 2024).

Both forms of linguistic parochialism reflect deeper sociopolitical tensions within Catalonia, where language is not merely a means of communication but a symbol of identity and political allegiance (Woolard, 2016). The challenge lies in balancing these competing attitudes to foster a cohesive society that respects and values its linguistic diversity.

In contrast, linguistic cosmopolitanism refers to attitudes that favor accommodation, bilingualism and linguistic diversity, promoting a harmonious coexistence of languages within the region (Trenchs-Parera & Newman, 2009). This perspective supports bilingualism and values proficiency in both Catalan and Spanish, recognizing the importance of each language in different spheres of life. For instance, Catalan is often seen as the language of cultural identity and regional pride, while Spanish serves as a bridge to the broader Spanish-speaking world and international communication (Ning, 2024a). This dual proficiency is encouraged through educational policies that ensure students achieve high levels of competence in both languages, preparing them for a multilingual and globalized society.

Linguistic cosmopolitanism looks beyond parochial in-group communities and favors bridging linguistic boundaries. It encourages interactions and exchanges between different linguistic groups, fostering mutual understanding and respect (De Costa & Jou, 2016; Newman *et al.*, 2008). This is evident in initiatives such as language exchange programs and cultural festivals that celebrate the linguistic diversity of Catalonia. For example, events like the 'Festa de la Diversitat' (Festival of Diversity) bring together speakers of various languages to share their cultures and languages, promoting a sense of community and inclusivity.

Chinese Immigrants in Catalonia: New and Special Speakers of Catalan

Among the immigrants in Catalonia, the community of Chinese origin is special since they are one of the largest immigrant communities while also being geographically, linguistically and culturally the most distant one. By 2023, there were already 61,864 Chinese immigrants residing in Catalonia without counting those who had obtained Spanish citizenship.

Many Chinese immigrants in Catalonia are involved in small businesses and entrepreneurship. They often run small shops and enterprises, particularly in urban areas like Barcelona. These businesses are typically characterized by small size, long working hours and the employment of family members or other employees of the same origin (Del Pozo, 2006). Some Chinese immigrants, especially those from the younger first generation and second generation, work in professional fields such as law, teaching, medicine or in multinational companies. Their monthly incomes are generally around 1,500 to 2,000 euros, which is close to the average per capita salary in Spain. Despite their socioeconomic class, their participation in broader social and political activities in Spanish society is relatively low (Li & Du, 2023).

First-generation Chinese immigrants usually face greater language barriers that hinder their integration into Catalan society. However, there are notable differences between first-generation and second-generation Chinese immigrants. The second generation tends to have a higher level of education, better language skills and a stronger sense of belonging to Spanish society compared to the first generation (Li & Du, 2023). This generational shift is gradually leading to improved social integration.

Another significant segment of the Chinese immigrant community in Catalonia consists of international students of Chinese origin. These individuals initially arrived to pursue undergraduate or graduate studies at Catalan universities. Many chose to remain in the region after completing their academic programs, seeking professional opportunities or further integrating into Catalan society (Ning, 2024b). Similarly to second-generation Chinese immigrants, these students typically possessed a high level of education and advanced linguistic competencies. Their multilingual abilities and familiarity with diverse cultural environments position them as active participants in social integration initiatives, which makes them new speakers of the Catalan language (Costa, 2015; Pujolar & Puigdevall, 2015), contributing significantly to fostering mutual understanding and enriching the sociocultural fabric of Catalonia.

Chinese immigrants in Catalonia usually have Mandarin and their regional varieties (if applicable) as their L1, and they often prioritize learning Spanish before Catalan due to its broader utility and prevalence in daily life and business across Spain (Solana *et al.*, 2012). Spanish is the dominant language in many social and professional contexts, making it a practical first step for integration. Additionally, many Chinese immigrants, especially those who came to carry out their studies in Catalonia, usually used Mandarin as a communication medium within the Chinese community in Catalonia, and arrived with some knowledge of Spanish (Ning, 2022, 2023, 2024b), either through initial language courses or formal education, which eased their transition. However, even when they have some knowledge of Spanish, acquiring Catalan still presents unique challenges. The language has distinct phonetic, grammatical and lexical features that differ significantly from Spanish and Mandarin. In the following sections, I will focus on the acquisition of Catalan by this community, beginning with a brief comparison between Mandarin and Catalan.

Acquisition of Catalan by L1 Mandarin Speakers: A Comparison of Mandarin and Catalan Grammar

The grammatical structures of Mandarin and Catalan are fundamentally different, reflecting their distinct linguistic roots and typologies. I will compare them from three aspects: morphosyntax, phonetics and phonology, and orthography.

Morphosyntax

Mandarin, a Sino-Tibetan language, is characterized by its simplicity in morphology and syntax. Thus, it is usually classified as an isolating language. It lacks inflectional morphology (Li & Bates, 1993), meaning that verbs do not conjugate for tense, mood or aspect. Instead, temporal and aspectual distinctions are often conveyed through context or auxiliary words. For example, the verb 吃, chī 'to eat' remains the same regardless of whether it is in the past, present or future tense.

Chinese also employs a subject-verb-object (SVO) word order, similar to Catalan, but relies heavily on word order and particles to indicate grammatical relationships due to its lack of inflection, as in:

(1) 我 明天 去 银行。

*I tomorrow go to bank

'Tomorrow I will go to the bank'.

(2) 我现在去银行。

*I now go to bank.

'I'm going to the bank now'.

(3) 我 已经 到 银行了。

*I already arrive at bank.

'I have already arrived at the bank'.

(4) 我 昨天 去了 银行。

*I yesterday go to bank.

'Yesterday I went to the bank'.

Table 22.1 An example of nouns inflected for gender and number

a boy	un noi	a girl	una noia
the boy	el noi	the girl	la noia
two boys	dos nois	two girls	dues noies
the boys	els nois	the girls	les noies

In contrast, Catalan exhibits a rich inflectional morphology. Verbs in Catalan conjugate according to tense, mood, aspect, person and number (Wheeler *et al.*, 1999), resulting in a complex system of verb forms. For instance, the verb *menjar* 'eat' changes to *menjo* 'I eat' and *menjaré* 'I will eat' according to the person and the tense.

Catalan nouns also inflect for gender (masculine and feminine) and number (singular and plural), which affects the form of articles and adjectives that agree with the nouns. Additionally, Catalan uses definite and indefinite articles, which change form based on gender and number, such as *el* ('the,' masculine singular) and *la* ('the,' feminine singular) (see Table 22.1).

Phonetics and phonology

The Catalan phonological system is by and large more complicated than that of Mandarin, with mid-open and mid-closed contrasts in vowels, vowel reduction and final consonant clusters. However, an aspect that may make Mandarin more difficult to acquire is the use of tones. Mandarin uses four primary tones to distinguish meaning, making tonal pronunciation crucial for comprehension (Zhang, 2020). The same syllable can have different meanings depending on the tone used, such as 妈 mā 'mother' versus 马 mǎ 'horse'. Catalan, on the other hand, does not use tones to differentiate meaning, relying instead on segmental phonology, stress and intonation patterns similar to other Romance languages.

Orthography

The orthography is also significantly different between the two languages. Mandarin uses logographic characters 汉字 Hanzi where each character represents a morpheme, while Catalan uses the Latin alphabet, with a phoneme-to-grapheme correspondence that is not completely regular but far more predictable than Chinese characters. During the reading and writing process, each word should be separated using space in Catalan, while Mandarin does not give space between each word, which means that word segmentation is an essential skill in reading Mandarin.

Overall, while both languages share an SVO sentence structure, their grammatical systems are markedly different. Mandarin's use of logographic characters, lack of inflection and reliance on word order and particles contrasts sharply with Catalan's Latin alphabet, inflectional morphology and agreement rules. These differences highlight the unique challenges and learning curves for speakers of each language when acquiring the other.

A Catalan Language Sample and Analysis

To elucidate the potential challenges and acquisition patterns of Catalan by Chinese multilingual adults, this analysis will utilize a short story as an example. The focus will be on examining the linguistic differences between their first language, Mandarin, their second language, Spanish, and the target language, Catalan. This comparative analysis will highlight the morphological, syntactic and pragmatic discrepancies among these languages. Additionally, it will identify common errors that Chinese learners are likely to produce during the acquisition process.

Language sample: A story in Catalan

En Pere va sortir de casa amb una motxilla i un llibre vell que havia trobat a l'àtic. El sol començava a despuntar darrere de les muntanyes, i l'aire era fresc i net. Mentre caminava pel bosc, va escoltar el cant d'un rossinyol que semblava saludar-lo. 'Avui serà un gran dia', va pensar en Pere, somrient. Quan va arribar al riu, es va asseure en una roca i va obrir el llibre. Però, quina sorpresa! Dins del llibre hi havia una nota misteriosa: 'Segueix el camí del roure fins a la clariana.' En Pere va decidir seguir les instruccions, sense imaginar-se que aquell dia canviaria la seva vida per sempre.

Translation in English

Pere left the house with a backpack and an old book he had found in the attic. The sun was beginning to rise behind the mountains, and the air was fresh and clean. As he walked through the forest, he heard the song of a nightingale that seemed to greet him. 'Today will be a great day', Pere thought, smiling. When he reached the river, he sat down on a rock and opened the book. But what a surprise! There was a mysterious note inside the book: 'Follow the oak path to the clearing'. Pere decided to follow the instructions, without imagining that that day would change his life forever.

Analysis of the Language Sample: Potential Errors and Patterns in the Acquisition by Chinese Multilingual Adults

Possible influences from Mandarin

Articles and gender agreement

The use of both definite articles (*el*, *la*, *les*, *en*) and indefinite articles (*un*, *una*) in this small story illustrates a complex system of number and gender agreement in Catalan. Mandarin, in contrast, does not employ articles; it relies on context or demonstratives to indicate definiteness. This fundamental difference may pose challenges for L1 Mandarin speakers learning Catalan, as they must acquire the concept of articles and their correct usage. Common errors may include the omission of articles or incorrect gender and number agreement.

Tense and conjugation

This language sample demonstrates the use of various tenses, including the indefinite past tense (*va sortir*), the imperfect past tense (*començava a despuntar*) and the perfect past tense (*havia trobat*). In Mandarin, aspect markers are used instead of conjugated verbs to indicate tense. This structural difference can make it challenging for L1 Mandarin speakers to understand and distinguish between Catalan tenses. Potential difficulties may include incorrect verb conjugation and confusion regarding the appropriate use of the indefinite, perfect and imperfect past tenses in different contexts, especially the distinction between indefinite and imperfect past tense.

Prepositions

In this very short story, we can find the use of six prepositions: *de*, *a*, *amb*, *per*, *en*, *sense*. Prepositions in Catalan have specific uses that do not directly translate to Mandarin. Furthermore, some prepositions have various uses in different contexts, making it difficult for L1 Mandarin learners to distinguish. Thus, during the acquisition process, they may be confused by the use of some similar prepositions such as *en* and *a*.

Reflexive verbs

Reflexive verbs, such as '*es va asseure*' in the language sample, do not exist in Mandarin. The use of reflexive pronouns *es*/*se*, when it should be *es* or *se*, and the contexts in which they should or should not be used, can vary significantly. Consequently, learners may struggle to grasp their correct usage. Common errors among L1 Mandarin speakers include the omission of *es*/*se* in reflexive verbs, addition of *es*/*se* in non-reflexive verbs, and confusion between *es* and *se*.

Possible influence from Spanish

As we have discussed before, Chinese immigrants in Catalonia always learned Spanish before Catalan, or at least acquired both languages simultaneously in this bilingual society. Thus, their Spanish knowledge usually plays a crucial role in the acquisition of Catalan. In this part, I will explain the possible influences from Spanish based on this language sample.

Apostrophe, contraction and accent

A notable orthographic difference between Spanish and Catalan is the use of apostrophes and contractions, as exemplified by a *l'àtic* and *pel bosc* in the language sample. *L'àtic* is the contracted form of the definite article *el* (masculine) or *la* (feminine) when preceding a noun starting with a vowel, while *pel* is the contraction of *per el*. In Spanish, *por el* remains separate. Another significant difference is that Catalan features two types of accents: the open accent (`), which corresponds to an open vowel, and the closed accent (´), which corresponds to a closed vowel. The vowels <e> and <o> can bear both types of accents, whereas <a> is always open and takes the open accent, as in *àtic*. In contrast, Spanish employs only one type of accent, making the distinction between open and closed accents potentially challenging for learners.

Weak pronouns

Hi havia in the story is used to indicate existence. Its counterpart in Spanish is *había* and the clitic pronoun *hi* does not exist in Spanish. This may lead learners to use *havia* in Catalan context and omit *hi*.

Similar lexicons

There are some similar lexicons in Spanish and Catalan, such as *motxilla* ('mochila' in Spanish), *llibre* ('libro'), *fresc* ('fresco') and *dia* ('día'). For learners with Spanish knowledge, there might be negative transfer, and they may use Spanish lexicons directly when producing Catalan.

Small differences in grammar rules

There are nuanced differences between Catalan and Spanish that may confuse learners. One example is *en Pere*. In informal or colloquial contexts in Catalan, it is customary to use a definite article before a person's name, with the article agreeing in gender. In Spanish, articles are not used before a person's name, which may lead learners to omit the article in Catalan contexts. Other examples from the language sample include *saludar-lo* (compared to *saludarlo* in Spanish), *quina sorpresa!* (compared to *¡qué sorpresa!* in Spanish) and *la seva vida* (compared to *su vida* in Spanish). These differences are likely to cause errors when learners produce Catalan.

Implications for Researchers

Until now, language acquisition studies primarily focus on one-language-dominated societies, and acquisition that happens in a bilingual society has not been fully studied. The situation we have addressed in this chapter is particular in that almost all the Catalan learners in Catalonia acquire Spanish before or simultaneously with Catalan in the bilingual context. Cross-linguistic influences from Spanish should always be taken into consideration when studying the acquisition patterns of Catalan, especially for learners with non-Romance L1, such as Mandarin speakers in our case. A similar situation can also be found in the North American context, where a language other than English has a large number of speakers (like Spanish in Miami) or even has co-official status (French in Quebec). Speakers discussed in this chapter can also be found in North America facing a new language acquisition situation, such as English and French, where their Spanish and Catalan knowledge will play a role alongside their L1 Mandarin. In this case, the sociolinguistic situation and learners' language and cultural backgrounds should be taken into consideration when studying this group of speakers.

Implications for Practitioners

This chapter also offers valuable insights for speech-language practitioners, particularly regarding adult language acquisition and development patterns. What we have addressed here highlights the complexity and dynamism inherent in language acquisition in multilinguals, where previously acquired languages interact and influence the acquisition of the additional language. When working with this group of speakers in North America or working in other bilingual contexts such as Miami and Quebec, practitioners should be aware of the unique acquisition patterns with possible transfers between two or more languages and avoid making decisions merely based on monolingual standards. Understanding that adults bring pre-established communication patterns and varying degrees of proficiency in multiple languages, practitioners can tailor their approaches to address specific challenges, such as interference from other languages and the need for explicit instruction in areas where transfer is less likely. Additionally, recognizing the role of social context and cultural background in adult language learning can help practitioners create supportive, engaging and culturally responsive learning environments and strategies that facilitate sustained language development.

Conclusion

Language acquisition is a multifaceted process at any stage of human development. The acquisition of an additional language is not merely an augmentation of the learner's linguistic repertoire. Rather, it involves a complex interplay of all previously acquired linguistic knowledge. Throughout this process, various factors, including social context, cultural background and affective factors, play pivotal roles. The insights gained from studying Chinese multilinguals acquiring Catalan in Catalonia can be extrapolated to similar bilingual societies in North America, where immigrants from diverse origins coexist, thereby fostering a multilingual environment. Some of the Chinese multilinguals with L3 Catalan may also be found in North America, acquiring English or other languages. Each of their previously learned languages, including Mandarin, Spanish and Catalan, may influence their language use, which will lead to a complex linguistic interplay and special linguistic patterns. This chapter aimed to shed light on the intricate dynamics of language acquisition by adults in multilingual settings. More studies in different contexts are needed to gain a better understanding of this intriguing yet crucial process.

Notes

(1) https://www.idescat.cat/poblacioestrangera/?b=0&nac=d407 (accessed on January 8th, 2025).

(2) The Common European Framework of Reference for Languages (CEFR) divides language proficiency into six levels: 1) beginner: A1 and A2; 2) intermediate: B1 and B2; 3) advanced: C1 and C2.

References

Andresen, J.T. and Carter, P.M. (2016) *Languages in the World: How History, Culture, and Politics Shape Language*. Wiley Blackwell.

Apaolaza, E.Z. (2015) Principios constitucionales sobre las lenguas en Francia (Constitutional principles on languages in France). *Revista de Llengua i Dret* 63, 92–112. https://doi.org/10.2436/20.8030.02.95

Besalú, X. and Besalú Costa, X. (2006) El plan para la lengua y la cohesión social (Plan LIC) del gobierno de Cataluña (The language and social cohesion plan from the Government of Catalonia). *Revista Interuniversitaria de Formación Del Profesorado* 20 (2), 45–68.

Branchadell, A. (2015) Language education for adult migrants in Catalonia: Nation-state ambitions without nation-state resources. In J. Simpson and A. Whiteside (eds) *Adult Language Education and Migration* (pp. 82–93). Routledge. https://doi.org/10.4324/9781315718361-6

Camps-Durban, E. (2022) Radios libres y normalización del catalán: medios comunitarios en la recuperación de una lengua minorizada (Free radio and standardization of the Catalan language: The role of community media in the reinvigoration of a minority language). *Comunicacion y Medios* 36 (46), 135–147. https://doi.org/10.5354/0719-1529.2022.65956

Caria, M. (2014) Alghero-L'Alguer o i catalani d'Italia (Alghero-L'Alghero or the Catalans of Italy). *Bollettino Dell'Atlante Linguistico Italiano* 38, 75–90.

Conesa, A. and Ibarz, R. (2015) El Consorci per a la Normalització Lingüística: "25 anys fent bategar el català" (The Consortium for Language Normalisation: "25 years making Catalan's heart beat"). *Llengua i Ús: Revista Tècnica de Política Lingüística* 56, 70–78. http://gencat.cat/llengua/liu

Costa, J. (2015) New speakers, new language: On being a legitimate speaker of a minority language in Provence. *International Journal of the Sociology of Language* 2015 (231), 127–145. https://doi.org/10.1515/ijsl-2014-0035

Crameri, K. (2008) *Catalonia: National Identity and Cultural Policy, 1980–2003*. University of Wales Press.

De Costa, P.I. and Jou, Y.S. (2016) Unpacking the ideology of cosmopolitanism in language education: Insights from Bakhtin and Systemic Functional Linguistics. *Critical Inquiry in Language Studies* 13 (2), 73–97. https://doi.org/10.1080/15427587.2015.1132628

Del Pozo, P.S. (2006) El comercio de los inmigrantes en el centro histórico de Barcelona en 2004 (Immigrants' trade in the historic centre of Barcelona in 2004). *Estudios Geográficos* 67 (261), 635–672. https://doi.org/10.3989/egeogr.2006.i261.35

Garvía, R. and Santana, A. (2020) The linguistic regime in Catalan Schools: Some survey results. *European Journal of Language Policy* 12 (1), 85–108. https://doi.org/10.3828/ejlp.2020.5

Kozhanovsky, A.N. (2024) Кастильский и другие: языковая ситуация в современной Испании (Castilian and others: The language situation in today's Spain). *Cuadernos Iberoamericanos* 12 (1), 189–209. https://doi.org/10.46272/2409-3416-2024-12-1-189-209

Li, L. and Du, X. (2023) La integración social de los inmigrantes chinos en la España contemporánea: un análisis desde el trabajo de campo en Barcelona (The social integration of Chinese immigrants in contemporary Spain: An analysis from fieldwork in Barcelona). *Ibero-América Studies* 6 (2), 16–28. https://doi.org/10.55704/ias.v6i2.03

Li, P. and Bates, E. (1993) Processing a language without inflections: A reaction time study of sentence interpretation in Chinese. *Journal of Memory and Language* 32 (2), 169–192. https://doi.org/10.1006/jmla.1993.1010

Muñoz, C. (2005) Trilingualism in the Catalan educational system. *International Journal of the Sociology of Language* 171, 75–93. https://doi.org/10.1515/ijsl.2005.2005.171.75

Newman, M. and Trenchs-Parera, M. (2015) Language policies, ideologies and attitudes in Catalonia. Part 1: Reversing language shift in the twentieth century. *Language and Linguistics Compass* 9 (7), 285–294. https://doi.org/10.1111/LNC3.12141

Newman, M., Trenchs-Parera, M. and Ng, S. (2008) Normalizing bilingualism: The effects of the Catalonian linguistic normalization policy one generation after. *Journal of Sociolinguistics* 12 (3), 306–333. https://doi.org/10.1111/j.1467-9841.2008.00369.x

Ning, R. (2022) Chinese graduate students in Catalonia: Learning Catalan within the social networks in a bilingual society. *Journal of Multilingual and Multicultural Development* 43 (10), 935–950. https://doi.org/10.1080/01434632.2020.1783543

Ning, R. (2023) Language attitudes and identity construction through minority language learning in a host country. In T. Mammadova (ed.) *Academic Mobility through the Lens of Language and Identity, Global Pandemics, and Distance Internationalization* (pp. 48–58). Routledge. https://doi.org/10.4324/9781003366942-6

Ning, R. (2024a) "No one speaks Catalan with me" — Chinese Learners of Catalan in Barcelona: Difficulties to learn a minoritized language in a bilingual society. In C. Lamar Prieto and Á. González Alba (eds) *Digital Flux, Linguistic Justice and Minoritized Languages* (pp. 41–59). De Gruyter. https://doi.org/10.1515/9783110799392-003

Ning, R. (2024b) Chinese graduate students in Catalonia: Motivation to learn Catalan in a bilingual society. *Journal of Multilingual and Multicultural Development* 45 (2), 475–488. https://doi.org/10.1080/01434632.2021.1902335

Oller, J.M., Satorra, A. and Tobeña, A. (2021) Parochial linguistic education: Patterns of an enduring friction within a divided Catalonia. *Genealogy* 5 (3), 77. https://doi.org/10.3390/genealogy5030077

Palau, A. (2011) Un dispositif réglementaire au service d'une politique d'unification culturelle et linguistique: Les modalités de la répression anticatalane sous le régime franquiste (A regulatory system at the service of a policy of cultural and linguistic unification: The modalities of Anti-Catalan repression under Franco's regime). *Textes & Contextes* 6, 1–19.

Peytaví Deixona, J. (2021) Catalan language in French Catalonia today: A case of revernacularisation? A path between identity recovery and linguistic heritage. *Journal of Multilingual and Multicultural Development* 42 (10), 969–981. https://doi.org/10.1080/01434632.2020.1827649

Pons, E. (2020) Language law and language policies. In J.A. Argenter and J. Lüdtke (eds) *Manual of Catalan Linguistics* (pp. 649–668). De Gruyter. https://doi.org/10.1515/9783110450408-027

Prieto, P., Borras-Comes, J., Cabre, T., Crespo-Sendra, V., Mascaro, I., Roseno, P., Sichel-Bazin, R. and del Mar Vanrell, M. (2015) Intonational phonology of Catalan and its dialectal varieties. In S. Frota and P. Prieto (eds) *Intonation in Romance* (pp. 9–62). Oxford University Press. https://doi.org/10.1093/acprof:oso/9780199685332.003.0002

Pujolar, J. and Puigdevall, M. (2015) Linguistic mudes: How to become a new speaker in Catalonia. *International Journal of the Sociology of Language* 2015 (231), 167–187. https://doi.org/10.1515/ijsl-2014-0037

Roller, E. (2002) When does language become exclusivist? Linguistic politics in Catalonia. *National Identities* 4 (3), 273–289. https://doi.org/10.1080/1460894022000026132

Solana, M.S., De, V., Luken, M., García, D.R., Àngels, Y. and De Sans, P. (2012) Conocimiento de las lenguas oficiales entre inmigrantes extranjeros en Cataluña, e implicaciones sobre su integración social (Official language knowledge among foreign-born immigrants in Catalonia, Spain, and implications for their social integration). *Migraciones* 32, 103–138.

Trenchs-Parera, M. and Newman, M. (2009) Diversity of language ideologies in Spanish-speaking youth of different origins in Catalonia. *Journal of Multilingual and Multicultural Development* 30 (6), 509–524. https://doi.org/10.1080/01434630903147914

Vernet, J. and Pons, E. (2011) The legal systems of the Catalan language. In M. Strubell and E. Boix-Fuster (eds) *Democratic Policies for Language Revitalisation: The Case of Catalan* (pp. 57–83). Palgrave Macmillan. https://doi.org/10.1057/9780230302426_3

Wheeler, M., Yates, A. and Dols, N. (1999) *Catalan: A Comprehensive Grammar*. Routledge.

Woolard, K.A. (2016) Introduction. In K. Woolard (ed) *Singular and Plural: Ideologies of Linguistic Authority in 21st Century Catalonia* (pp. 1–18). Oxford University Press. https://doi.org/10.1093/acprof:oso/9780190258610.001.0001

Zhang, H. (2020) Teaching Chinese tones. In C. Shei, M.E. McLellan Zikpi and D. Chao (eds) *The Routledge Handbook of Chinese Language Teaching* (pp. 166–179). Routledge.

23 Afterword

Understanding the Power of Linguistic Variation

Benjamin E. Munson and Elizabeth Ancel

Introduction

This chapter provides a commentary on the topic of this book, linguistic variation and linguistic diversity. This topic is of great practical relevance to many professional communities, including speech-language pathologists (SLP). SLP is the academic and professional field of the authors of this afterward. We believe that linguistic variation is fundamentally fascinating, as it reveals much about the origins of human language and how languages change. It is also fascinating because it reveals much about differences in the values and ideologies held by different professional communities and by the public at large. By bringing together scholars whose work integrates empirical and critical perspectives, this book reinforces the emerging community of 'applied sociolinguists', that is, speech-language-hearing disorders researchers and practitioners whose work addresses – and is informed by – scholarship on linguistic diversity, linguistic variation, sociocultural linguistics and cultural critique.

Applied sociolinguistic perspectives are particularly useful in understanding the ways that linguistic variation has been treated by applied fields like SLP. Much research in SLP endeavors to develop assessment methods that minimize the likelihood of mischaracterizing an individual's language as being indicative of a disorder and, hence, needing treatment. This can happen when an individual uses a language variety that is not widely understood, that is used by people who do not hold positions of power in a particular society, or which differs from the language of powerful groups in ways that are superficially like the language of people in powerful groups with identified communication disorders. Critical perspectives can help understand why such situations arise, and how social, cultural and political forces can contribute to the maintenance of procedures that procedurally mischaracterize the language of certain groups of people (Nair *et al.*, 2024; Yu *et al.*, 2021). For the purposes of this piece, critical perspectives refer to the family of qualitative analyses that were designed to understand how social, cultural and political forces shape issues that are so complex that they cannot be understood fully through experimental studies on individuals, or studies on discrete subgroups of a population (Thompson, 2017). Critical analyses endeavor to understand how social forces work together to inhibit social change and, in turn, how undoing those social forces promotes change and progress. Given this focus, critical theories differ in the dimensions of culture that they focus on. The remainder of this essay argues that social forces drive discussions of linguistic variation that serve to maintain inequities across racial identity, gender, sexuality, and social class within and across societies.

This commentary provides an opportunity to rethink some previous work – including some research and scholarship described in this book's chapters – in light of the new perspectives from applied sociolinguistics, particularly those that emerge from critical scholarship. We believe that fully appreciating the consequences of linguistic variation can only be achieved if one understands the contexts in which variation arises, and hence this commentary includes a discussion of that. We also believe that an understanding of the individual and societal treatment of linguistic variation must involve a discussion of the logical opposite of linguistic variation, that is linguistic homogeneity. This essay describes each of these in turn. We end with a discussion of how this information can aid readers in achieving the stated goal of this volume to '[enhance…] understanding of linguistic diversity and its practical applications.'

Terminology: Thinking Critically

Prior to addressing the primary goals of this commentary, we address the issue of terminology. One challenge to this book's authors, these writers included, is the lack of universally agreed upon terminology for describing linguistic variation. One of the most widely used terms in scholarship on linguistic variation and in the public, *dialect*, has connotations that can both *bias* and *constrain* discussion. We avoid the term dialect in this essay because it is often used to identify languages and communities of language users as being inherently less valuable than languages and language communities associated with 'standard' or 'real' languages. This sentiment is captured in the widely cited witticism popularized by the linguist Max Weinreich, who is reported to have said, 'a language is a dialect with an army and navy [אַ שפראַך איז אַ דיאַלעקט מיט אַן אַרמיי און פֿלאָט],' quoting an audience member from a lecture he gave (Maxwell, 2018). This quote illustrates the sentiment, widely shared among applied sociolinguists, that the distinction between a language and a dialect is largely of the power and prestige of the communities of users. The role of power in determining the status of a language is one reason why seemingly objective methods for determining this, like looking at whether the language can be widely understood by people who use an ostensibly different language, are problematic (Gooskens & Van Heuven, 2021).

Instead, we use the term *language variety* to describe distinct ways of using language by different groups of people who can otherwise understand each other. This is consistent with the title of this book and does not carry the same negative connotations as dialect. For example, the first author of this chapter could be described as knowing and using at least two distinct regional varieties of American English: the variety associated with his birthplace, Western New York State, and the variety associated with the location where he has lived the longest, Minnesota. The view of languages and varieties as modular entities is consistent with the use of the term *code-switching*, which refers to the process of using different distinct languages or varieties in different communicative contexts.

However, we concede that variety, like dialect, has the problem of assuming that languages, dialects and varieties are discrete entities. The term *translanguaging* was developed in part as an alternative to this view (Creese & Blackledge, 2015; Li, 2018). Translanguaging reflects the reality that all language users command a set of different ways of using language. These are sometimes called *languaging practices*, which we use in the remainder of this chapter. For example, the first author of this commentary's languaging practices include the use of phonological features that are associated with Western New York State. These include a tense, raised TRAP vowel and a raised PRICE vowel in certain phonological contexts. These are used alongside other pronunciations of the TRAP and PRICE vowels that are not consistent with Western New York, including ones that are associated with Minnesota. Each of these pronunciations – those that are associated with Western New York and those that are associated with Minnesota – are associated with different *social meanings* (Babel, 2025; Beltrama, 2020; Campbell-Kibler, 2010; Eckert, 2012), which themselves differ across contexts. For example, using these regionally marked vowels outside the region in which they originated could be used to emphasize the talker's *disaffiliation* with the local variety and, by extension, the local culture and community. The first author does not switch between these varieties but instead uses different aspects of them strategically to convey information about himself, though often without explicit awareness of having done so. The translanguaging framework is important for understanding the power associated with different varieties of language and different languaging practices.

The issue of terminology is important because it conveys and reinforces notions about the very nature of language. The term code-switching implies the existence of discrete, distinct codes that one selects among when communicating. The translanguaging approach emphasizes the functions of different forms of language, regardless of whether they are from a specific code like a regional variety. This, in turn, invites a deeper understanding of the origins and functions of the use of different languaging practices.

Language Change and Linguistic Variation

Many of the chapters in this volume emphasize the practical challenges that linguistic variation poses for clinical and educational practices. Language variation is an object of study to be understood, appreciated and honored, as many of the chapters also emphasize. Language is inherently dynamic. Language change happens for myriad reasons, including the instability inherent in any complex system that is subject to competing demands. Consider sound change, such as the change in the pronunciation of the word *knight* from a pronunciation of /knixt/ in Middle English to its current pronunciation of /nʌɪʔ/ in many varieties of English. Sound change happens in part because of the competition between the principle that speech production should minimize articulatory effort, with the principle that talkers should maximize sounds' perceptual distinctiveness. These two constraints are often in direct conflict: maximizing perceptual distinctiveness often requires extra articulatory effort. Languages differ in the ways that these tensions are resolved, and these resolutions can change over time, thus changing languages' sound structure (Ohala, 1993). Similar forces affect the composition of the lexicon, syntax and word meaning. Even in isolated, linguistically homogeneous environments, language change is expected and, hence, is normal.

One widely accepted explanation for the development of distinct languages and language varieties is that they are the consequence of language evolving differently between geographically or socially distinct language communities. For example, the contemporary Romance languages arose in geographic communities that used Latin as their everyday language because they were part of the Latin-speaking Roman Empire and were administered by people in communication with Latin-speaking Rome. In these various geographic communities (which correspond to, among other places, modern-day France, Italy, Portugal, Romania and Spain), Latin evolved uniquely, but the extent of language change was constrained by the need to maintain communication with other Latin-speaking areas in the Roman Empire and with the Roman colonizers. The collapse of the Roman Empire removed the pressure to maintain a common language with others in the then-former Roman Empire. Language change continued in these communities. At some point, the languages were different enough that communities that used one could not understand communities that used others, and the distinct Romance languages can be said to have been formed.

Language change of the sort described in the previous paragraph is often accompanied by language contact. Language communities in different parts of the former Roman Empire interacted with people who used Germanic, Slavic or Celtic languages, which influenced each other's trajectory of change. For example, French was affected greatly by contact with Germanic and Celtic languages (Hélix, 2011), which may have led to French having front-rounded vowels unattested in most other Romance languages. In contrast, another Romance language, Romanian, was affected by contact with Slavic languages, which led to the incorporation of Slavic-origin words, like the Romanian word *a iubi* for *to love*.

One particularly striking example of language change arising from contact concerns the formation of creole languages. When there is extensive contact between two groups of people speaking different languages, creole languages form to enable communication between those two communities. One historically significant example of creole language formation in the United States concerns the development of African American Vernacular English (AAVE). AAVE developed in communities of Black people who had been kidnapped from Africa and brought to colonial America and the Caribbean to provide slave labor for the white colonists. Groups of Black Africans were often intentionally grouped by their captors so that few individuals shared a common language with one another, thus making it difficult for enslaved people to collaborate to escape slavery. The language that developed in these communities evolved into AAVE. The cultural and historical significance of AAVE is one of the reasons why its name has been debated. For example, the term African American Language (AAL) removes the words 'Vernacular' and 'English,' thus rejecting the negative connotations associated with the word 'vernacular' and the association with English, the language of those who kidnapped and enslaved Black people. In the remainder of this essay, we use AAVE because of its status as the most widely used label in scholarly studies. Studies of the development of AAVE actively debate the role of enslaved people's first languages on the structure of AAVE, but the consensus is that creolization played an important role (Rickford, 1998).

This description of language evolution in the previous paragraph is a great simplification and is presented here to emphasize that **language variation is normal** because **language change is normal**. Indeed, **to expect language to be uniform would be to deny fundamental facets of what it means to be human**. The linguistic landscape reflects the history of human migration, connection, distance and contact. It can reflect resistance and resilience, as in the case of AAVE. It is a proverbial living artifact of human history. Given this, it is natural to view the preservation of linguistic diversity as critical to preserving human history. This point has been made recently in work on language planning, that is, governmental and non-governmental activities to ensure the maintenance and use of different languages and language varieties (Bernini, 2014; Rajagukguk *et al.*, 2022).

The Opposite of Variation

A discussion of linguistic diversity would not be complete without a discussion of its logical opposite, linguistic homogeneity. Why would a linguistically diverse group of people use a single language? For example, in the United States, why is English – a language that was not present in that part of the world prior to the 17th century – used so frequently? There are at least two answers to this general question. The first of these is pragmatic: a common language allows for official interactions to take place without having to spend resources providing access to speakers of a variety of languages. This represents what some scholars call 'classic' language planning policy (Jernudd & Nekvapil, 2012; Réaume & Pinto, 2012) in which the languages that are supported are those that in turn support nation-states.

Classical language policy can be seen as the linguistic situation in France. Both historically and currently, France is linguistically diverse. The language that most people call French is one of many languages in France, which also includes the Occitan languages in Southern France and the Picard language of the Northwest, among others. Despite this linguistic variation, the sole official language of France is French. The reason for this is clear given what we know about the origins of linguistic diversity, as described in the previous section: French was the language used by the most powerful class of people in the French state. The French government was built in such a way that using French was required to participate in official state functions in France. One can argue that having a single national language is an efficient and cost-effective way for a linguistically diverse country to interact. Learning a common language could be seen as a necessary investment of an individual's time to participate in official functions.

The second reason, though, is arguably more ideological, and that is the idea that some languages are inherently better than others, sometimes referred to as *standard language ideology*. Standard language ideologies are described in Milroy (2001), who defined them as systems for the *imposition* of uniformity on an otherwise variable behavior. Milroy argues that these ideologies drive many people who use certain widely spoken languages, like English, to believe that there is a canonical, 'correct' form of a language, and that this form should be the only one that is promoted and upheld. At times in history, this view has been explicitly labeled as reflecting 'common sense' and hence not needing an explicit, evidence-based justification. This sentiment runs counter to volumes of research showing that languages that do not meet these standards of correctness are governed by the same complex grammatical principles that govern all the world's languages. Given this, all languages and varieties should be regarded as equally 'correct' to those who use them. Despite this public knowledge, standard language ideologies continue to be endorsed widely, as seen in the formation of educational policies surrounding language teaching (Cushing, 2023).

The role that standard language ideologies play in educational settings was recently discussed by MacSwan (2020). MacSwan critiqued the use of the term *academic language*, which is sometimes used to describe the variety of language taught and used in educational settings. The term academic language is meant to convey the seemingly pragmatic approach to language uniformity described earlier, as a tool to allow a group of teachers and learners that use different varieties and languaging practices outside of school to communicate and learn in classrooms. MacSwan argues that discourse on academic language has evolved such that it is often discussed as being the only variety that can be used to adequately teach concepts as complex as those taught in school. Hence, while academic language could be framed as a pragmatic solution to the challenges posed by educating a linguistically diverse group of learners, it has evolved to be a mechanism for enforcing the use of a restricted, 'standard' set of linguistic codes in schools.

The problems with standard language ideologies described in the previous paragraphs are perhaps eclipsed by the critique that the existence of standard languages reflects systemic discrimination, as standard languages are almost always the varieties and languaging practices that are used by people who hold official power. In the United States, this group comprises primarily the white people who colonized North America, rather than the Indigenous people who lived in North America since the Paleolithic period, or the Black people forcibly brought to North America and enslaved to provide labor for white people. Given this, standard language ideologies in the United States serve to reinforce racism (Figueroa, 2024; Kosse & Tripp, 2025). A related argument is presented in detail in Flores and Rosa (2015), who discuss the use of 'appropriateness' criteria to determine the language varieties and languaging practices that should be taught in schools. Flores and Rosa argue that these approaches disproportionately penalize the language of racialized groups of learners and hence represent the maintenance of the linguistic forms prized by standard language ideologies.

While knowledge of language varieties is important, it is not the only tool needed to prevent the mischaracterization of language. Indeed, standard language ideologies frame all languages other than the 'standard' as being inherently less worthy. If deeply internalized, these ideologies could cause someone – perhaps a member of the language community itself – to both acknowledge that a variety is systematic and principled, but 'errored' because it deviates from the standard. Moreover, adherence to the pragmatic sentiment that standard languages are needed for the smooth functioning of multilingual communities might see the use of a certain language variety not to be sufficiently pro-social, even if the use is regarded as not inherently incorrect. A further complicating factor is that the lack of shared, society-wide terminology for describing varieties and the lack of a wide understanding of the functions of language variation makes it difficult for practitioners to fairly determine the language that an individual uses in all spheres of their daily lives. That is, it is not always practically possible to ask people about varieties used in their daily lives. While some individuals have an acute awareness of this, this awareness exists despite the ways that standard language ideologies are imbricated in institutions like schools and governments. In short, standard language ideologies greatly complicate the task of differentiating difference from disorder.

Promoting the maintenance of linguistic variation is one way to push back on standard language ideologies. It has the additional benefit of maintaining the historical record that linguistic variation reflects. Bernini (2014) outlines principles that could be used to aid in the preservation of linguistic variation. These include plans to explicitly document and promote the *status* and *prestige* of different varieties and to plan for their continued acquisition. These principles, while an important first start, still reflect an understanding of varieties as discrete entities. Moving forward, applied sociolinguistics must devise ways of preserving linguistic variation that reflect the realities of language use that motivated the development of translanguaging frameworks.

Critically Engaging with Variation

Understanding status and prestige, and the motives for adopting languaging practices from different varieties requires applied sociolinguists, including SLPs, to understand why different varieties and different languaging practices are used within and across different individuals and communities. Some cases of this are straightforward: a person who uses both English and Spanish will likely not use Spanish when conversing with people who are believed not to know Spanish. The straightforwardness of such cases belies the daunting complexity of real-world linguistic variation. Consider again the example of the first author's variable use of different ways of producing the TRAP and PRICE vowels. The use of these was described earlier as conveying a sense of affiliation or distance from an audience. That is, it is not simply the case that the first author uses one set of vowels when speaking to Western New Yorkers and another set when talking to Minnesotans. Rather, these different ways of speaking are deployed to convey various types of information about the talker himself and his perceived relationship to both his audience and the topic under discussion. Third-wave sociolinguistics research has documented meticulously the different social meanings associated with different language forms and languaging practices.

Social meanings are generally not codified institutionally the way that the grammars of 'standard' languages are. Hence, they can be very fluid.

For example, the production of an especially loud, especially fronted /s/ can convey the very specific social meaning of 'fierceness' in the context of a drag performance (Calder, 2019) but give the impression of the talker being younger in a different setting (Mack & Munson, 2012). In short, as emphasized by Babel (2025), who said '[s]ocial meaning resides in the ways that people perceive linguistic behavior as patterned and predictable, depending on their experience with, stereotypes about, and understanding of different groups.' Third-wave sociolinguistics has the potential to enrich the work of applied fields like SLP. Practitioners seeking to understand the motives and origins of different languaging practices in individuals receiving evaluation or treatment must be aware of the fluid nature of social meaning. This will likely require an SLP to be a keen observer of languaging practices in the communities in which they, and their (potential) clients, live. This requires SLPs to enrich their skill set to include ethnographic and experimental sociolinguistic methods.

For SLPs, understanding linguistic variation has been central to preventing the mischaracterization of language variation as a language disorder. As professionals, SLPs are tasked with determining whether an individual's language usage is sufficiently different from 'typical' language to constitute the need for intervention focused on communication goals. A canonical example of this concerns AAVE in the United States. Many linguistic forms that are normal in AAVE superficially resemble forms that are used by individuals with language disorders who speak other varieties, including those varieties that resemble the 'standard' variety described in the previous section. For example, AAVE uses a null copula in many utterances, such as *he an expert*, noted by Bender (2001). This is the normal way for someone using AAVE to convey that a person (in this case referred to with the pronoun *he*) holds a particular attribute (in this case, being *an expert* at something). This same sentence would be consistent with the production of a child with Developmental Language Disorder (DLD, that is, difficulty learning language without an obvious medical or psychosocial cause) who is acquiring a variety in which the same information would be conveyed with the sentence *he's an expert*.

A child who is exposed to a 'standard' variety in which *he's an expert* is the typical form produced by an adult would be said to have made an error in saying *he an expert*. A child who is exposed to AAVE in which *he an expert* is the typical form produced by an adult would not be said to have made an error. A great deal of research in SLP has focused on reducing the likelihood that a normal pattern (like AAVE *he an expert*) is mistakenly identified as an error. Hence, the determination of what constitutes 'typical' language for children is influenced by the SLPs' knowledge and understanding of language variation. An SLP who is unaware of the normal pattern in AAVE would have no reason to believe that the utterance *he an expert* represents anything other than an error. Fortunately, many detailed linguistic descriptions of AAVE exist. Many other varieties, including those described in chapters in this book, do not have similarly rich descriptions that are easily available to practitioners like SLPs. The descriptions in this book are a powerful and useful resource for reducing the likelihood that normal variation will be misidentified as representing a disorder.

Understanding the power associated with different language varieties is another tool to improve services (Tripp & Munson, 2023). In the educational sphere, the power associated with different language varieties is evidenced by their acceptability as a sufficiently 'academic' means of communication. Simply acknowledging the existence of different language varieties does not change the fact that specific language varieties are favored in instructional settings and deemed to be more necessary for educational and vocational purposes. However, favoring a specific language variety over others in instruction reinforces the stigmatization of language varieties that are *not* the focus of instruction as varieties that are lesser, improper or otherwise inappropriate for academic settings. In the case of AAVE, high school-aged speakers of AAVE reiterated the negative stigma associated with AAVE and expressed stereotypes about speakers of AAVE as being 'ignorant' or 'uneducated' (Baker-Bell, 2013). To improve instruction, then, requires the critical evaluation of which language varieties are reinforced by practices in SLP, and which are not. If the mission of SLP is to holistically improve communication outcomes, this necessarily involves acknowledging *and* giving power to the language varieties used by the populations we serve.

Planning for the Future

This final section considers how the information in this afterward and this book can inform theoretical and practical work moving forward. Such recommendations are both easy and difficult to write. They are easy in the sense that much work needs to be done, and previous scholarship has provided clear directions for this work. They are difficult, however, in that many issues related to the mistreatment and mischaracterization of linguistic variation reflect broader cultural and political factors that are deeply embedded in societies.

One general recommendation is for scholars to embrace participating in the public sphere and conducting activism. As described by Ball (2021) and Bassett (2020), the failure of scientists to engage in these activities is likely one reason why science-based policy recommendations, like the public health measures promoted during the COVID-19 pandemic, were not uniformly adopted. They are also based on the incorrect assertion that political and social factors are inherently nonscientific. The behaviors of individuals and groups of people are governed by the laws and principles that affect any multidimensional dynamical system, just as the physical world is. Hence, scholarship in and engagement with society, politics and culture is well within the scope of science. This argument is described in greater detail in Pierrehumbert *et al.* (2000), Munson (2025) and in recent work using the *Diversity Science* framework (Plaut, 2010).

How might this work be deployed? A recurring theme in this afterword has been the role of power on the use and treatment of different language varieties. Indeed, talking about variation without talking about power is at best incomplete, and at worst is truly harmful. Moreover, talking about power without talking about the origins and justifications of power is equally problematic. Scholarship on standard language ideologies, and on language and power more generally, can help speech and language practitioners like SLPs understand the broader individual and social consequences of facilitating – or failing to facilitate – different varieties of language. This could involve the explicit acknowledgment of when their work focuses exclusively on providing people the language skills associated with accessing power by facilitating the languaging practices that are used by those in power, when they are exercising power. Doing so can be seen as endorsing the standard language ideologies described earlier, a point made recently by Farrugia-Bernard (2018). An argument can be made that these ideologies promote linguistic discrimination against people whose languaging practices differ from those in power.

The explicit consideration of language and power can also help practitioners like SLPs understand the functions of those practices. Some languaging practices exist specifically to resist the dominant power structures. Consider the use of Cantonese in Hong Kong. Cantonese is the historical language of Hong Kong and areas surrounding it. It is not mutually intelligible with the variety of Mandarin used by the central government of the People's Republic of China [PRC], which began to gradually assume power in Hong Kong after the end of British colonization in 1997. In 2019, there was a wave of pro-democracy protests in Hong Kong, protesting a PRC-backed bill to suppress political discourse. During these protests, Cantonese was used strategically by Hong Kong activists, both to convey a sense of solidarity among themselves and to make their communication less easily understood by Mandarin-speaking individuals, including police (Tong, 2024). While this example is somewhat far afield from the issues that SLPs face, it serves as a valuable reminder that some languaging practices and language varieties are used specifically to resist power. The same general sentiment is true of many languaging practices in the United States, including the use of AAVE. Because some languaging practices and language varieties exist to resist power structures, bringing those practices into official structures like schools and clinics comes with potential complications and risks.

What, then, would be a useful solution to the practical problems that practitioners face? One possible solution is to use plain language. Plain language is a version of language that is designed to be maximally accessible, that is, to be as easily understood as possible by as wide a group of people as possible. Plain language is discussed extensively in law, where it is thought to be a method to ensure the broadest engagement with laws and the legal system as possible (Adler, 2012). It has since been applied to medicine, finance and science. Plain language avoids low-frequency words whenever possible (i.e. using *hard* rather than *herculean*, or *smooth muscle cancer* instead of *leiomyosarcoma*) and complex syntax, especially when their use would render a message ambiguous. The use of plain language in official capacities, including education and medicine, has the potential to address many of the issues that SLPs face, as it would officially separate the language varieties and languaging practices needed to participate in official functions, like excelling at school and work, from those needed to participate in social functions, like participating in civil rights protests. Promoting plain language is an almost utopian ideal and, as such, it has more of the character of an aspiration than a plan. It also comes with the risk that the version of plain language that is devised is not, in fact, universally accessible, but is more accessible to groups who already have power because it resembles their language. However, as an aspiration, plain language can shape work in the shorter term. Other shorter-term work in SLP attempts to circumvent the challenges of disentangling disorder from linguistic variation by capitalizing on the fact that language abilities draw on more general, language-neutral cognitive-linguistic and perceptual skills. Work in this vein, in which non-linguistic measures are used for assessment, has shown great promise (e.g. Ebert *et al.*, 2014; Ebert & Pham, 2019).

In the most general sense, though, practitioners like SLPs can continue to carry the proverbial torch represented by this book and celebrate linguistic diversity. Linguistic diversity is an essential component of being human. It provides a living record of the past and resources for navigating the diverse worlds in which we live. Any effort to erase linguistic diversity denies humanity that history and that function. Any practitioner whose job is to facilitate language should have those undeniable facts in mind in everything they do.

References

Adler, M. (2012) The plain language movement. In L. Solan and P. Tiersma (eds) *The Oxford Handbook of Language and Law* (pp. 67–83). Oxford University Press.

Babel, A. (2025) A semiotic approach to social meaning in language. *Journal of Sociolinguistics* 29, 59–73.

Baker-Bell, A. (2013) "I never really knew the history behind African American Language": Critical language pedagogy in an Advanced Placement English Language Arts class. *Equity & Excellence in Education* 46, 355–370.

Ball, P. (2021) Science is political, and we must deal with it. *The Journal of Physical Chemistry Letters* 12, 6336–6340.

Bassett, M. (2020) Tired of science being ignored? Get political. *Nature* 586, 337–338.

Beltrama, A. (2020) Social meaning in semantics and pragmatics. *Language and Linguistics Compass* 14, e12398.
Bender, E.M. (2001) Syntactic variation and linguistic competence: The case of AAVE copula absence. PhD Dissertation, Stanford University, Stanford, CA.
Bernini, A. (2014) Preserving languages beyond the political dimension: Some proposals for dialect planning. Darnioji Daugiakalbystė [Sustainable Multilingualism] 4, 14–24.
Calder, J. (2019) The fierceness of fronted /s/: Linguistic rhematization through visual transformation. *Language in Society* 48, 31–64.
Campbell-Kibler, K. (2010) The sociolinguistic variant as a carrier of social meaning. *Language Variation and Change* 22, 423–441.
Creese, A. and Blackledge, A. (2015) Translanguaging and identity in educational settings. *Annual Review of Applied Linguistics* 35, 20–35.
Cushing, I. (2023) Policy mechanisms of the standard language ideology in England's education system. *Journal of Language, Identity & Education* 22, 279–293.
Ebert, K.D. and Pham, G. (2019) Including nonlinguistic processing tasks in the identification of developmental language disorder. *American Journal of Speech-Language Pathology* 28, 932–944.
Ebert, K.D., Kohnert, K., Pham, G., Disher, J.R. and Payesteh, B. (2014) Three treatments for bilingual children with primary language impairment: Examining cross-linguistic and cross-domain effects. *Journal of Speech, Language, and Hearing Research* 57, 172–186.
Eckert, P. (2012) Three waves of variation study: The emergence of meaning in the study of sociolinguistic variation. *Annual Review of Anthropology* 41, 87–100.
Farrugia-Bernard, A. (2018) Speech-language pathologists as determiners of the human right to diversity in communication for school children in the US. *International Journal of Speech-Language Pathology* 20, 170–173.
Figueroa, M. (2024) Language development, linguistic input, and linguistic racism. *Wiley Interdisciplinary Reviews: Cognitive Science* 15, e1673.
Flores, N. and Rosa, J. (2015) Undoing appropriateness: Raciolinguistic ideologies and diversity in education. *Harvard Educational Review* 25, 149–171.
Gooskens, C. and van Heuven, V. (2021) Mutual intelligibility. In M. Zampieri and P. Nakov (eds) *Similar Languages, Varieties, and Dialects: A Computational Perspective* (Studies in Natural Language Processing) (pp. 51–95). Cambridge University Press.
Hélix, L. (2011) *Histoire de la Langue Française* [History of the French Language]. Ellipses.
Jernudd, B. and Nekvapil, J. (2012) History of the field: A sketch. In B. Spolsky (ed.) *The Cambridge Handbook of Language Policy* (pp. 16–36). Cambridge University Press.
Kosse, M. and Tripp, A. (2025) White supremacist themes in linguistics. In O. Robinson and E. Moriarty (eds) *A Crip Linguistics Reader*. Gallaudet University Press.
Li, W. (2018) Translanguaging as a practical theory of language. *Applied Linguistics* 39, 9–30.
Mack, S. and Munson, B. (2012) The influence of/s/quality on ratings of men's sexual orientation: Explicit and implicit measures of the 'gay lisp' stereotype. *Journal of Phonetics* 40, 198–212.
MacSwan, J. (2020) Academic English as standard language ideology: A renewed research agenda for asset-based language education. *Language Teaching Research* 24, 28–36.
Maxwell, A. (2018) When theory is a joke: The Weinreich witticism in Linguistics. *Beiträge zur Geschichte der Sprachwissenschaft* 28, 263–292.
Milroy, J. (2001) Language ideologies and the consequences of standardization. *Journal of Sociolinguistics* 5, 530–555.
Munson, B. (2025) Taking up the mantle: How speech scientists can fight linguistic discrimination. *Perspectives of the ASHA Special Interest Groups* 10 (4), 1309–1322.
Nair, V.K.K., Brea, M.R. and Yu, B. (2024) Decolonizing speech language "Pathology": Critical foundational concepts for research, pedagogy and praxis. *Journal of Critical Study of Communication and Disability* 2, 71–94.

Ohala, J.J. (1993) Sound change as nature's speech perception experiment. *Speech Communication* 13, 155–161.

Pierrehumbert, J., Beckman, M.E. and Ladd, D.R. (2000) Conceptual foundations of phonology as a laboratory science. In N. Burton-Roberts, P. Carr and G. Docherty (eds) *Phonological Knowledge: Conceptual and Empirical Issues* (pp. 273–304). Oxford University Press.

Plaut, V.C. (2010) Diversity science: Why and how difference makes a difference. *Psychological Inquiry* 21, 77–99.

Rajagukguk, R., Malems, T. and Ginting, M. (2022) Preserving linguistic diversity: Strategies for language preservation and cultural heritage safeguarding. *Jurnal Ilmu Pendidikan Dan Humaniora [Journal of Studies in Education and the Humanities]* 11, 221–236.

Réaume, D. and Pinto, M. (2012) Philosophy of language policy. In B. Spolsky (ed.) *The Cambridge Handbook of Language Policy* (pp. 37–58). Cambridge University Press.

Rickford, J. (1998) The creole origins of African American Vernacular English: Evidence from copula absence. In S. Mufwene, J. Rickford, G. Bailey and J. Baugh (eds) *African American English* (pp. 154–200). Routledge.

Thompson, M.J. (2017) Introduction: What is critical theory? In M. Thompson (ed.) *The Palgrave Handbook of Critical Theory*. Political Philosophy and Public Purpose (pp. 1–14). Palgrave Macmillan.

Tong, C.T.M. (2024) Cantonese as a protest language in Hong Kong: 1967, 2014, and 2019. In J.-F. Dupré (ed.) *The Politics of Language in Hong Kong* (pp. 43–62). Routledge.

Tripp, A. and Munson, B. (2023) Acknowledging language variation and its power: Keys to justice and equity in applied psycholinguistics. *Applied Psycholinguistics* 44, 495–513.

Yu, B., Epstein, L. and Tisi, V. (2021) A DisCrit-informed critique of the difference vs. disorder approach in speech-language pathology. In R. Horton (ed.) *Critical Perspectives on Social Justice in Speech-Language Pathology* (pp. 105–128). IGI Global.

Index

For Product Safety Concerns and Information please contact our EU Authorised Representative:

Easy Access System Europe

Mustamäe tee 50

10621 Tallinn

Estonia

gpsr.requests@easproject.com

www.ingramcontent.com/pod-product-compliance
Ingram Content Group UK Ltd.
Pitfield, Milton Keynes, MK11 3LW, UK
UKHW021012120926
8556IPUK00039B/1077
9781800412637